COPING WITH DEPRESSION

From Catch-22 to Hope

COPING WITH DEPRESSION

From Catch-22 to Hope

Jon G. Allen, Ph.D.

*Helen Malsin Palley Chair in Mental Health Research and
Professor of Psychiatry, Menninger Department of Psychiatry and
Behavioral Sciences at the Baylor College of Medicine
Senior Staff Psychologist, The Menninger Clinic,
Houston, Texas*

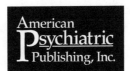

American
Psychiatric
Publishing, Inc.

Washington, DC
London, England

Copyright © 2006 American Psychiatric Publishing, Inc.
ALL RIGHTS RESERVED

Manufactured in the United States of America on acid-free paper
09 08 07 06 05   5 4 3 2 1
First Edition

**WM
171
A425c
2006**

Typeset in Adobe's Janson Text and HelveticaNeue.

American Psychiatric Publishing, Inc.
1000 Wilson Boulevard
Arlington, VA 22209–3901
www.appi.org

Library of Congress Cataloging-in-Publication Data
Allen, Jon G.
    Coping with depression : from catch-22 to hope / by Jon G. Allen.—1st ed.
      p. ; cm.
    Includes bibliographical references and index.
    ISBN 1-58562-211-7 (pbk. : alk. paper)
      1. Depression, Mental—Etiology. 2. Depression, Mental—Treatment.
    I. Title
      [DNLM: 1. Depressive Disorder—etiology. 2. Depressive Disorder—therapy.
    WM 171 A425c 2006]
    RC537.A44 2006
    616.85'27—dc22
                                                                    2005027488

British Library Cataloguing in Publication Data
A CIP record is available from the British Library.

For Clifford

There was only one catch and that was Catch-22, which specified that a concern for one's own safety in the face of dangers that were real and immediate was the process of a rational mind. Orr was crazy and could be grounded. All he had to do was ask; and as soon as he did, he would no longer be crazy and would have to fly more missions. Orr would be crazy to fly more missions and sane if he didn't, but if he was sane he had to fly them. If he flew them he was crazy and didn't have to; but if he didn't want to he was sane and had to. Yossarian was moved very deeply by the absolute simplicity of this clause of Catch-22 and let out a respectful whistle.

"That's some catch, that Catch-22," he observed.

"It's the best there is," Doc Daneeka agreed.

—Joseph Heller, *Catch-22*

CONTENTS

Part I
GROUNDWORK

Part II
DEVELOPMENT

Part III
PRECIPITANTS

FOREWORD

The problem with the disorder of depression is that despite many years of effective research culminating in a good understanding of the illness and successful treatments, it is still underestimated in the public's and in policy makers' understanding. Rates of depression are ever increasing, particularly in younger cohorts—and still only a minority of those with the disorder seek treatment, with few having access to the most effective treatments. So although research into the disorder has done its job well, the communication about and the understanding of depression is still only partial—which means that a treatable disorder is still responsible for a good deal of misery, unproductiveness, and failed family relationships. Often for a substantial part of a lifetime, a large number of people, particularly women and those who are underprivileged, suffer needlessly from this illness. For this reason, Dr. Jon Allen's book is much needed and its timing is opportune. This book is masterful in its capacity to render a disorder with complex roots and varied treatments easily understandable—a skill no doubt learned by the author over his years of conducting psychoeducational treatments with severely depressed patients. The book's particular strength is in its message of hope about prevention and treatment, a message critical for those who experience depression, whether firsthand or witnessing it among those close to them.

Depression is complicated. Its acknowledged causes are biopsychosocial, and it has a developmental or life-history trajectory. Thus, a large and varied number of factors in combination need to be understood to fully grasp how physical, mental, and social bases culminate in a disorder of clinical intensity. This understanding is no mean feat for experts in the field, but the task is daunting for the layperson. Yet this book manages to straddle the world of the mental health expert and the layperson in an elegant and accessible summary of the scientific knowledge.

Coping With Depression provides a deceptively easy journey through the various elements that make up the vulnerabilities and provoking stressors of the disorder. This book not only makes the message simple, clear, and coherent, but uses language to highlight some of the traps and pitfalls of depression. Encompassed by the catch-22 analogy, these traps and pitfalls have provided barriers to the recognition, acceptance, and treatment of depression. And there are many traps and pitfalls embedded in the disorder of depression. For example, those vulnerable to depression experience an unequal amount of external stress and yet are the very people who have less internal and external resources for dealing with it. Features of the disorder (such as social withdrawal and hopelessness) are more likely to impede help seeking and treatment compliance. Solutions through support seeking are hijacked by mistrust, hostility, or felt stigma that accompany the illness. And perhaps the biggest trap: that the word for depression simultaneously conveys an everyday emotional state and a serious clinical disorder. All these conspire to make the depressed person misunderstood, isolated, and overwhelmed.

The book provides a comprehensive explanation and description of depressive disorder in its different forms. In a wonderfully even-handed manner, Dr. Allen achieves a natural-feeling balance among the psychological, social, and biological components of depression without betraying any partisanship to contributing disciplines, measures, or treatments. In the current academic and political climate, genetic, biological, and pharmacological influences in vogue are in danger of monopolizing the paradigm. Yet Dr. Allen consistently shows how social disadvantage, early life trauma, and attachment problems set the trajectory of lifetime depressive disorder. He shows how social environments can conspire to damage the individual, how personal characteristics amplify their impact, and how biological factors dictate the transmission mechanisms.

Dr. Allen is indeed an expert. He integrates his substantial clinical, academic, and educational experience in clinical disorders with thoughtful interpretations of his experiences. His careful attention to language in communicating to his many patients over the years has fine-tuned a talent for communication.

My own contact with Dr. Jon Allen began in the 1990s, when he was based at the Menninger Clinic in Kansas, and part of the Child and Family team directed by the UK clinician and researcher Professor Peter Fonagy. This fascinating and creative period for research was exemplified in the eclecticism of the group. Influences from psychology, psychoanalysis, sociology, and biology combined a range of methodologies that tracked the natural histories of individuals previously treated in the Clinic—many with traumatic and adverse backgrounds—to look at the psychological disorders they encountered in consequence. Dr. Allen openly absorbed the numerous scientific and theoretical influences in play, not only from around the United States but also from the United Kingdom and elsewhere. He quickly developed a mastery of the intensive biographical interviews developed in the United Kingdom by George Brown and his team, of which I was a part. These interviews were distinct in their subtle attention to context and meaning and emphasis on the role of social adversity. These interviews became integrated into the life-history approaches developed for this project. I was privileged to be a part of the ensuing discussions and training sessions held between our two groups on both sides of the Atlantic; indeed, I remember it as a truly creative and instructive collaboration absorbing much of the best of social science and clinical research in the 1990s.

I hope that books such as *Coping With Depression* will rekindle the commitment of science to include personal experience and social context in its investigations, not falling prey to the potential reductionism of the biological paradigm. This book is a template for how different levels of experience can be encompassed and communicated comprehensively and sensitively.

Dr. Allen ends his exposition of depression by talking about hope. Hope is necessary to so many aspects of well-being and to achieving contentment and success in life—and its absence is why depression is so malignant a disorder. But *Coping With Depression* shows how depression and hope can coexist, and it gives practical guidance for how the latter can triumph. The book is thus an instruction in how to live well.

Antonia Bifulco, Ph.D.
Professor in Health and Social Care
Royal Holloway, University of London

September 2005

ACKNOWLEDGMENTS

Those who have lived with depression are the true experts, and I have been privileged to have many such experts as my teachers. I learned many years ago that the best way to understand psychiatric disorders is to teach those who have them—and to be educated in the process. I have been taught, and I have learned how to teach. Thus my main debt is to the patients in my educational groups as well as those who have worked with me in psychotherapy. Their patience, honesty, openness, imaginativeness, and critical thinking have contributed immeasurably to my grasp of this often crippling illness. I am particularly grateful to those patients who have kept in touch with me over the course of many years; knowledge of their recovery has been invaluable in inspiring hope, which I can thereby pass on to others.

The clinical work reflected in this book was made possible by an extraordinarily supportive institution, The Menninger Clinic, which has been my professional home for three decades. The humane spirit of the clinic, coupled with a climate of intellectual inquisitiveness, has made it possible for clinicians and patients to collaborate in furthering our collective understanding of psychiatric disorders and how best to treat them. In recent years, this whole enterprise was challenged by the need to relocate the clinic from Topeka, Kansas to Houston, Texas for the purpose of forming a partnership with the Baylor College of Medicine. I could not have written this book without the devotion of all my colleagues who sustained the clinic through this daunting transition and without the administrative support I received from Ian Aitken, Efrain Bleiberg, Richard Munich, and Stuart Yudofsky to create a position in which I could continue my work. Richard Munich also played a major substantive role in this book by drawing my attention to the importance of agency in psychiatric illness and helping me articulate it. In addition, I am grateful for the support of the Helen Malsin Palley Chair in Mental Health Research and to Peter Fonagy, director of the Child and Family Program, whose intellectual leadership and bright spirit have played a paramount role in my professional development over the past decade.

Being a member of the newly formed Menninger Department of Psychiatry and Behavioral Sciences at the Baylor College of Medicine has been a boon in writing this book. I have been particularly fortunate to rely on the medical expertise of my psychiatrist colleagues, Norma Clarke, Florence Kim, and Lauren Marangell, who have generously reviewed and helped me refine the sections of this book on neurobiology and medical matters. Many other colleagues with specialized expertise have graciously reviewed and critiqued various parts of the manuscript; I thank Throstur Bjorgvinsson, Carolyn Cochrane, John Hart, Toby Haslam-Hopwood, Peter Fonagy, Lisa Lewis, Richard Munich, Cheryl Scoglio, Carla Sharp, and Melinda Stanley for their expert help and suggestions. I also thank Roger Verdon for his thoughtful editorial counsel and Cassandra Shorter for her invaluable help with literature searches and acquiring references. I am also grateful to my wife, Susan, for her critical reading of parts of the manuscript, but especially for her unflagging devotion, which makes all my endeavors possible.

Finally, I thank Robert E. Hales, M.D., Editor-in-Chief, and John McDuffie, Editorial Director, of the Books Department at American Psychiatric Publishing, Inc., for their enthusiasm, encouragement, and expert guidance throughout the planning and writing of this book and its companion, the second edition of *Coping With Trauma*. Yet again, I am grateful for Ann Eng's expert editorial direction in the final production.

INTRODUCTION

I began teaching patients about depression in the context of conducting educational groups on psychological trauma throughout The Menninger Clinic, and then developed an educational program devoted solely to depression for patients in the Professionals in Crisis Program. I discovered fairly quickly that if I merely told patients about all the things they could do to lift their depressed mood, I was dead in the water; they just tuned me out. They explained why these various things I had recommended didn't work all that well. I listened. I learned that I could be far more helpful by acknowledging the limitations of treatments for depression and by helping patients understand the multitude of reasons for their difficulty recovering. Then they listened.

My approach to educating patients about depression is based on one fundamental premise: depression is one of the leading causes of disability worldwide; therefore, although the vast majority of people do recover from depression, it cannot generally be easy to do so. This soberly realistic approach to patient education has the merit of helping depressed patients feel less guilty for their inability to recover quickly, and it helps to deter them from giving up too quickly on treatments that can be helpful in the long run.

Recovering from depression generally is not easy, and neither is facing the seriousness of the illness. Despite a decade of schooling and many years of clinical practice thereafter, I did not fully appreciate the plight of the depressed person until I began working with patients in educational groups and delved into the voluminous professional literature. The stark reality is a far cry from the popular stereotype, which holds that depression is an acute illness: something bad happens, you get depressed, and then you recover fairly quickly—perhaps with the aid of antidepressant medication. True, depression can be a relatively time-limited response to stressful events, and a significant number of persons do respond relatively quickly and fully to treatment. But that is not the norm, and I am assuming that anyone perusing this substantial book with "catch-22" in the title is having a hard go of it.

Understanding *why* it can be so hard to recover from depression may make the recovery process less painful. Many persons who struggle to recover from depression add insult to injury. They criticize themselves for their difficulty recovering: "I should be able to snap out of it, but I can't—I'm weak." This book counters that self-criticism. When you understand the challenges of the recovery process, you will be able to adopt a more compassionate attitude toward yourself.

If you had a heart attack, you would need to learn about your heart and circulatory system to be able to best take care of yourself. If you develop diabetes, you will need to learn about blood sugar, insulin, and diet. If you are overweight, you need to learn about nutrition and exercise. So it is with depression. You will do best if you have the most current knowledge about the nature of depression, its causes, and its treatment. A glimpse at the table of contents will alert you to the extensive ground this book covers, but much of this territory can be viewed through the lens of two simple ideas: catch-22 and stress pileup.

CATCH-22

Depression is a difficult problem. Why might it take so long to recover? Why might recovery be so difficult and painful? If you are having a hard time climbing out of depression, you might have been given some or all of this advice: Be active. Have fun. Think positively. Don't isolate yourself from other people. This is good advice, and you have probably been trying to follow some or all of it. Here's the rub: *all the things you need to do to recover from depression are made difficult by the symptoms of depression.*

You should maintain your physical health by eating and sleeping well, but depression leads to lack of appetite and insomnia. You should be active—even exercise—but one of the main symptoms of depression is lack of energy. You should have fun, but depression erodes your capacity for pleasure. You should think realistically, but depression spawns negative thinking and brings back bad memories. You should socialize with others, but you feel like withdrawing, and you might encounter subtle rejection when you do attempt to interact with others. So all the good advice might seem to boil down to this: Don't be depressed!

The fundamental catch-22: to recover from depression you must have hope, but depression spawns hopelessness. The *Shorter Oxford English Dictionary* defines "catch-22"[1] as a condition that precludes success or a dilemma in which the victim cannot win. Lest my attention to catch-22 add fuel to hopelessness, we must distinguish between difficult and impossible; hope lies in this difference. The reason catch-22 makes recovery difficult rather than impossible is that impairment associated with depression is a *matter of degree*. Fortunately, we are not dealing with black and white but with shades of gray—sometimes dark grays. For example, you will need to be motivated to recover, but depression depletes your energy. Being depressed, you have less energy, but you still have *some* energy and *some* motivation—at least *some of the time*. These degrees of preserved functioning provide some leverage over depression in each domain of the catch-22: you can get some sleep, you can eat some, and you can get yourself going to some degree.

I think *underestimating* the difficulty of recovering from depression contributes to hopelessness. If you think recovery should be easy, you will feel like a failure for being unable to just snap out of it. If you don't recognize catch-22, you might be setting unrealistic goals for yourself. Failure to reach goals is depressing. If you understand that catch-22 can make recovery slow and difficult, you might take some satisfaction in small steps toward improvement. Over time, these small steps lead toward recovery. When you acknowledge and appreciate small successes, you begin to overcome the continual feeling of failure.

During an educational group for hospitalized patients, when I asserted that recovering from depression is difficult but not impossible, one participant rightfully protested: he had been so depressed that it was utterly impossible for him to recover *on his own*. He had been virtually paralyzed. Now I introduce this caveat: in maintaining that it is difficult but not impossible to recover, I point out that it can be impossible to recover without help. Fortunately, all sorts of help are available, and the more you know about them, the more leverage you'll have over your depression. Part V of this book ("Coping With Catch-22") is intended to help you find that leverage.

STRESS PILEUP

This book takes a developmental approach. For some persons, depression seems to come out of the blue. For most persons, however, depression signals the breaking point after a pileup of stress that can accumulate over the lifetime. This book draws your attention to this developmental process for two reasons: first, if you can understand what led up to your depression, you will be in a better position to recover and remain well; second, when you understand the reasons for your depression, you will have more compassion for yourself. I don't mean to imply that all the adverse developmental factors I describe apply to each depressed individual; rather, I have included diverse contributions to the development of depression so that you are likely to find some information about all those that pertain to you.

I have organized this book chronologically, considering how you get into depression through stress pileup over the course of your lifetime and then how you can get out from under the pileup and stay out. I start, however, by laying the groundwork in the first three chapters. Chapter 1 ("Depression") describes different forms of depression; Chapter 2 ("Between a Rock and a Hard Place") documents the seriousness of the illness; and Chapter 3 ("Agency and Elbow Room") emphasizes the need for you to take an active role in recovering.

The next three chapters begin addressing stress pileup. Chapter 4 ("Constitution") reviews different sources of biological vulnerability to stress; Chapter 5 ("Attachment") considers the role of insecure attachment in depression; and Chapter 6 ("Childhood Adversity") delineates the contribution of stress early in life to the development of depression. The accumulation of biological vulnerability and early life stress can render you more susceptible to the precipitants of depressive episodes in adulthood. Chapter 7 ("Stressful Events") considers the role of external stress, and Chapter 8 ("Internal Stress") highlights the role of emotional conflicts in the last straws of stress pileup. Then we get into the illness itself. As I view it, although you might want to keep going in the face of stress pileup, your brain and body ultimately go on strike. Chapter 9 ("Brain and Body") construes depression as a physical illness, and Chapter 10 ("Related Disorders") considers additional psychiatric illnesses that frequently accompany depression.

Continuing the developmental progression, having considered the pathways into depression, we need to think about how to recover and remain well. Helpfully, yet confusingly, clinicians have developed a wealth of treatment approaches. You will need to prioritize by figuring out where best to direct your efforts; the last part of the book is intended to help you do so. I've organized these chapters from the simple (but not easy) to the complex: Chapter 11 ("Health") describes behavioral approaches to enhancing your physical functioning; Chapter 12 ("Flexible Thinking") summarizes cognitive therapy techniques developed to counter negative thinking; Chapter 13 ("Supportive Relationships") reviews interpersonal and psychodynamic therapies intended to address problems in attachment relationships; and Chapter 14 ("Integrating Treatment") evaluates the effectiveness of antidepressant medication in relation to various forms of psychotherapy. I conclude with some reflections on hope in Chapter 15 ("Hope").

READING THIS BOOK

You won't need any technical background to understand this book; your personal experience will do. I'm addressing the reader as "you," with the person struggling with depression in mind. Yet I intend this book for a wider audience: not just those who have depression but all those who care for them—loved ones and mental health professionals alike. In short, I wrote the book for anyone seeking a comprehensive understanding of depression and its treatment.

However, if you are severely depressed, reading this book will confront you with catch-22: you have a lot to learn, but you might have difficulty concentrating, and you may have difficulty remembering what you have read. I've packed a great deal of information into this book, and I intend it to be intellectually challenging in stimulating new ways of thinking. Here, as elsewhere, there is only one way around catch-22: take it slowly, proceeding by small steps. I have organized the book to be conducive to this approach, breaking down each chapter into short sections. You will be able to tell easily from the chapter titles, headings, and subheadings what you wish to read and prefer to skip. Later material builds on earlier material, so I designed the book to be read front to back. If you are eager to get straight to recovering, there's no harm in diving right into the last part on coping—or starting with the last chapter on hope, for that matter. As I will be emphasizing throughout this book, you are a free agent.

• Part I •

GROUNDWORK

```
┌─────────────────────────────────────┐
│  ┌──────────────────────────────┐    │
│  │                              │    │
│  ├──────────────────────────────┤    │
│  │                              │    │
│  │   •  C h a p t e r   1  •    │    │
│  │                              │    │
│  └──────────────────────────────┘    │
└─────────────────────────────────────┘
```

DEPRESSION

A true wimp of a word. That's how author William Styron characterized depression in his poignant memoir, *Darkness Visible:*[2]

> When I was first aware that I had been laid low by the disease, I felt a need, among other things, to register a strong protest against the word 'depression'.... 'Melancholia' would still appear to be a far more apt and evocative word for the blacker forms of the disorder, but it was usurped by a noun with a bland tonality and lacking any magisterial presence, used indifferently to describe an economic decline or a rut in the ground, a true wimp of a word for such a major illness... for over seventy-five years the word has slithered innocuously through the language like a slug, leaving little trace of its intrinsic malevolence and preventing, by its very insipidity, a general awareness of the horrible intensity of the disease when out of control. (pp. 36–37)

Depression connotes the commonplace; few of us could lay claim to never having been depressed. Yet those who have been depressed in the ordinary sense might mistakenly assume that they know what it is like to be ill with depression; in actuality, they cannot comprehend it. Styron explained, "Such incomprehension has usually been due not to a failure of sympathy but to the basic inability of healthy people to imagine a form of torment so alien to everyday experience" (p. 17). *Depression* misleads us in its blandness. Endeavoring to describe the indescribable, Styron refers to helpless stupor, immobilized trance, anguish, a leaden and poisonous mood, an insidious meltdown, an immense and aching solitude, unrelenting pain, and despair beyond despair. He underscored the uncommonness of the experience:

"Mysteriously and in ways that are totally remote from normal experience, the gray drizzle of horror induced by depression takes on the quality of physical pain" (p. 50).

ORIENTATION

I've introduced this chapter by emphasizing the sheer severity of depression, distinguishing between the kind of *depressed mood* that all but the most stalwart among us experience from time to time and *depressive illness* that warrants a psychiatric diagnosis and treatment. Yet depressive illness varies along a continuum of severity and comes in different forms. Our starting place is mapping out the diagnostic territory of depression. We must, as it were, begin by understanding our opponent. Modern psychiatry has been at this task for more than a century, so we have plenty of ground to cover.

I am launching this book with a necessarily complicated chapter, and I want to provide some orientation so you don't get bogged down at the very start of the journey. As you're likely to know all too well from direct experience, anxiety and depression are close companions, often running together in a blur. But we can sharpen our understanding of depression by distinguishing it from anxiety, and I start there. Then I describe *major depression*, the defining and most extensively researched form of the illness. Next, with forewarning of a somewhat encyclopedic rendering, I distinguish several diagnostic variants of the illness, which revolve around severity and duration of symptoms. I also distinguish several way stations along the course of the illness. The detail in these two sections on variations in depression and course of illness may be more or less relevant to your personal concerns, and you have little to lose by skimming them if you are so inclined. But don't miss a central point: low-grade or "minor" symptoms short of major depression are clinically significant, because they potentially erode your quality of life, undermine your functioning, and render you more vulnerable to more severe depression. Take them seriously, and aspire to overcome them as best you can.

Having mapped out the diagnostic territory, I elaborate a major thesis of this book: depression is best understood from a developmental perspective. Gaining a clearer idea of how you got into depression will help you get out of it and stay out of it. However, staying out of depression necessitates that you learn to use the feelings of depression as signals of overload, which brings us to a paradoxical topic: the potential adaptive functions of depression. Yet, as this whole book will attest, I have no intention of looking at depression through rose-colored glasses, and I conclude with Styron's comments on the need to take the seriousness of depression seriously.

ANXIETY AND DEPRESSION

At the beginning of the twentieth century, writing about his "philosophic pessimism and general depression of spirits," philosopher-psychologist William James[3] gave this account:

> I went one evening into a dressing-room in the twilight to procure some article that was there; when suddenly there fell upon me without any warning, just as if it came out of the darkness, a horrible fear of my own existence.... [Identifying with an epileptic patient in an asylum] I became a mass of quivering fear. After this the universe was changed for me altogether. I awoke morning after morning with a horrible dread at the pit of my stomach, and with a sense of the insecurity of life that I never knew before, and that I have never felt since. It was like a revelation; and although the immediate feelings passed away, the experience has made me sympathetic with the morbid feelings of others ever since. It gradually faded, but for months I was unable to go out into the dark alone. (p. 6)

Close companions as they are to depression, I give anxiety and fear their due throughout this book. Anxiety and depression often feed into each other, and sometimes it's hard to tell them apart. In the language of academic psychology, here's the basic contrast:[4] anxiety is an excess of negative emotion, and depression is a deficiency of positive emotion (see Figure 1–1). If this distinction doesn't make immediate sense, bear with me.

NEGATIVE EMOTIONALITY

Let's start with anxiety. Think of a spectrum of negative emotion ranging from 0 to 10. At the low end of this spectrum—0 to 1—you'd feel calm, relaxed, and content. Slightly higher up, you'd become more alert. In the middle—4 to 6—you'd feel tense or anxious, maybe jumpy and irritable. Somewhat higher—7 to 8—you might feel downright afraid. At the extreme—9 to 10—you'd feel panicky or terrified.

Negative emotion, although unpleasant, serves a positive function: it affords sensitivity to threat and promotes avoidance. Responding to danger, you are physiologically energized so as to take vigorous action, such as fleeing or fighting. Negative emotion also promotes learning: you learn to steer clear of anything that has caused physical or emotional pain.

In thinking about the adaptiveness of emotion, however, it's helpful to distinguish between *states* and *traits*. Although a burst of fear or anger (a *state*) can be adaptive, prolonged negative emotion (a *trait*) can be corrosive. By virtue of genetic makeup and stressful early experience, some persons are characteristically prone to negative emotions such as anxiety, distress,

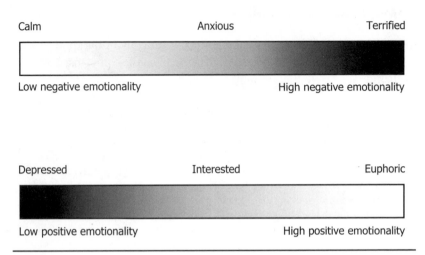

FIGURE 1–1. Anxiety versus depression.

irritability, and guilt feelings. When it's relatively pervasive, negative emotionality becomes a personality trait.

We refer to individuals who worry needlessly as "neurotic," and negative emotionality is labeled *neuroticism* in personality research.[4] Tending toward neuroticism myself, I don't take this epithet as a great insult; I'm generally sympathetic with it. In addition to distress proneness, neuroticism includes a tendency to be introspective and to ruminate as well as an inclination to focus on negative aspects of oneself and the world. Being a personality trait, neuroticism comes in all degrees. Persons characterized by a high degree of neuroticism are especially sensitive to stress. Given that depression is a response to prolonged stress, neuroticism puts us at higher risk for depression.[5]

POSITIVE EMOTIONALITY

Depression would seem to be a clear case of negative emotion, but it's not. Rather, the core of depressed mood is the loss of your capacity to experience positive emotions such as interest, excitement, and joy. Styron characterized his depression as dank joylessness. Here's one of my favorite ideas: decades ago, psychologist Paul Meehl[6] speculated that depression results from a lack of cerebral joy juice.

If you're not too depressed to do so, think of the excitement you have felt when you anticipated doing something you really enjoyed. The positive emotion of excitement serves an adaptive function: whereas negative emotions push you away from whatever might be bad for you, positive emotions draw you toward whatever might be good for you. For example, you eagerly anticipate a delicious meal. Negative emotions lead you to avoid punishment; positive emotions lead you to approach reward.

When you're depressed, you have no interest in anything, and you may just sit in a chair or stay in bed. The things that you ordinarily enjoy—gardening, listening to music, reading, movies, sports, and dinner with your friends—no longer provide any pleasure. You have no interest in doing them. Nothing matters, and you can't look forward to anything. Others urge you to relieve your depression by engaging in pleasurable activities. You have undoubtedly tried this, to little avail. You're confronted with catch-22: to get over depression, you must experience pleasure; because you're depressed, your capacity for pleasure is diminished.

Going beyond the idea of cerebral joy juice, neuroscientist Jaak Panksepp[7] identified a *seeking* system in the brain that propels us into rewarding activity. Seeking is energizing: positive emotion is associated with an outward focus and active engagement with the environment, including the social environment. When you're feeling good, you're more inclined to socialize, and socializing is a major source of positive emotional experience. Thus, the personality trait of positive emotionality is *extraversion*, the counterpart to neuroticism.[4] Extraverts not only are gregarious but also are inclined to seek out stimulating and rewarding experiences more generally. If you are an extravert by temperament, you'll become more introverted when you get depressed, and you'll return to being more extraverted when you recover.

A DUAL CHALLENGE

Most depressed persons struggle with the combination of too much negative emotion and too little positive emotion. If you're depressed, you have been contending with extreme stress, and you're likely to feel anxious, to worry, or even to feel frightened—perhaps even having uncanny experiences akin to those William James described. You might also feel frustrated and irritated at the obstacles you've encountered. You might feel hostile or resentful toward others who have played an active role in your troubles.

Anxiety and depression feed into each other. Anxiety fuels depression because it wears you out and saps your energy, not to mention also robbing you of pleasure and enjoyment. Depression also contributes to anxiety; for example, you may become more anxious when you must face a social obligation or work situation that you feel you cannot handle because you're so depressed.

Depression and anxiety present a double-whammy: both promote *disengagement* from the environment in general and from other people in particular. Being depressed, you have little incentive to be with other people, because the pleasure is not there. Being anxious, you may be inclined to withdraw from other people. Engaging in social contacts that don't demand a great deal of interaction may provide a middle ground (see Chapter 13, "Supportive Relationships").

Given the likelihood of having to struggle with both depression and anxiety, you have two challenges. On the one hand, being depressed, you need to activate yourself—to develop more energy and interest in things. On the other hand, being anxious, you need to deactivate yourself—to feel more calm and relaxed. Controlling depression and anxiety is quite a balancing act. If you can get yourself absorbed and engaged in relaxing activities, you might be able to accomplish both at the same time. If these relaxing activities involve some contact with other people, so much the better.

I discuss stressful experience and anxiety throughout this book in the context of the development of depression, the neurobiology of depression, and psychiatric disorders that often accompany depression. For now, we focus on depression in its purer forms.

MAJOR DEPRESSION

The diagnostic criteria for a *major depressive episode* require that the symptoms be present every day for most of the day for at least 2 weeks.[8] Table 1–1 displays the symptoms of major depression, which cause significant distress or impairment in your social or occupational functioning. If you have experienced a major depressive *episode*, it's likely that a diagnosis of major depressive *disorder* will be made. However, major depressive episodes also may occur in the context of other psychiatric disorders (e.g., bipolar disorder) or general medical conditions (e.g., stroke or hypothyroidism); such alternatives must be ruled out to make a diagnosis of major depressive disorder (see Chapter 10, "Related Disorders").

What is depressed in depression? Positive emotion. The diagnosis of a major depressive episode entails depressed mood or loss of interest or pleasure in activities—a low level of positive emotionality. Yet the diagnosis goes beyond depressed mood: a whole *syndrome*—a cluster of symptoms that go together—must be present. Specifically, five of the nine symptoms listed in Table 1–1 must be present. As you know if you've experienced it, major depression affects your *whole being*—your physical functioning, way of thinking, view of yourself, and relationships. One potentially confusing point: the physical symptoms typically include sleeping too little (insomnia)

TABLE 1–1.   Symptoms of major depression

Depressed mood
Diminished interest or pleasure in activities
Significant decrease or increase in weight or appetite
Insomnia or hypersomnia
Motor agitation or retardation
Fatigue or loss of energy
Feelings of worthlessness or excessive guilt
Diminished ability to think or concentrate; indecisiveness
Recurrent thoughts of death; suicidal thinking or behavior

and poor appetite, often associated with weight loss. Yet a substantial minority of depressed persons experience the opposite pattern, *atypical symptoms:* sleeping too much (hypersomnia), overeating, and weight gain.

VARIATIONS IN DEPRESSION

VARIATIONS IN SEVERITY

Researchers have marked off different levels of depression along a continuum of severity, and persons who struggle with severe depression move from one level to another. We can distinguish two levels of symptoms that are less severe than major depression: subthreshold symptoms and minor depressive disorder. In addition, we can identify particularly severe signs: melancholic and psychotic features.

   We can best think of depression as one illness that varies in degrees, both in children[9] and adults.[10] Degrees of depression take three forms. First, each of the symptoms of depression varies from mild to severe. Second, you might have any number of the nine symptoms. Third, depression varies in duration, ranging from a brief episode to chronic depression. Different diagnoses reflect different combinations of severity and duration. In this section I start by distinguishing different levels of severity and duration, and then I discuss several diagnostic variants (see Table 1–2):

• *Subthreshold*[11] or *subsyndromal*[12] depression is not precisely defined but involves one or more symptoms of mild depression that are not sufficient to warrant a diagnosis. You might be at the subthreshold level prior to sliding into a major depression. You'd be at the subthreshold level in the course of recovery when you feel better but don't feel like you're back to

TABLE 1–2.   Diagnostic variants

Major depressive episode	At least 2 weeks of five or more severe symptoms
Chronic major depression	Major depression for at least 2 years
Dysthymic disorder	Symptoms less severe than major depression for at least 2 years
Double depression	Major depressive episodes superimposed on dysthymic disorder
Depressive personality disorder	Enduring depressive personality pattern (e.g., gloomy, critical, pessimistic)
Seasonal affective disorder	Recurrent depressive episodes at a particular time of year (typically winter)

your usual self. Or you might remain at the subthreshold level without experiencing a major depressive episode. These mild symptoms are not insignificant: they're best viewed as an active phase of depressive illness; they're associated with significant problems in functioning;[13] and they're associated with a heightened risk of lapsing into a more severe level of illness (e.g., back into a major depression).

- *Minor depressive disorder*[8] includes the same criteria as major depression but fewer active symptoms: at least two, but fewer than the five required for major depression. These symptoms must include either depressed mood or diminished pleasure or interest in activity (the core mood symptoms) as well as significant distress or impairment in functioning.
- *Major depression* is the severest level of depression in terms of intensity if not duration. Yet there are degrees of severity within this condition: each symptom may be more or less severe, and you might have any number of symptoms from five to all nine.
- *Melancholia,* a condition recognized for two millennia, is a particularly severe form of major depression.[8] Melancholic features include especially severe mood disturbance: loss of pleasure in all, or almost all, activities or lack of reactivity to ordinarily pleasurable stimuli (e.g., not feeling much better—even temporarily—when something good happens). In addition, three or more of the following symptoms characterize melancholia: distinct quality of depressed mood (e.g., different from that following a major loss), depression regularly being worse in the morning, early morning awakening, marked agitation or retardation of activity, significant anorexia or weight loss, and excessive or inappropriate guilt.
- *Psychotic features*[8] entail a loss of contact with reality. Psychotic symptoms include hallucinations (unrealistic perceptions) and delusions (unrealistic beliefs). For example, the psychotically depressed person might have

auditory hallucinations, such as voices that berate the person for short-comings or sins. Or the depressed person may have delusions of guilt (e.g., feeling responsible for world tragedies). When psychotic features are present, treatment must be tailored accordingly (see Chapter 14, "Integrating Treatment").

VARIATIONS IN DURATION

The experience of depression can range from hours to years, and protracted depression typically waxes and wanes in severity over time. Thus all combinations of severity and duration are possible. Two forms of severe depression vary in duration:

1. Combining high severity and long duration, a diagnosis of *chronic major depression* requires that full criteria for major depressive episode have been met continuously for at least 2 years.[8]
2. At the other end of the duration spectrum, a pattern of *recurrent brief depression* also has been identified.[14] This pattern entails brief episodes—typically 1–3 days—of major depressive symptoms that recur at least monthly for more than a year.

DYSTHYMIC DISORDER

Dysthymia refers to a prolonged disturbance (*dys*) of mood (*thymia*). The criteria for diagnosing dysthymic disorder[8] are similar to those for major depression, but the severity of the symptoms is less whereas the duration is longer: depressed mood for most of the day, more days than not, over a period of *at least 2 years*. The diagnosis requires that, while the person is depressed, at least two of the following symptoms also be present: poor appetite or overeating; insomnia or hypersomnia; low energy or fatigue; low self-esteem; poor concentration or difficulty making decisions; and feelings of hopelessness.

To meet criteria for dysthymic disorder, you must not have had a symptom-free period of 2 months or more over the course of the illness, and you must not have had a major depressive episode during that period. Here's a danger with dysthymic disorder, especially when you develop it early in life: you might resign yourself to depression as being "just the way I am," or you might have become so accustomed to it that you don't even recognize that you are depressed—like a fish not knowing what water is. Although the symptoms of dysthymia are less severe than those of major depression, dysthymia is a serious condition associated with considerable suffering and impairment of functioning.[15] Dysthymia in childhood or adulthood also significantly increases the risk of developing a subsequent major depressive episode.[16]

You should not resign yourself to chronic, low-grade depression: many persons with dysthymia respond well to treatment. To date, there is some evidence for the effectiveness of psychological treatment and more evidence for the effectiveness of antidepressant medication.[17] Consider this heartening conclusion from a naturalistic study of patients who had developed dysthymia at an average age of less than 13 years and who received specialized care:[18] "3 of 4 patients immersed in gloom for much of their lives achieved for the first time good to superior levels of functioning that were maintained for an average of 5 years" (p. 508).

DOUBLE DEPRESSION

Many persons with a history of dysthymia go on to develop major depression, in which case they're considered to have *double depression*—major depression on top of dysthymia.[19] Given the compounding of chronic depression with episodic severe symptoms, double depression is a particularly serious condition.[20] Persons with double depression who recover from major depressive episodes are likely to return to being dysthymic, but ongoing dysthymia after a major depressive episode presents a high risk for relapse into major depression as well as portending a faster time to relapse.[21] Plainly, although it's more difficult to do, you're advised to aspire to recovering fully from a major depressive episode rather than settling for a return to a baseline of dysthymia. To reiterate, like major depression, dysthymia is treatable.

DEPRESSIVE PERSONALITY DISORDER

Depressive personality disorder is diagnosed when depressed mood has become woven into the personality. Criteria for the diagnosis include joyless, unhappy mood; low self-esteem; self-criticism; brooding and worrying; negativism and criticism of others; pessimism; and proneness to guilt feelings.

Because both involve chronic, low-grade depression, it is challenging to distinguish between depressive personality disorder and dysthymia;[22] thus the diagnostic manual[8] provisionally includes depressive personality in an appendix as a disorder in need of further study. Although many persons with chronic depression have both depressive personality disorder and dysthymia, a sufficient proportion of individuals have one without the other to justify distinguishing the two.[23,24] Depressed mood is more prominent in dysthymia than in depressive personality disorder, and a substantial minority of persons with depressive personality disorder do not experience the pronounced mood disturbance. Yet depressive personality disorder is no less serious: like dysthymia, depressive personality disorder is associated with significant impairments in functioning, and it increases the risk of developing major depression.

SEASONAL AFFECTIVE DISORDER

Seasonal affective disorder (SAD)—winter depression—has been recognized since the 1980s.[25] SAD is diagnosed when the onset and remission of depression occur consistently at a particular time of year. Most commonly, the depression begins in the fall or winter and ends in spring. To make the diagnosis, this pattern must be recurrent, with all or most episodes occurring at the same time of year. In addition, the association of depression with a specific time of year must not be based on seasonal stress (e.g., routinely starting school or being out of work at that time of year). SAD is associated with the atypical pattern of depressive symptoms: sleeping too much, overeating, weight gain, and craving carbohydrates.[8]

The physiological basis of SAD remains to be determined; factors being investigated include genetic vulnerability, disturbances in circadian rhythms, disruptions in the sleep–wake cycle, and altered serotonin neurotransmission.[26] Because most seasonal depressive episodes occur in the winter and resolve in the spring, the shortened period of light is suspected to be the primary trigger. Accordingly, light therapy (exposure to bright light for 30–120 minutes daily, typically in the morning) has proven to be an effective treatment, and antidepressant medication also is helpful.[27] Given the potential benefit of light therapy for those with SAD, it's worthwhile to determine if there is a seasonal pattern to your depression.

COURSE OF ILLNESS

Like other illnesses, depression has a course, a pattern of progression over time. A fever has a waxing and waning course; it gets worse, then better, then worse again. As illustrated in Figure 1–2, clinicians distinguish among the "five Rs" in charting the course of depression:[28,29]

1. *Response* to treatment is the point at which significant improvement short of return to wellness is observed.
2. *Remission* is a resolution of symptoms; the illness is assumed to be active but suppressed (e.g., by medication).

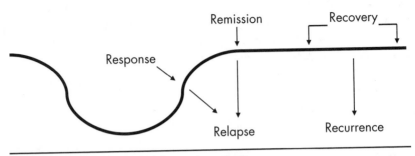

FIGURE 1–2. Course of a depressive episode.

3. *Relapse* is a return of more severe illness during a period of response or remission; during these periods of response and remission, the vulnerability to relapse remains high, because the illness remains active.
4. *Recovery* follows a significant period of remission. After recovery, the likelihood of returning symptoms is substantially lower than during remission. How long the symptom-free period should be before you are considered recovered is not sharply defined. Depression researchers use a range from 2 to 6 months to define recovery, but even a 4-week period of wellness is a good indication of recovery, because it indicates a substantially lowered likelihood of relapse.[30]
5. *Recurrence* is a return of illness after a period of recovery. The illness is assumed to have been in abeyance, such that a recurrence is considered to be a new episode, potentially with different triggers or causes.

To illustrate the five Rs most simply, I've depicted the course of depression in Figure 1–2 as a single dip from wellness into major depression back to wellness. Although this pattern fits some persons, many others experience waxing and waning symptoms—hills and troughs with some canyons—over long periods, potentially extending over much of a lifetime. With or without signs of illness, *vulnerability* to depression can evolve over the lifetime.

DEVELOPMENTAL PERSPECTIVE

For some persons, a depressive episode in adulthood can seem to come out of the blue. Others may struggle with varying degrees of depression over much of their lifetime. More often than not, adulthood psychiatric disorders are preceded by childhood and adolescent disorders. A landmark study of individuals followed from birth to age 26 revealed that half of the 26-

year-olds with psychiatric disorders had a diagnosable disorder at 11–15 years of age and three-quarters had a disorder before age 18.[31] Usually, the disorders were the same; for example, childhood or adolescent depression preceded adulthood depression.

Even when major depression first erupts in adulthood, it's often possible to identify a developmental history that contributes to vulnerability. Although Styron's depression emerged de novo at age 60, he traced its origins to his early sorrow at the death of his mother when he was 13, and he noted that suicide had been a recurrent theme in his books; three of his major characters killed themselves.

I devote Part II of this book to developmental origins of depression, which I construe broadly as stress pileup over the lifetime (see Figure 1–3). I believe that taking seriously whatever factors may have rendered you vulnerable will mitigate self-criticism and help you develop a more compassionate attitude toward yourself as you struggle with depression. Furthermore, appreciating the factors that render you vulnerable can help you care for yourself and increase your resilience.

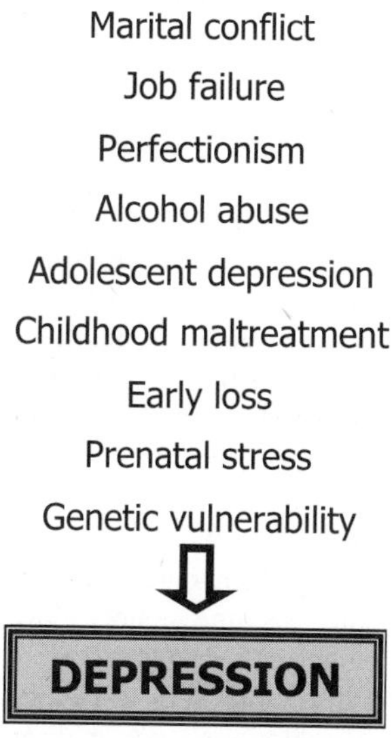

Marital conflict

Job failure

Perfectionism

Alcohol abuse

Adolescent depression

Childhood maltreatment

Early loss

Prenatal stress

Genetic vulnerability

⇩

DEPRESSION

FIGURE 1–3. Example of stress pileup over the lifetime.

Source. Adapted with permission from Allen J: "Depression," in *Coping With Trauma: Hope Through Understanding.* Washington, DC, American Psychiatric Publishing, 2005, p. 155. Used with permission. Copyright 2005 American Psychiatric Publishing.

Consider the complex developmental trajectory that can eventuate in major depression.

Amanda, a woman in her early 50s, entered the hospital after a serious suicide attempt in which she had consumed a pint of gin in combination with tranquilizers and sleeping pills. She said she'd just wanted peace—to go to sleep, perhaps forever. When she entered the hospital, she was ill in many respects, not just feeling depressed. She couldn't sleep and she could hardly eat. She was out of shape, having been physically inactive for months. She said she felt exhausted and just "sick."

Amanda's suicide attempt and run-down condition presented a stark contrast to most of her adult life. She had coped effectively with a traumatic childhood; when she was 8 years old, her mother died after a prolonged illness, and her father's occasional alcohol use gradually escalated into a pattern of alcoholism. He was often away from home, and he was irritable and withdrawn when he was around. Fortunately, Amanda's aunt lived only a block away, and she took over Amanda's care, including her emotional needs, during her mother's illness and after her death. Amanda's father remarried a few years after her mother's death, and Amanda's stepmother quickly became jealous of Amanda's close relationship with her aunt. Her stepmother became increasingly cold and hostile, at times both emotionally and physically abusive. One time in a fit of rage, she tore up Amanda's favorite picture of her mother, plunging Amanda into despair and fueling her resentment.

Amanda was blessed with many assets, which included artistic talent, good intelligence, a warm personality, and a remarkable capacity to persist at challenges. As her home life became more stressful, she plunged into schoolwork and consistently earned good grades. She routinely participated in school activities and art fairs. She made friends and earned the admiration of teachers, thriving on their frequent praise. She won a scholarship to college and she seized the opportunity to leave home, moving to another state. Amanda anticipated that leaving home would be a great emotional relief, and it was. Yet she had not anticipated the impact of losing the considerable support network she'd developed, and she slowly began to struggle with sadness and depression akin to what she had felt in childhood after her mother's death.

Amanda relied on her determination to get her through the transition to college. By the end of her freshman year, she was achieving good grades and gaining some recognition from teachers. She developed a close relationship with another student in her dorm who became her confidant. She also stayed in contact with her high school friends. She continued making use of her talents, pursuing a double major in art and secondary education.

Over the course of many years, Amanda had nurtured a strong desire to have a family of her own—a loving home akin to the one she had lost when her mother became ill. She began dating in her sophomore year and fell in love with one of her classmates in her senior year. She graduated and found a position as a high school art teacher, a career she had maintained throughout her adult life. A few years after graduating, she married and, over the course of the next several years, she had three children. Except for periods of maternity leave, she taught school as well as taking the main responsibility for raising her children. Her husband, a high school math teacher, was very engaged with the family, although he was extremely busy with coaching as well as teaching.

Amanda had been highly successful on many fronts: despite the loss of her mother and the painful relationships with her father and stepmother, she consistently sought out close relationships—defying her stepmother to visit her aunt, developing friendships, connecting with her teachers, finding a devoted husband, and maintaining affectionate relationships with her children. In addition, she developed her academic and artistic talents into a stable career in which she could nurture adolescents, being especially attentive to those who, like herself, needed special attention.

Yet Amanda's life was fraught with strain. She exemplified what we have come to call the "run-run-run/go-go-go lifestyle" that contributes to stress pileup.[32] She and her husband held high standards for themselves: both had demanding careers; both were devoted to their children; and both were torn between work and family, often feeling they could never do enough on either front. "Leisure" and "relaxation" were hardly in their vocabulary. The stress mounted. Their middle child, a son, had been hyperactive virtually all his life and—to his parents' chagrin—was getting into increasingly serious trouble in the school district in which they both worked. Amanda's father, struggling with chronic depression and alcoholism—and smoking two packs a day—developed heart disease. Amanda took a great deal of responsibility for his welfare, an ongoing stress compounded by their antagonistic relationship. The added stress began taking its toll. As she had earlier in life, Amanda experienced bouts of depression. She pushed herself to keep going and did not seek professional help. She mistakenly regarded her depression as a natural consequence of her difficult life circumstances.

As the years wore on, Amanda often felt she was being "run ragged." Inclined to worry as well as feel extremely responsible, she was characteristically highly anxious—her husband described her as high-strung. Furthermore, feeling burdened by high demands with no periods of relief, she began following in her father's footsteps, drinking more regularly—a stiff drink or two before dinner and sometimes another before bedtime to help her wind down and go to sleep.

In the months before her suicide attempt, the chronic strain increased further as Amanda grappled with additional stressors. After many years in a first-rate art program that she had developed, she was abruptly moved to a new school as a result of reorganization—an administrative decision that she felt to be arbitrary and ill considered. Although she had no serious complaints about the new school, her program had been dismantled, and she had lost the daily support of several close colleagues as well as having her relationships with treasured students disrupted. Her drinking escalated; unbeknownst to her, it was worsening her depression while it temporarily dampened her anxiety. Her energy was decreasing, and her anxiety now was intermingled with irritability. Her relationship with her husband was deteriorating. Although their children were now older and there were now ample opportunities for recreation, she lost interest in doing things with her husband, and he increasingly found things to do with friends, leaving her alone. She resented his absences; he resented her lack of interest in doing anything with him and worried about her drinking. They began to argue.

Several months after Amanda moved to her new school, her son—now in his late 20s—was arrested for stealing. Although she had worried for years about his getting into trouble, this event came out of the blue. She was shocked, irate, and humiliated. Then came the last straw. After drinking in the evening, she developed a headache and discovered she was out of aspirin. She drove to the pharmacy. It was dusk; she was slightly intoxicated, and she was preoccupied about an argument she had had with her husband about her son. A few blocks from home, she nearly hit a girl on her bicycle. The girl swerved just in time but fell off her bike; she was badly scraped but not seriously injured. The girl was frightened and upset and, by the time Amanda got out of the car to check on her, the girl was outraged: "You could've killed me!" She was right.

Amanda went through a kaleidoscope of emotions in the aftermath of this near miss. At first profoundly relieved, she quickly became horrified, playing through in her mind numerous scenarios involving what could have happened—maiming or killing the girl. In a daze, she proceeded to the pharmacy, bought the aspirin, and returned home. Then she began to worry and ruminate. Should she have contacted the girl's parents? Did the girl get her license plate? Would they try to find her? Would she be arrested for driving while intoxicated? Her ruminations turned to self-recrimination— not just for this incident but for what she began to see as her many failings over the previous several months. She couldn't calm down; on the contrary, she was becoming more and more agitated. She was too ashamed of what she had done to reach out for help. She wanted peace.

Amanda had been in the habit of mixing alcohol and sleeping medication to knock herself out. At the end of her rope, she wanted to knock herself out for a long time—perhaps for good. She wasn't thinking clearly. Alone in her home, she finished the pint of gin and took all her remaining sleeping medication—with a handful of aspirin for the headache. Soon after she nodded off, her daughter called and was alarmed to find Amanda to be groggy and incoherent. By sheer luck, her daughter knew that her father was at a neighbor's; she was able to get in touch with him, and he got Amanda to the emergency room.

When she had recovered, Amanda was horrified by her suicide attempt, feeling profoundly ashamed. She had no desire to die, but this event only compounded the stress and deepened her depression. It was at that point— for the first time in her life—that she sought professional help.

Looking back over her life, Amanda was able to see emotional warning signs of the trouble to come. Hindsight is always better than foresight. With professional help, Amanda was able to learn a great deal from this near tragedy. Ideally, we might use feelings of depression as a signal before they evolve into illness.

ADAPTATION GONE AWRY

Depression is an illness, and we don't usually think of illnesses as being beneficial. However, we have two reasons for wondering if there might be some adaptive value to depression—if we heed the signs. First, as Darwin[33] identified more than a century ago, a wide range of distressing emotions evolved as adaptive responses to environmental challenges. Second, although most of us do not become ill with depression, virtually all of us have some capacity to feel depressed.

We can easily understand how fear and anger are adaptive emotions; they evolved as part of the fight-or-flight response.[34] Fear and anger are self-protective: almost instantaneously, when you are threatened or attacked, your sympathetic nervous system is activated, and your body gears up for vigorous action. You fight back in anger or flee in fear. It's not so easy to understand how depression could be adaptive. What good is depression? What purpose could it serve to be stalled? Depression seems to be the antithesis of coping.

Three theories have been proposed to address the adaptive aspects of depression: conservation-withdrawal, incentive disengagement, and involuntary subordination. Each of these theories suggests that depression might serve some useful purpose. Yet, when it goes too far—becoming an illness—depression backfires as an adaptation. To make use of depression, it is necessary to develop tolerance for depressive feelings so as to avoid depressive illness. I discuss depression tolerance after reviewing the three theories about depression's adaptive functions.

CONSERVATION-WITHDRAWAL

When you are facing stressful challenges, it's natural to cope by trying harder—exerting more effort, perhaps pushing yourself to the limit or beyond. When it fails to resolve the problem, however, such extra effort merely adds to stress pileup. Many persons who spiral into depression have been exerting increasing effort as they've been running out of energy. The gap between exertion and energy widens and, ultimately, they crash into depression. Depression thus stops them in their tracks.

Here's a simple idea about the adaptive functions of depression: when stress is overwhelming, your body shuts down at some point to prevent itself from *completely* burning out. You run out of gas before you burn up your engine. More technically, this adaptation has been called the *conservation-withdrawal reaction*.[35] The model is the infant whose prolonged crying leads to sleep. This example illustrates how shutting down can be protective when heightened activity (crying) is ineffective. Analogously, depression has been likened to hibernation;[36] you conserve energy until the situation becomes more favorable for active coping.[37]

The conservation-withdrawal hypothesis is appealing, but there is a major problem with it: the baby who cries herself to sleep may have conserved her energy and awakened restored and refreshed; but depression isn't restful. More than anyone, the depressed person needs rest. A temporary depressive retreat might help. Yet depression doesn't provide the needed rest, respite, and conservation. Depression is a protracted high-stress state. If it's a conservation-withdrawal reaction, the conservation has gone awry. Depression is draining, wearing, and tiring. But let's not give up on the idea that depression might be self-protective in some sense, even if it backfires to some degree.

INCENTIVE DISENGAGEMENT

We generally value persistence and admire people who don't give up in the face of obstacles. We are taught that giving up is a bad thing. However, persistence in the face of insurmountable obstacles is stressful and futile, like banging your head against a wall. I think giving up is an underrated coping strategy. The challenge is to know *when* to give up.

Giving up on highly valued goals is extremely difficult; we need some means of disengaging. Psychologist Eric Klinger[38] proposed that depression is a stop mechanism that diminishes the reward value of the blocked goal. Psychiatrist Rudolph Neese[39] put it simply: "Depression inhibits futile efforts" (p. 17). However, Neese recognized catch-22: "Failure to disengage can cause depression and depression can make it harder to disengage" (p. 17). Thus depression also can keep you stuck and, by undermining your ability to experience anything as potentially rewarding, it can block your interest in moving on to more attainable goals.

INVOLUNTARY SUBORDINATION

One connotation of being "depressed" is being pushed down—*oppressed.* Think of depression as a reaction to feeling overpowered—overpowered by stress, by events, by obstacles, or by other persons, whether it involves feeling dominated and inadequate, outclassed and inferior, excluded and being an outcast, or the extremes of being abused, tormented, or battered.

Here's the adaptation: when you are overpowered, fighting back might get you hurt; giving up might be the most self-protective thing you can do. Psychologist Paul Gilbert[40] construed depression as an *involuntary subordi-*

nation strategy, a reflexlike emotional response that enforces passive surren-
der when aggressive confrontation would place the individual in harm's
way. Depression communicates to the potentially overpowering competi-
tor: "I give up; I'm out of action."

In Gilbert's view, depression is not a conscious strategy; it is an automatic biological adaptation. Yet it goes too far, as research on the *learned
helplessness* model of depression illustrates.[41] When subjected repeatedly to
inescapable electric shock, many animals were traumatized: they would lie
down and give up, showing signs of depression. When the experimenter
subsequently made it possible for them to escape, the animals remained depressed and did not learn; they had learned to be helpless. These animals
were overpowered, and they gave up.

You can imagine how depression would protect you from getting into
more danger, for example, if you are overpowered in an abusive relationship
and fighting back would only result in your getting hurt worse. Yet depression goes too far. You may give up on everything and, as the learned helplessness experiments illustrate, you may remain depressed even when you
are no longer in danger and in a position to do something to overcome the
oppression.

DEPRESSION TOLERANCE

These three theories suggest that depression has a purpose, although it is
overdone. When the adaptation becomes an illness, depression has gone
too far; it undermines coping. After you have recovered and before you become ill, you can learn to use depressive *feelings* as a signal that you are over-
loaded, perhaps feeling overwhelmed and overpowered. You cannot reach
your goals, and somehow you must do something differently. However, if
you keep pushing yourself to no avail, the *illness* of depression will stop you
in your tracks.

Viewed as a signal, depression should be heeded. Being able to tolerate
depressive feelings is an important strength: you can allow yourself to feel
the feelings and understand where they are coming from. Think of this aspect of depression as being akin to physical pain. Depression is a signal.
Your body is telling you it cannot keep going in the face of challenges,
stresses, and obstacles. The capacity to face depression and to bear it is
therefore adaptive.[42] It is an indication that your goals and strategies—perhaps along with your stressful lifestyle—need to be reconsidered.

Psychotherapist Philip Martin[43] best captured the adaptive functions of
depression in his masterful little book, *The Zen Path Through Depression*. He
argued that by slowing you down, depression provides you an opportunity

to become more aware of your plight. In urging readers to hear the message depression conveys, he counseled:

> When we are lost in the woods, we can stop, look at our situation, and see where we are. And when we are in the midst of depression, we can stop and look at where we are and how we came to be here.... Although it is often painful and frightening to approach depression, we can do so. We can stand and not run. We can even allow it in and let ourselves learn what it has to tell us. (pp. 2–3)

Of course, it's best to attend to depressive feelings sooner rather than depressive illness later. As I view it, failing to heed the yellow light, you can run through the red and crash into illness.

SERIOUSNESS

We are off to a rather heavy start: I have highlighted the sheer seriousness of the illness of depression, and I continue this theme in the next chapter. Plainly, I am making no effort to cheer you up. When you're seriously depressed, all such efforts are bound to fail—or to disappoint, if you're temporarily seduced into an unrealistic view of the illness.

After he became depressed, William Styron[2] read extensively about the illness during his more lucid periods. He described a lot of the literature as "breezily optimistic, spreading assurances that nearly all depressive states will be stabilized or reversed if only the suitable antidepressant can be found; the reader is of course easily swayed by promises of quick remedy" (p. 13). But he characterized books that claim an easy fix to be "glib and most likely fraudulent" (p. 10). Without disparaging treatment, which ultimately led to his recovery, Styron proposed that the "most honest authorities face up squarely to the fact that serious depression is not readily treatable," that depression is best situated "squarely in the category of grave diseases," and that "the wisest books...underscore the hard truth that serious depressions do not disappear overnight" (pp. 9–11).

In educating patients about depression, I strive for a balanced view, maintaining that you have solid reasons for hope while acknowledging the seriousness of the illness. Here's one fundamental facet of that balance: the vast majority of patients with major depression recover, but recovery can take a considerable period of time and effort—as Styron's well-balanced account attests.

Chapter 2

BETWEEN A ROCK AND
A HARD PLACE

All but the most undaunted optimists know what it feels like to be depressed. Who hasn't been in a funk for a few hours, a few days, or even a few weeks? No wonder we're likely to equate depressive illness with transient depressed mood. The availability of antidepressant medication contributes to the stereotype of depression as an acute problem: surely you should recover after taking Prozac for a few weeks! This popular misconception fits hand in glove with the current healthcare system in the United States, as psychiatrist Robert Michels[44] described:

> Depressed persons who see psychiatrists or other mental health professionals are more likely to receive a diagnosis of depression but not to receive the long-term care required. Here the problem is that the system wants depression to be an acute disease with no need for long-term treatment and with treatment selected by cost without regard for patient acceptability or adherence. Unfortunately, the depression that patients have is often not the same as the depression that is acceptable to the world of managed care, and the most appropriate treatment courses are not necessarily the shortest or the least expensive. (p. 52)

This chapter addresses several facets of the seriousness of depressive illness, underscoring the potential need for extensive treatment as Michels described it. Even if you know in your heart how serious depression is, you might find the evidence I am about to review startling. I don't intend to alarm you but rather to inform you: you must face the reality of the illness so as to obtain proper treatment.

I begin this chapter by reiterating my plea to face the seriousness of the illness rather than minimizing it. Then I summarize some key research evidence supporting this plea: depression is common; it impairs your functioning; you are likely to need a considerable period of time to recover; the illness can become chronic; and you will remain vulnerable to relapse and recurrence. I have included some statistics to buttress these points in case you or someone you know needs convincing. If you find the detail tedious, you can breeze through it, but don't gloss over the latter part of the chapter, which addresses one important reason for these grim findings: depression is notoriously undertreated, and you should know that proper treatment hastens recovery and decreases the likelihood of recurrence. Thus I conclude the chapter by reminding you that you are not a statistic: the illness is serious, but *you can do something about it.*

THE ROCK AND THE HARD PLACE

When you're depressed, you're caught between a rock and a hard place:

> The rock: It's not that serious—If you'd just [do X], you would snap out of it.

> The hard place: Depression is a serious, persistent, mental-physical illness.

Let's first consider the rock. Many persons who have struggled for a long time to overcome depression have been urged by others, "If you'd just [eat right, go out and exercise, have more fun, stop isolating yourself, quit wallowing, etc.], you wouldn't be depressed." Or consider this line of reasoning: depression is just a mental problem, so you should just change your mind! I have come to think of "just" as a fighting word—it's inflammatory to persons who have struggled for a long time to fight their way out of it with limited success. There's no single, simple solution to persistent depression. You must work on several fronts. Recovery can be a long slog, even if you are able to put effort into it.

I focus primarily on the hard place, because it's more realistic. Depression is a serious illness, recovery may take a lot of time, and you remain vulnerable to recurrence. This is a hard place indeed, but sitting on the rock is potentially crazy-making: you should be able to snap out of it, but you cannot. Therefore you conclude that you are lazy, inadequate, a wimp, or some other depressing idea.

To say that depression is a persistent illness does not mean that you are destined to be severely depressed continuously. You may spend quite a lot of time, however, at different levels of depression, ranging from mild to more severe. I use the term *persistent* to emphasize the fact that you remain vulnerable to recurrence, particularly in the face of significant stress. In this respect, depression is much like other chronic physical illnesses, such as hypertension or diabetes. The main implication of *persistent* is this: you will do best if you obtain adequate treatment and take care of yourself over the long haul, making use of all the help you need to do so when you need it.

DEPRESSION IS COMMON

If you are depressed, you are likely to feel alone. In part, you might feel alone because you're inclined to withdraw and isolate yourself from others. In addition, you may feel that others don't understand what you're going through. You might be thinking that others cope with problems much better than you do and that your depression is a sign of your personal failure.

Ambitious studies beginning in the 1980s have shown that depression is extremely common.[45] For example, the National Comorbidity Survey revealed that, at any given time, 5% of persons in the U.S. population have a major depressive episode.[46] This same study showed that 17% of the population reported having had an episode of major depression at some time in their lifetime. Consistently, studies show that women are about twice as likely as men to develop depression, and this is also a worldwide finding. In the National Comorbidity Survey, for example, 4% of men reported current depression and 13% reported a lifetime history of depression—a high prevalence by any standards. Yet women showed an even higher rate: about 6% reported current depression and 21% reported a lifetime history. The reasons for these gender differences have been studied actively, and I discuss them in Chapter 4 ("Constitution").

Considerable concern has been raised about the apparently increasing prevalence of depression among children and adolescents.[45] Such findings are worrisome not only because of the personal suffering involved but also because of the developmental implications. Depression early in life can hamper the development of needed coping skills, increase the likelihood of more serious later disturbance, heighten the risk of exposure to stress, and set the stage for recurrence of depression later in life.[47] These concerns highlight the importance of early intervention.

DEPRESSION IMPAIRS FUNCTIONING

The diagnosis of any psychiatric disorder entails clinically significant distress or impairment in social, occupational, or other important areas of functioning.[8] Emotional distress—depressed mood—is central to the definition of depression. Yet as you know from personal experience, impaired functioning also comes with this territory, as it would with any other serious illness. This impaired functioning is one reason we must take depression seriously as an *illness.*

When we consider that depression includes a wide range of symptoms that can affect your whole being, it is not surprising that depression can interfere with everything from work and leisure to interpersonal relationships.[48] As you would expect, the more severe the symptoms, the greater the impairment in functioning is likely to be.[49] Even subthreshold symptoms (falling short of the criteria for minor or major depression) are associated with some impairment of functioning. Such symptoms call for continued treatment. You might also be mindful as you recover from depression that improvement in functioning typically lags behind improvement in symptoms;[48,50] you need to feel better before you can get back on your feet.

To underscore my point that you are not alone if you are feeling handicapped by depression, I describe the results of two major research efforts.

MEDICAL OUTCOME STUDY

If you have any doubt that depression is a real illness, consider the results of Psychiatrist Kenneth Wells and colleagues' Medical Outcome Study.[13] This study compared depression with five other chronic medical conditions: hypertension, arthritis, diabetes, heart disease, and lung disease. The authors carefully assessed limitations of functioning in several domains: performing work, engaging in regular daily activities, and participating in social activities such as visiting friends or relatives. They also kept track of days spent in bed and levels of bodily pain.

The findings of this study are striking: for most domains of functioning, depression is *more* debilitating than most chronic general medical conditions. Only serious heart disease was associated with more days spent in bed, and only arthritis was associated with more bodily pain. The authors conducted the study to help identify the most cost-effective care. Not surprisingly, they found that the lowest costs (in the general medical sector) were associated with the poorest treatment outcomes, whereas the highest costs (in psychiatry) were associated with the best outcomes. Their finding that patients continued to struggle with symptoms and impairment—to greater or lesser degrees—over the course of a 2-year follow-up underscores the point that we cannot regard depression as an acute illness but rather must provide adequate treatment over the long haul.

GLOBAL BURDEN OF DISEASE

Perhaps most striking in documenting the seriousness of depression are the findings of the World Health Organization's Global Burden of Disease study.[51,52] As a measure of impairment, the researchers constructed an index of disability-adjusted life years, based on the years of life lost due to premature death combined with years of living with disability. They compared various psychiatric and general medical conditions; the level of disability caused by major depression was ranked equivalent to blindness or paraplegia.

In 1990, depression was found to be the fourth leading cause of disability worldwide, responsible for more than 1 in every 10 years of life lived with disability. Moreover, depression was the leading cause of disease burden in both developing and developed countries for women, and the authors[51] concluded that "while programmes to reduce the unacceptably high burden of poor reproductive health must remain a high priority for years to come, women's psychological health also deserves much more attention" (p. 25). Furthermore, anticipating an increase in depression in coming decades, the authors projected that by 2020 depression will be the second leading cause of disability, only surpassed by ischemic heart disease.

RECOVERY TAKES TIME

Depression is a painful illness that can cause a great deal of disruption to your life. Naturally, you want to recover quickly. You may have heard or read about other persons who bounced back quickly from an episode of depression, perhaps with the help of medication. You might be thinking, "Why can't I just snap out of it like everyone else does?" This view is depressing and adds insult to injury. A sense of inadequacy or failure might have preceded your depression; feeling like a failure for not recovering quickly will compound it. In addition, this view is based on a misunderstanding of the potential seriousness of depression.

Some persons do recover quickly from a major depressive episode, but most do not. In the early part of the twentieth century, the eminent German psychiatrist Emil Kraepelin[53] observed that episodes of mood disorder typically lasted from 6 to 8 months. A number of recent systematic research programs around the world have confirmed Kraepelin's observations that the typical duration of an episode of major depression is several months.[54-57]

One of the most ambitious and informative studies conducted on the course of depression is the Collaborative Depression Study[55,58,59] funded by the National Institute of Mental Health. Participants were several hundred men and women who sought treatment for an episode of major depression at treatment centers in five U.S. cities: Boston, Chicago, Iowa City, New York City, and St. Louis. These participants have been followed up for more than two decades. Keep in mind that these patients were severely depressed; a large majority of participants were *hospitalized*. Moreover, this naturalistic study did *not* include any special treatment interventions; many participants did not obtain adequate long-term care.

In the Collaborative Depression Study, the point of recovery from the episode was defined as beginning with the first of 8 consecutive weeks with either no symptoms or mild symptoms coupled with no impairment of functioning.[58] Consistent with other studies, the median time to recover (i.e., the point by which half the patients had recovered) was 5 months, once the person had entered the study. Of course, there are substantial individual differences in time to recovery, and as time goes on, a greater proportion of patients will recover. For example, 31% of patients had recovered by 2 months, 67% by 1 year, 88% by 5 years, and 94% by 15 years.[60] To reiterate: *several months to full recovery from an episode of severe major depression is typical*. Moreover, this several-month period to recovery often followed a long bout of illness—typically several months—prior to patients seeking treatment at the research site.

Several factors are associated with slower recovery: greater length of the current[61] or prior episodes;[55,59] greater severity of the current episode;[56,62] concomitant general medical conditions[63] or psychiatric conditions such as substance abuse and anxiety;[62] lack of social support;[56,63] and ongoing life stress during the period of recovery.[63] Conversely, positive life changes during the episode can speed recovery.[56]

Regardless of how long it takes, recovery will be gradual, occurring in small steps. Although you may take several months to recover fully, you won't spend all these months at the most severe level, at which you meet full criteria for major depression. The median time participants spent at full criteria in the Collaborative Depression Study was 4 weeks.[58] Fortunately, as your symptoms abate, the likelihood that you will recover increases substantially.

DEPRESSION CAN BECOME CHRONIC

Although the time to recovery may be agonizingly slow, the findings on recovery are encouraging: the vast majority of persons do recover. Yet there remains a small minority of persons who fail to recover after 2 years and whose depression may be considered *chronic*. If you have been struggling for years to recover from depression, you should know that you are not alone. The prevalence rate of chronic depression in the general U.S. population is estimated to be 3%–5%.[64] You should know, however, that persons with chronic depression can recover. One study of persons who had been continuously ill for the first 5 years found that 35% recovered in the next 5 years.[55] On average, 9% recovered each year. Thus even persons who have struggled continuously with depression for years should not give up hope of recovery.

Chronic depression isn't necessarily continuous; symptoms wax and wane. Unfortunately, however, persons with a history of severe major depression are likely to be battling symptoms of depression much of the time. A careful examination of weekly levels of depressive symptoms over a 12-year period in the Collaborative Depression Study[65] showed that patients experienced *some level* of depression the majority of the time (59% of weeks). The severity of symptoms varied: participants spent 15% of the time in major depression, 27% of the time with significant symptoms that fell short of full criteria for major depression, and 16% of the time with minor symptoms. Yet many of these patients were not obtaining adequate treatment.

DEPRESSION IS RECURRENT

Sadly, research findings clearly indicate that depression is often a recurrent illness. The Collaborative Depression Study of hospitalized patients provided the most systematic evidence on the likelihood of recurrence after recovery.[66] As time went on, the likelihood of recurrence increased. For example, after recovery from the initial episode, 25% of the participants had a recurrence within the first year, 42% by 2 years, and 60% by 5 years. Moreover, the more recurrences you have, the shorter the time interval from one to the next. This pattern of recurrence can begin early in life: a study of female high school seniors showed that those who had an episode of major depression in adolescence had a 70% risk of recurrence within the next five years.[67] Thus adolescent depression is a harbinger of depression in young adulthood.

The most substantial factor increasing the risk of relapse is continuing to experience *some symptoms of depression*—residual symptoms or partial remission.[68] Persons in the Collaborative Depression Study with subthreshold depressive symptoms—even if they were relatively mild—relapsed three times faster to major depression than those who had been symptom free. Moreover, well intervals are many times shorter for those with sub-threshold symptoms. Importantly, the subthreshold symptoms that portended recurrence are relatively mild: not feeling your usual self and having one or more mild symptoms increases your risk.

The risk of recurrence also increases directly with the number of prior episodes.[66] As the current diagnostic manual[69] summarizes: "At least 60% of individuals with Major Depressive Episode, Single Episode, can be expected to have a second episode. Individuals who have had two episodes have a 70% chance of having a third, and individuals who have had three episodes have a 90% chance of having a fourth" (p. 372). Yet the longer you are able to stay well, the lower your chances of recurrence.[70] The Collaborative Depression Study found that the probability of recurrence decreases significantly for each successive 6-month interval after recovery.[66]

Many other factors besides number of previous episodes have been shown to predict recurrence: environmental stress,[63,70] absence of social support,[70] substance abuse,[60,71] anxiety disorder,[60] and personality disturbance.[55,72] In addition, several factors were associated with a higher risk of recurrence in the study of adolescent women:[67] history of family violence, prior psychiatric disorder, and episodic life stress.

DEPRESSION IS UNDERTREATED

As I have documented, depression is a serious illness that often requires a long period of healing. Yet many persons endure long periods of depression owing to inadequate treatment. The first step to adequate treatment is a correct diagnosis. There's a big problem at the starting gate: failure to diagnose depression is common, even for persons who come for emergency treatment after a suicide attempt.[73]

Treatment is also likely to be inadequate.[60,74] A minority of patients are likely to receive medication,[75] and a minority of those who do are likely to receive an adequate dosage.[76,77] Patients in specialty mental health care are more likely than those in primary medical care to be receiving appropriate treatment.[78] The Collaborative Depression Study showed that 50% of patients who had been depressed for 2 years received no treatment or minimal treatment; 50% who had a recurrence of illness had not been treated in the month prior to the recurrence; and 60% of those who had a recurrence and remained ill for more than 1 year had no treatment or minimal treatment.[64] Even at the severest levels of depression, as many as 40% of patients were receiving no medication.[65]

Even when patients seek treatment and take medication, they are likely to discontinue too soon. Often after some improvement or failure to improve, patients stop taking their medication,[58,79] which greatly increases the likelihood that they will relapse into severe depression. One study showed that only 30% of patients filled more than three prescriptions for antidepressant medication, and failure to continue on medication was associated with relapse.[71] Undertreatment with medication also is associated with a briefer time to recurrence of a new episode of illness.[66,80]

The reasons for undertreatment of depression are complex, involving both practitioners and patients.[78] Depressed persons might not recognize that they are ill, and if they do recognize it, they may feel too ashamed to seek treatment. Alternatively, they may not be able to afford treatment. Catch-22 also plays a role here: given the potentially long road to recovery, patients must maintain motivation and exert effort to persist in treatment; a continuing depression will interfere with doing so. Remaining at least somewhat depressed, patients can be discouraged and give up too soon. In addition, even when they seek treatment, their depression might not be properly diagnosed; moreover, even when depression is diagnosed, the practitioner might not provide optimal treatment. Unsurprisingly, a number of efforts to enhance treatment in community settings have shown that better care results in better outcomes.[81–83]

TREATMENT HASTENS RECOVERY

I have underscored the seriousness of depression: it's prevalent, episodes are long, and it involves significant impairment in functioning. No wonder that depression is one of the most disabling diseases. Yet as I have just indicated, this rather dismal picture is compounded by the sad fact that the vast majority of persons with depression do not receive adequate treatment. Herein lies hope: obtaining adequate treatment—and persisting in it—will enhance both the likelihood and the rate of recovery.

Ample research indicates that treatment of depression with medication and therapy leads to improvement within 1–3 months[55,64] and shortens the duration of major depressive episodes.[84] The Collaborative Depression Study showed that transitions into wellness were nearly double for those patients receiving adequate dosages of medication compared with those who received lower dosages.[79]

Although medication is very likely to lead to some improvement, many patients recover partially rather than fully, and ongoing symptoms leave a person especially vulnerable to relapse.[11] Accordingly, it is best to aspire to full recovery for the sake of maximizing your functioning and remaining well. Some patients who show only partial response to antidepressant treatment may be helped to recover fully with the addition of psychotherapy.

Thus, as I review at length in Part V ("Coping With Catch-22"), you can improve your chances of full recovery by working actively on a number of fronts.

YOU ARE NOT A STATISTIC

I have highlighted two facets of the seriousness of depression: the intrinsic seriousness of the illness and the all-too-common failure to obtain adequate treatment. I've emphasized the seriousness of the illness not to demoralize you further but rather to reassure you that, if you are having difficulty recovering, it's a reflection of the intrinsic seriousness of the illness rather than being an indication of some personal failing. Minimizing the challenges of recovering from depression is demoralizing; you can't just "snap out of it"—although you wish you could more than anyone else does.

The sobering statistics I've quoted on the prevalence of depression, the duration of episodes, and the chronicity of the disorder in part reflect a cascade of problems.[85] To reiterate: depressed persons may not recognize that they are ill; if they do recognize it, they may not seek treatment; if they do seek treatment, they may not be diagnosed; if they are diagnosed, they may be undertreated; if they are adequately treated, they may not fully respond; and if they do respond, they may experience a relapse or recurrence.

Here's where you have some leverage. The statistics can reassure you that you are not alone in having difficulty with this illness. But you are not constrained by the statistics. You can do something about your illness. Knowing what you're dealing with and understanding how to cope with depression, you can improve your odds of recovering fully and remaining well. But you must take an active role in this process, which brings us to the topic of agency.

Chapter 3

AGENCY AND ELBOW ROOM

Imagine sitting in your kitchen when, out of the corner of your eye, you spot a small crumb moving across the floor. Looking more closely, you see an ant tugging it along. The ant, not the crumb, is the agent. *Agency* is your capacity to initiate action for a purpose. In reading this book, you are exercising agency; you're *doing* something about your depression, learning more about the illness for the purpose of coping more effectively.

I am employing agency as a central concept throughout this book, because agency plays a fundamental role in depression. Consider this vicious circle: in the face of stress pileup, you feel overpowered, helpless, and trapped; your agency is undermined, leading you to feel depressed; and your depression further undermines your agency by interfering with your ability to cope actively with the stress. Below, a common scenario unfolds.

Beth had struggled to put herself through college by working nights and weekends, only to find herself struggling yet again to find employment after she graduated. Following her passion, she had majored in anthropology. She had intended to apply for graduate school, but she needed to begin working to pay off her student loans. Being unable to find work in her educational field, she took a clerical job. As the months rolled by with little prospect of finding work more consistent with her interests, she became increasingly frustrated and demoralized. Conflicts in her relationship with her live-in boyfriend compounded her distress. Despite considerable talents and a likeable personality, she had felt unattractive and unworthy since adolescence, and she had formed a relationship with a young man who was often emotionally unavailable and sometimes downright callous. Having a low opinion of herself, she felt she deserved no better. She felt trapped in a dead-end job and an unsatisfying relationship.

Having become progressively more fed up with her job, Beth quit abruptly after she received a routine supervisory evaluation that included some minor criticisms that she felt were unjustified. Week after week, she was unable to find another job. The financial pressures of supporting herself—much less meeting her loan payments—continued to mount. She became increasingly irritable and frustrated with her boyfriend's inattentiveness. A minor disagreement escalated into a major fight, and she demanded that he move out.

Beth had felt increasingly trapped in her dead-end job and unfulfilling relationship, feeling helpless to do anything to improve her lot. She had taken some action in quitting her job and ending her relationship. Yet she felt even more helpless in being unemployed, and she also felt abandoned and alone after her boyfriend left. She spiraled into more severe depression. She began to spend much of the day in bed. When she wasn't in bed, she zoned out watching daytime television. She lacked the energy or confidence to look for work. She felt too ashamed to make contact with friends and family members, although they would have been glad to offer support. She was berating herself for being such a failure, and she feared that her parents would criticize her for quitting her job.

Feeling defeated, Beth had given up; her helplessness evolved into hopelessness. Her depression undermined her agency; she retreated from the world and was unable to cope. Fortunately, Beth's older sister recognized that she was seriously depressed and insisted that she seek treatment. Contrary to Beth's fears, her parents were supportive, and her friends were sympathetic. Over the next several months, as she felt less alone and began to recover from her depression; her agency was restored, and she was able to begin moving forward again.

Beth's plight illustrates the essence of catch-22: you require agency to cope, but depression undermines agency. In profound depression—when you're essentially bedridden, for example—your agency is almost completely abolished. Then you need help, and others must step in. More commonly, depression diminishes your agency rather than completely abolishing it. You're depressed to some degree, but you still have some capacity to take action on your own behalf—some elbow room.[86]

Part V of this book ("Coping With Catch-22") addresses the role of agency in recovering from depression and remaining well, indicating how you can use your remaining elbow room as leverage over your symptoms. However, we have much ground to cover beforehand. Understanding how you got into depression can help you find your way out and avoid getting back into it. If you weren't already convinced, I hope I have persuaded you in the first two chapters that you must take depression seriously as an illness. In this chapter, I elaborate this thesis: *illness imposes constraints on agency*.

I am emphasizing agency for two reasons: first, I want to encourage active coping; second, I want to discourage self-blame. Many depressed persons add insult to injury by blaming themselves for their depression and for their difficulty recovering. Feeling guilty only compounds their depression. I'm striving for a delicate balance and putting you on a tightrope: to the extent that your illness constrains your agency, you can absolve yourself of responsibility for your plight; to the extent that your agency is preserved, you must take responsibility for your plight. You can fall off one side of the tightrope by condemning yourself for difficulties that are beyond your control; you can fall off the other side by failing to take whatever steps are possible to help yourself.

This chapter proceeds as follows. First, I elaborate the concepts of agency and constraints. Second, I examine the potential role of agency in generating the stress that leads into depression. Third, I consider the balance of agency and constraints in the illness of depression. Fourth, I tackle the problems of responsibility and blame. I conclude by noting how the theme of agency versus constraints will play out through the rest of this book.

AGENCY VERSUS CONSTRAINTS

To reiterate, an agent is an originating cause.[87] Agents initiate action—intentional, goal-directed behavior. Agency implies will, autonomy, freedom, choice, and responsibility. At the most basic level, theoretical biologist Stuart Kauffman[88] defined an autonomous agent as an entity "able to act on its own behalf" (p. x). He equated agency with life, including all free-living cells and organisms in this definition—from bacteria on up. From Kauffman's standpoint, the ant is a high-level agent!

However, we are interested in human agency. You're a *conscious* agent. As psychiatrist Daniel Stern[89] put it, you have a "sense of authorship" of your own actions (p. 71). Moreover, you are a *self-conscious rational* agent: you are aware of acting on the basis of certain reasons.[90] A caveat: you're *potentially* self-conscious and rational. You're not always aware of reasons for your actions, and much of the time as you go about your daily activities you need not reason deliberately about what you are doing. Yet when you run into trouble, you must become more self-aware so as to enhance your agency and thereby exert greater control over your actions. That is the point of reading this book and gaining greater insight into your depression.

To sharpen the concept of agency, consider its opposites. Agency entails voluntary action; its contrary includes involuntary responses such as reflexes. You can't help being startled by a sudden loud noise—you don't act; you react. Agency entails activity; its converse is passivity. Agency entails power and control. When your agency is undermined, you feel powerless and out of control—acted upon rather than acting on your own behalf.

Traumatic events ranging from tsunamis to assaults are extreme examples: they are overpowering, and they are traumatizing largely by virtue of undermining your agency, rendering you helpless.

SELF-EFFICACY

Psychologist Albert Bandura's[91] pioneering research on agency underscores the importance of *beliefs*: "Among the mechanisms of personal agency, none is more central or pervasive than people's beliefs in their capability to exercise some measure of control over their own functioning and over environmental events.... Efficacy beliefs are the foundation of human agency" (p. 10). Bandura and colleagues' research[92] showed that children who did not believe in their own efficacy—power to produce intended effects—were more prone to depression. For example, children who believed themselves to be incapable of academic and social success were more depressed and less successful in those domains; these beliefs became self-fulfilling prophecies. Lack of self-efficacy promoted depression; depression contributed to failure; and failure added to depression. Moreover, problems managing emotions compounded the children's difficulty. Those who perceived themselves as unable to regulate their emotions also were more vulnerable to depression. Thus agency pertains not only to your ability to exert influence over the outer world but also your capacity to influence your own state of mind.

I emphasize the connection between interpersonal relationships and depression throughout this book, and I want to underscore the role of agency here. Our capacity to exert influence over each other is a central domain of agency. Not surprisingly, Bandura found that children who believed they lacked social self-efficacy were more prone to engage in problematic social behavior, such as aggressiveness and disruptiveness. These children's poor sense of agency, as well as the negative consequences of their social behavior, contributed significantly to their depression. These findings are important in light of the role of social support in buffering depression.[93] Yet Bandura[92] emphasized the role of agency in social support: "Social support is not a self-forming entity waiting around to buffer harried people against stressors. People have to go out and find, create, and maintain supportive relationships for themselves. These interpersonal attainments require a strong sense of social efficacy" (p. 259).

CONSTRAINTS

To varying degrees, constraints limit your agency.[94] Your agency can be constrained by anything that limits your range of choices or possibilities

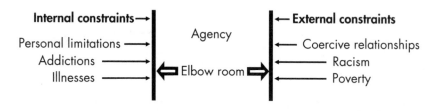

FIGURE 3-1. Agency and elbow room versus some constraints.

(see Figure 3–1). Constraints abound. Pure freedom of action—agency without limit—is an impossibility. You make choices continually, but you cannot choose to do absolutely anything. You always choose among a limited set of possible alternatives. When you think about it, most things are beyond your control. Your environment imposes innumerable constraints: you are born at a particular time into a particular culture and a particular family, potentially affected by social constraints such as poverty, racism, and sexism. Factors within you impose constraints: your natural talents are limited, or you might be constrained by injuries or disabilities. Your genetic makeup might limit how much stress you can tolerate without becoming depressed.

Constraints generally prevent you from taking action. Yet your agency also can be diminished when you are *forced to act* in ways that go against your will. Such forces also act as constraints, limiting your freedom. You can be psychologically pressured, threatened, or coerced into doing something you do not want to do. Some of the worst trauma, for example, entails being forced into participating in abusive or violent situations—or being prevented from doing something to stop them.[95] Ironically, your agency also may be constrained from within: you might feel forced into action by an internal compulsion, such as an addiction. You can feel helpless when you can't stop yourself from doing something you don't want to do. To reiterate, all these constraints are potentially depressing to the degree that they undermine your agency.

A MATTER OF DEGREE

Agency isn't an all-or-none phenomenon; it's a matter of degree (see Figure 3–2). If we put agency on a spectrum, involuntary behavior and passive helplessness would be at the low end. An example of the latter: you're stopped at an intersection and rammed by a truck. At the high end we'd put self-conscious rational agency: taking a broad range of factors into consideration, you deliberate, make a decision, and act on it. In the middle range

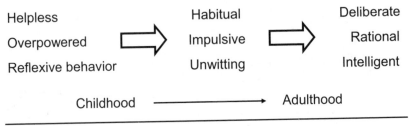

FIGURE 3-2. Increasing degrees of agency.

of agency, where we typically operate, we are more or less aware of what we're doing. When we act on the basis of habits or routines, we're exercising agency—engaging in goal-directed action—even though we're not thinking about what we're doing. We are also in the middle range when we behave impulsively—we're active agents but not as self-conscious and deliberate as we might be. When we're young, we're active agents but limited in knowledge and capacity to deliberate about what we're doing. As philosopher Alain de Botton[96] commented, "We are all made to live before we can even begin to know how" (p. 155). When we have developed the capacity to do so, we need to step up the degree of agency if our habits, routines, or relatively mindless actions get us into trouble. Then we need to maximize our agency by putting our *intelligence* to work, using our past experience to guide our present actions on the basis of what we anticipate their future consequences to be.[97]

AGENCY IN BECOMING DEPRESSED

We tend to think of the environment as an independent influence over our actions. Our environment affords opportunities and imposes constraints. Yet the perspective of agency draws our attention to the *active role we play in shaping the environment* that, in turn, exerts such a powerful influence on us.[98] As Bandura stated, social support isn't just out there to buffer us; we must create, maintain, and actively reach out for it. Agency creates environmental opportunities. Joining organizations creates opportunities for friendships. Getting a good education creates opportunities for jobs. Similarly, agency creates environmental constraints. For example, after you decide to take a job, you must accommodate to all the constraints it imposes, like having to get up on time.

Psychologist Arnold Buss[99] neatly delineated three ways in which your agency shapes your social environment: selection, evocation, and manipulation. Of course, you don't choose the family you're born into or the schools you attend in your early years. Yet, as you grow older, you increasingly *select* your social environment. You might pick a school to enroll in and a town or city to live in. You pick friends and romantic partners. In addition, as an agent, you automatically *evoke* reactions from your social environment. For example, highly active or aggressive children evoke controlling responses from parents and teachers. Ambitious students evoke competitiveness from their peers. Dominant individuals evoke peers' efforts to cut them down to size. Finally, you actively and intentionally *manipulate* your social environment, purposefully exerting an influence on the behavior of others. For example, you might employ social strategies such as using your charm, trying to reason with another person, giving them the silent treatment, or ranting and raving until you get your way.

I have used the term *stress pileup* to characterize the role of environmental stress in depression. Yet, from the agency perspective, you consider your active role in piling up stress. I don't want to overstate this point: much of the stress that contributes to depression is unavoidable—traumas, losses, and hardships too numerous to contemplate.[93] In chapters to come, I emphasize a number of biological vulnerabilities and social stressors in early life that are outside the realm of agency. Yet a substantial amount of stress that contributes to depression is at least partly *self-generated*, a result of the depressed person's actions.[100] To take a line from author Richard Rhodes,[101] "All stories are ultimately the same story: someone falls into a hole and has to find a way to get out" (p. 54). Understanding whatever active role you played in falling into the hole of depression can help you climb out of it and stay out of it in the future.

No doubt, you became depressed against your wishes. Whatever active role you played in becoming depressed was unintentional. Yet we must bring this active role to light. As described at the beginning of this chapter, Beth didn't quit her job or dump her boyfriend for the purpose of piling up stress, much less to plummet herself into depression; yet these actions unwittingly put her deeper into the hole.

The following example illustrates how unconscious conflicts can play a role in actions that escalate stress.

Craig entered the hospital in a state of suicidal despair after reaching a level of utter desperation with his escalating anxiety. He had gone into investment banking with his high-powered brother, Tom. Tom had criticized and dominated Craig since their childhood and, rubbing salt into the wound, Tom was the family "star" and the favorite son. Craig had long resented Tom and, indeed, was quite often infuriated with him. In the business context, Craig's resentment was understandable; he was a talented and highly successful investor in his own right, but Tom insisted on making all the major decisions. Moreover, Tom was far more conservative than Craig, a source of ongoing tension between them.

Several years into the partnership, Tom developed cancer, which increasingly curtailed his day-to-day involvement with the business. Unbeknownst to Tom, Craig went out on a limb, making a huge investment that went sour. In a frantic effort to recoup his losses before Tom found out, Craig began making a series of increasingly risky investments, only digging himself deeper into the hole. In effect, he had slipped from investing to gambling.

Throughout this process, Craig had seen himself as the victim of circumstances, stressed out and having panic attacks. In the course of his psychotherapy, Craig came to see how his resentment toward Tom played a significant role in his squandering the funds of the firm. Craig saw himself as an agent in the development of his anxiety and depression. In hindsight, he could see his pattern of reckless investing as an *aggressive action*. Of course, his evolving illnesses—anxiety and depression—eroded his capacity to make sound decisions, increasingly constraining his agency.

Craig found psychotherapy to be hard work. Circumstances required that he do this hard work when he was depressed, although some degree of recovery was necessary before he was able to become fully engaged. Not surprisingly, Craig found the process of exploring his conflicts with Tom—and especially his self-destructive retaliation—to be extremely painful; he faced it squarely but reluctantly. Yet recognizing his unconscious motivation and the role of his unwitting actions in the development of his depression was essential, because it put Craig in a position to avoid recreating the same stressful situation in the future and risking a recurrence of depression.

To repeat, you do not create interpersonal conflicts, work yourself to the bone, or sacrifice your own health for the *purpose* of becoming depressed, just as the prospective alcoholic doesn't start drinking for the purpose of developing alcoholism. Yet, looking back and taking stock of your life, you could see your depression as an *unwitting* creation; an agent was involved, namely, you. Your *actions* may have played *some* part in piling up stress, although that was not your intention. Once stress pileup has put your mind, brain, and physiology into what psychiatrist Aaron Beck[102] aptly called the *depressed mode*, you're ill; then your agency is further constrained.

ILLNESS

Illness runs counter to agency: it's not something you *do*; it invades, overtakes, happens. We naturally associate illness with something gone wrong in our body—something out of our control. Our intuitive concept of illness is *disease*, "a particular destructive process in the body, with a specific cause and characteristic symptoms."[103] Is depression really an illness—a disease?

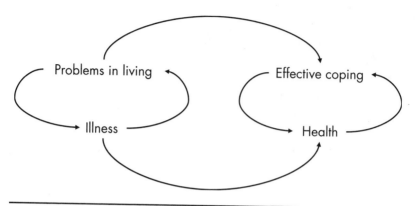

FIGURE 3-3. From vicious circles to benign circles.

Decades ago, psychiatrist Thomas Szasz[104] notoriously declared: "Mental illness is a myth. Psychiatrists are not concerned with mental illnesses and their treatments. In actual practice they deal with personal, social, and ethical *problems in living*" (p. 262; emphasis mine). Sadly, Szasz was mistaken: mental illness is no myth. Yet Szasz helpfully drew our attention to problems in living; this is where agency and elbow room come in: we play an active role in our problems in living. Contrary to Szasz, I want to have it both ways: mental illness is true illness, and mental illness relates to problems in living. I envision a vicious circle (see Figure 3–3): problems in living contribute to mental illness and mental illness contributes to problems in living. We typically face a chicken-and-egg problem in trying to figure out how the cycle got going. Regardless, the challenge is to turn the cycle around, moving from problems in living to effective coping and from illness to health: just as problems in living and illness reinforce each other, so do effective coping and health.

DEPRESSION AS DISEASE

Mental illness is no myth. With increasing success and sophistication, the field of biological psychiatry is applying the model of disease to an ever-expanding array of psychiatric disorders. Burgeoning research demonstrates the neurobiological basis of depression along with many other psychiatric disorders such as bipolar (manic-depressive) disorder, schizophrenia, obsessive-compulsive disorder, posttraumatic stress disorder, and substance dependence. For decades, researchers have been documenting substantial genetic contributions to depression. The effectiveness of antidepressant medication also attests to the biological basis of depression. More recently, with the advent of neuroimaging, researchers are linking symptoms of depression to patterns of activity in different areas of the brain. I discuss these biological matters in more detail in subsequent chapters.

These dramatic advances in biological psychiatry can tempt us to explain everything in terms of neurophysiology. As you will see throughout this book, I am firmly committed to making full use of biological knowledge in understanding depression. Yet if we embrace biological psychiatry exclusively, we run the risk of dehumanizing psychiatric problems and taking the whole person—the agent—out of the picture.[105]

Not infrequently, when I am describing the stress pileup model of depression in educational groups, a patient protests: "But my doctor says I have a chemical-imbalance depression!" Rightly so, in the sense that we know depression is associated with alterations in brain chemistry. Yet that does not mean that psychological stress has played no part in the illness; on the contrary, we can view the "chemical imbalance" as partly a *consequence* of psychological stress. The biological perspective is essential, but it's only one perspective. I'm encouraging you to juggle multiple perspectives. Of course, if you're seriously depressed, you're likely to need help on the biological front, for example, from antidepressant medication. Yet going solely down the biological path can leave you feeling helpless if your depression doesn't respond to biological treatment or if you feel utterly dependent on medication. Also, the biological perspective alone doesn't fully explain how you got into depression.

A potential trap: if it's biological, it's out of my control. *All* action, from reading this book to playing tennis, has a biological basis. Biology per se is not contrary to agency; it's the basis of agency. Rather, *disordered* biological structure and function, such as occurs with disease, constrains agency to varying degrees. If you're debilitated by the flu, you cannot go to school. If you're depressed, you may not be able to go to work.

DEPRESSION AS A SOCIAL ROLE

Without discarding the biological-disease perspective, consider a contrasting psychosocial perspective on illness. A half-century ago, sociologist Talcott Parsons[106] introduced agency into the domain of medicine by construing illness as a *social role*: "The role of the sick person is a socially structured and in a sense institutionalized role" (p. 455).

Parsons made three crucial points. First, being ill, you're legitimately excused from social and occupational obligations. Second, being ill, you also incur obligations: to remain legitimately excused, you must seek and cooperate with treatment so as to become well as soon as possible. In doing so, you are accepting agency for your illness, a crucial foundation of recovery, as my colleague, psychiatrist Richard Munich, proposed.[107] I consider Parsons' third point to be the single most important matter for depressed patients and their family members to understand: "The sick person…cannot reasonably be expected to 'pull himself together' by a mere act of will" (p. 456). Plainly, while according agency a crucial role in recovery, Parsons recognized that illness constrains agency: *you cannot recover by a mere act of will.*

Don't lose sight of Parsons' last point as I nudge you toward adopting greater agency for your illness. Think of it this way: you cannot recover by one monumental act of will, but you can recover by *many acts of will* over an extended time period. Recovery is especially difficult, of course, when you are affected by depression, which saps your energy—catch-22. Moreover, recovering on your own can be well nigh impossible; then you'll need help from others. Effective agents avail themselves of help when they need it.[108]

To summarize, depression will constrain your agency to varying degrees, depending on the severity of the illness. Despite your depression, you remain a free agent, to some degree. You can make choices—not any imaginable choice, but some choices. Even when you're profoundly depressed, you might be in a position to sit up in bed or get out of bed. You must distinguish between *difficult and painful choices* and *no choice*.[109] When you've become ill, the challenge is to use whatever agency remains to get well and to *increase* your range of freedom and choice. You can use elbow room to expand elbow room, building agency on agency; the more you recover, the easier it becomes to recover further.

RESPONSIBILITY AND BLAME

Considering the role of agency in depression opens the door to a blaming attitude, and I have opened two doors. First, I've proposed that you may have played some active role in the development of your depression; you might read this as implying that it's your fault that you got depressed. Second, I've proposed that, despite being depressed, you have some remaining agency—elbow room—to work your way out of it. You might read this as implying that it's your fault you're still depressed.

As Figure 3–4 depicts, I emphasize agency to empower you, not to blame you. I'm convinced that we must think clearly about agency for the sake of addressing the problem of blameworthiness for depression.[105] Persons with psychiatric disorders in general and depression in particular often feel misunderstood and unjustifiably blamed for their illness-related behavior if not for their illness itself. Such blame is one of the elements contributing to stigma. Moreover, even if you don't feel blamed by others, you might blame yourself.

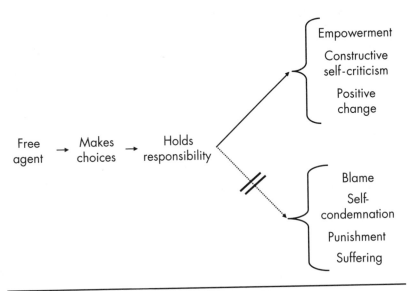

FIGURE 3–4. Agency and empowerment versus blame.

AGENCY AND MORAL JUDGMENT

When our actions have an adverse impact on others, we enter the domain of *moral* judgments, potentially moving from responsibility to moral blame. Contemporary philosopher Daniel Dennett[110] defined a responsible *moral agent* as one who "chooses freely for considered reasons and may be held morally accountable for the acts chosen" (p. 268). Philosopher Thomas Nagel[111] spelled out this relation in more detail:

> We cannot evade our freedom. Once we have developed the capacity to recognize our own desires and motives, we are faced with the choice of whether to act as they incline us to act, and in facing that choice we are inevitably faced with an evaluative question. Even if we refuse to think about it, that refusal can itself be evaluated.... The applicability to us of moral concepts is the consequence of our freedom—freedom that comes from the ability to see ourselves objectively, through the new choices which that ability forces on us. (p. 118)

As you well know from having struggled with depression, to the extent that you are perceived as a free agent—making choices and thereby held responsible for your depressive withdrawal—you have been judged and perhaps been resented, criticized, and blamed. Even if you have been spared from others' criticism, you might have berated yourself.

Recognize that depression is one instance of a problem that has long bedeviled the social view of psychiatric disorders. Are these true illnesses or moral failings? Alcoholism is the most glaring example: disease or sin?[112] Here's a counterpart with depression: illness or laziness? You might be surprised to learn that the concept of illness has a moral edge to it. Look up "ill" in the dictionary, and you'll find these archaic connotations: "morally evil, wicked, depraved."[113] In this sense, we continue to refer to some persons as "ill tempered" or "ill willed." With these condemnatory connotations in the background, it's no wonder that modern psychiatry considers itself enlightened in regarding psychiatric disorders as brain diseases rather than moral failings. Yet as author Andrew Solomon[114] astutely explained in his masterful autobiography, *The Noonday Demon*, pinning all the blame on the brain won't do:

> The word *chemical* seems to assuage the feelings of responsibility people have for the stressed-out discontent of not liking their jobs, worrying about getting old, failing at love, hating their families. There is a pleasant freedom from guilt that has been attached to *chemical*. If your brain is disposed to depression, you need not blame yourself for it. Well, blame yourself or evolution, but remember that blame itself can be understood as a chemical process and that happiness, too, is chemical. Chemistry and biology are not matters that impinge on the 'real' self; depression cannot be separated from the person it affects. (pp. 20–21)

I have no desire to escape the moral arena by deflecting all attention onto the brain. On the contrary, we must take this bull by the horns. That's because, short of being unconscious, you are an agent. The stakes are high. Sacrificing agency to chemistry or biology for the sake of circumventing value judgments is a costly maneuver; helplessness is a high price to pay. Gaining a sense of power over illness demands agency, and agency comes with inescapable moral evaluations.

STRIVING FOR BALANCE

Being unable to escape value judgments, it is crucially important to judge carefully and knowledgably. Keep in mind two principles: agency is a matter of degree, and agency is constrained by illness, chemistry and all. Hence, to get the moral perspective right, *we must evaluate the degree to which illness constrains agency for any given person at any point in time.*

Given our limited—albeit growing—understanding of the extent of biological disease in psychiatric disorders, properly estimating the degree of agency is no small challenge. Consciously or unconsciously, patients, family members, and mental health professionals make more or less educated guesses about the extent to which illness and disease constrain agency, and moral judgments accompany these estimations. For example, being depressed, you might retreat to your bedroom rather than joining a family gathering. Some family members might view your withdrawal from a moral perspective, feeling hurt and being critical, believing that you don't care enough about being with them to make the effort. Other family members, considering your behavior from the perspective of illness or disease, might be more sympathetic, believing you don't have the energy because you're so depressed. Such judgments are difficult to make—even for the depressed person. You might wonder, along with your family members, if you had a choice, or whether you made the best choice. Not an easy call.

Walking a tightrope in relation to agency, you can make two serious mistakes: taking responsibility for things you cannot control, and failing to take responsibility for things you can control. The venerable serenity prayer captures the challenge: "Grant me the serenity to accept the things I cannot change, the courage to change the things I can, and the wisdom to tell the difference." Striving to get the extent of agency and responsibility right, you need knowledge as well as wisdom. Yet, with limited biological knowledge, you and everyone else inevitably must resort to guessing about the extent of biological disease in your depression, the extent of constraint on your agency.

Here we might be guided by a broad historical trend in neurobiological research on psychiatric disorders, which increasingly reveals the extent of disordered biological structure and function associated with depression. Historically, we have tended to underestimate the role of disease, erring in the direction of blaming persons for actions over which their control was more limited than we knew. With the advent of new knowledge, we are in a better position to develop a more balanced view.

Consider how knowledge of recent research findings might make a difference in the following situation. A wife who feels burdened with household responsibilities on top of a demanding job increasingly resents her depressed husband's lack of participation in managing the family finances. As I describe in Chapter 9 ("Brain and Body"), researchers are now linking major depression to compromised functioning of the prefrontal cortex,[115] an area of the brain that not only regulates emotional distress but also plays a prominent role in executive functioning—deliberating, planning, decision making, and complex problem solving.[116] Would appreciating the role of impaired brain functioning in depression influence his wife's judgments and feelings about her husband's ostensible abdication of responsibility? Would this knowledge also temper his self-criticism?

In trying to judge the extent of agency and illness, only one thing is certain: we'll get it wrong if we think in terms of absolutes—either agency without constraint or no agency at all.

COMPASSIONATE CRITICISM

Here's the tightrope you walk: can you increase your sense of agency—and responsibility—for your depression without invoking blame and condemnation? I'm not suggesting that you should avoid all criticism; on the contrary, I'm encouraging a self-critical perspective. The challenge, as with all criticism, is to engage in *constructive criticism* for the purpose of beneficial change.

Being morally responsible for actions with harmful results implies that you reevaluate and change; it does *not* require that you suffer or be punished as a consequence.[90] Sometimes self-reproach and guilt feelings can motivate constructive change. Yet many persons struggling with depression already feel a crushing sense of guilt and shame—taking upon themselves the harshest moral connotations of illness. Excruciating shame will undermine your agency rather than enhance it. Ideally, by appreciating the extent—and the limits—of your agency in your illness, you will feel challenged, not reproached.

I used to think that my mother's injunction, "Just do your best!" was very permissive and forgiving. Now I realize it sets a very high standard. We don't always do our best and, to that extent, we leave ourselves open to criticism. If self-criticism influences you to improve, so much the better. You do need to push yourself to get out of depression; you're always going against the grain in making the effort. Yet I think a generally compassionate and encouraging attitude toward yourself will help prevent your self-criticism from turning into destructive self-blame.

LOOKING AHEAD

I advocate the concepts of agency and constraints to help you develop a balanced view of your depression. Fully acknowledging the constraints—factors beyond your control—will help you adopt a compassionate attitude toward yourself. I emphasize several areas of constraints in the chapters to come: constitutional factors such as genetics; childhood adversities such as loss and trauma; changes in brain activity associated with depressive illness; and ways the various symptoms of depression will interfere with your efforts to recover.

Yet if you only paid attention to the constraints, you would be left feeling helpless and hopeless. Thus you need to make room for agency. Perhaps you have done some things, unwittingly, that have increased your vulnerability to depression. I consider how external and internal stresses contribute to depression; both involve some balance of agency and constraints. Most important, difficult as it may be, you can *do something* to pull yourself out of depression. The constraints of depression make exerting your agency challenging, but your remaining agency gives you some elbow room to exert leverage over your depressive symptoms. You must strike a balance; as Solomon[114] put it, "If you push yourself too hard, you will make yourself worse, but you must push hard enough if you really want to get out" (p. 102). Fortunately, recovering from depression restores your agency, putting you in a better position to do whatever you must to maximize your chances of remaining well.

Next, some biological constraints.

• Part II •

DEVELOPMENT

Chapter 4

CONSTITUTION

This chapter launches our exploration of the development of depression by starting at the beginning: your biological constitution. I consider constitutional factors for two reasons: first, to emphasize the physical basis of depression; second, to help you develop a more forgiving attitude toward yourself as you appreciate that some factors beyond your control may have contributed to your depression. But here's my main point: *biology is not destiny*. Beginning in the womb, biological and environmental factors interact to influence the course of development and, as you mature, you exert increasing influence over your development through your exercise of agency. Yet your constitution imposes constraints on your development, and I examine four potential sources of constraint here: genetic risk, prenatal stress, temperament, and gender.

GENETIC RISK

We know that depression runs in families, but this observation does not distinguish between genetic and environmental influences. Researchers have employed several methods to tease apart the genetic and environmental contributions. For example, studies comparing monozygotic (identical) and dizygotic (fraternal) twins examine the extent to which greater genetic relatedness is associated with higher concordance for depression. Adoption studies allow researchers to separate genetic makeup from the childrearing environment, for example, to determine if the child's outcome is better predicted by the biological parents' characteristics (implying a genetic contribution) or the adoptive parents' characteristics (implying an environmental contribution). More precise still are molecular genetic studies, which relate different variants (alleles) of specific genes to risk for depression. Converging findings from all these methods have confirmed a genetic basis for depression, although the genetic contribution appears to be more substantial for more severe depression and most substantial for bipolar disorder.[117, 118]

The fact that depression has a genetic basis is not likely to be news to you. Thus my main goal is to address an alarming misunderstanding: *genetic determinism*, the idea that certain genes cause psychiatric disorders, directly and inevitably. You might think depression is inherited like eye color. There are rare conditions, such as Huntington's disease, in which a tight link exists between carrying specific genes and developing a disorder. In the realm of psychiatric disorders, however, genetic makeup is not destiny. Rather, a multitude of genes are involved, and genetic makeup potentially confers an increased *susceptibility* to depression; whether this susceptibility is translated into illness depends on a host of other factors I describe throughout this book.

If you find the following technical material daunting, keep in mind that I am merely making three simple points: your fate is not cast in stone in your genes; genetic predispositions interact with environmental influences; and genetic makeup predisposes you to other factors, such as personality characteristics, that also influence your risk for depression. All of us grow up with some combination of risk and protective factors.

WHAT GENES DON'T DO

Genes do not directly produce psychiatric disorders like depression; nor do they cause any other pattern of behavior. The pathways from genetic influences to behavior are mind bogglingly complex, and the following sketch of gene function aims mainly to dispel the gross oversimplifications that lead us to fear that our destinies are inscribed in our genes.[119]

Genes are sections of DNA located on chromosomes within the cell nucleus. All the cells of a given individual share the same complement of genes, although different genes are active in different types of cells. All the individuals in a particular species have the same complement of genes, but many genes have slightly different forms (alleles) that contribute to the differences among individuals within a given species (e.g., sex, eye color, height, various behavioral characteristics, and susceptibility to different diseases).

Genes play a specific role in cells: their DNA sequences contain *information* that RNA transcribes in the process of protein synthesis. Proteins, not genes, are the essential constituents of cells and therefore of life. As science historian Evelyn Fox Keller[120] epitomized, "DNA makes RNA, RNA makes proteins, and proteins make us" (p. 54). Proteins are the basis of cells' structure and functioning; they include enzymes, the catalysts that enable the cell to synthesize various molecules. Of particular interest to psychiatry, genes provide information for the synthesis of neurotransmitters, hormones, and cell membrane receptors, enabling neurons to communicate with each other and thereby to create patterns of brain activity that support experience and behavior (see Chapter 9, "Brain and Body").

By providing a template for protein synthesis, genes play a fundamental role in development and reproduction. Owing to the magnificently faithful copying process, the genetic code ensures regularity in the creation of cells, tissues, organs, and organisms, and the genetic code also enables individuals to reproduce, such that their offspring's cells can synthesize the same proteins. It is tempting, but misleading, to think that the genes contain something like a blueprint or program for constructing the body. The activity of any given gene is influenced by the activity of myriad other genes and proteins, such that the process of protein synthesis is extremely fluid and flexible. As Keller[120] summarized,

> The gene can no longer be set above and apart from the processes that specify cellular and intercellular organization. That gene is itself part and parcel of processes defined and brought into existence by the action of a complex self-regulating dynamical system in which, and for which, the inherited DNA provides the crucial and absolutely indispensable raw material, but no more than that. (p. 71)

The role of genes is not limited to stabilizing organism construction and reproduction. Cells are continuously synthesizing proteins, and genes must be continually turned on and off so these proteins are synthesized at the proper rate and time, depending on the needs of the cell. Thus the cell's operation depends on a subset of genes being *expressed* (actively transcribed in the synthesis of proteins) at a given point. Gene expression is determined by a multitude of factors.

We can therefore think of gene–environment interactions occurring at different levels. A particular gene's activity is affected by activity of neighboring areas of DNA, including other genes. Thus a gene is influenced by its local environment—surrounding areas within the nucleus. Genes also are involved in synthesizing proteins that influence the expression of other genes. Signals coming from the cytoplasm outside the nucleus as well as signals from outside the cell also affect gene expression. The environment outside the organism ultimately has an impact at the cellular level, influencing gene expression. For example, encountering psychological stress or taking antidepressant medication ultimately affects the activity of genes, the synthesis of proteins, and the cells' interactions with each other.

GENETIC SUSCEPTIBILITY TO ENVIRONMENTAL STRESS

Genes don't operate in a vacuum, nor do individuals. We think in terms of susceptibility to illness because genetic factors often influence the risk of becoming depressed *in reaction to stressors*.

A landmark study by psychiatrist Kenneth Kendler and his colleagues[121] illustrated how environmental stress interacts with genetic susceptibility in relation to depressive episodes. These researchers studied onsets of major depression in female–female twin pairs (monozygotic and dizygotic); they included more than 2,000 individuals. Although genetic risk increased the likelihood of depression in both the presence and absence of recent environmental stress, those individuals at higher genetic risk had a greater likelihood of becoming depressed in response to an environmental stressor. As the authors succinctly put it, "Genes have an impact on the risk of major depression in part by altering the individual's sensitivity to the depression-inducing effect of stressful events" (p. 834).

A group of researchers in New Zealand elegantly demonstrated how the interaction between a specific gene and environmental stress can contribute to depression.[122] These researchers focused on a gene that affects the levels of the neurotransmitter serotonin in the synaptic clefts (see Chapter 9, "Brain and Body"). They found that individuals with the short allele of this gene showed increased susceptibility to depression in the face of environmental stress in adulthood. Moreover, they found that childhood maltreatment was associated with adulthood depression *only* for persons with this genetic vulnerability (i.e., the short allele).

DEVELOPMENTAL CASCADES

We have seen that the genetic contribution is best construed as an increased susceptibility to depression in response to environmental stress. Yet this finding represents only the tip of the iceberg with respect to genetic contributions to depression; genetic makeup also influences the other factors that play a role in depression.

Genetic factors play a role not only in *response* to stress but also in the likelihood of *exposure* to stress. Kendler and colleagues[123] discovered a genetic risk for exposure to stressful events such as robbery, assault, illness, injury, marital problems, and financial problems. They proposed that genetically influenced personality traits (e.g., impulsivity, low frustration tolerance, and propensity to take risks) increase the likelihood of getting into stressful situations. Thus genetic factors can play a part in self-generated stress if they contribute to putting yourself in a high-risk environment. Here, as everywhere, we have an intermingling of genetic constraints and individual agency.

Genetic factors also play a role in protective factors. For example, genetic factors make a substantial contribution to the likelihood that an individual will have adequate social support.[124] Again, the likely explanation for this finding is personality: individuals who are more outgoing, for example, are likely to create a network of social support, and genetic makeup plays an important part in this personality characteristic.

Thus far, we have examined only a small set of factors that play a role in depression. As subsequent chapters show, throughout the course of development a wide range of risk and protective factors come into play in creating vulnerability to depression. I want to underscore here that the influence of genetic factors does not ordinarily erupt spontaneously later in life in response to stress. The genetic contributions to personality, exposure to stress, availability of social support, and susceptibility to depression influence all aspects of development all the way along.

PRENATAL STRESS

Plainly, stress pileup can begin at any point in life; of concern is recent research on depression that suggests stress pileup can begin in the womb.[125] As I discuss in Chapter 6 ("Childhood Adversity"), a number of researchers have begun examining the impact of maternal depression on infant behavior and development. These researchers noticed that newborns of depressed mothers showed signs of stress, raising the possibility that prenatal influences may have played a role in the newborns' condition.

Psychologist Tiffany Field[126] observed that, shortly after birth, infants of chronically depressed mothers show limited attentiveness and responsiveness, fussiness, disorganized sleep, and elevated stress hormones. Indeed, these infants appear to have a depressive profile of behavior and physiology that mirrors that of their mother. These observations of newborns prompted examination of fetuses of pregnant women who were depressed to determine whether the effects could be measured prenatally. In the second trimester, fetuses of depressed mothers showed higher levels of activity as well as increased reactivity to stimuli; they also showed lower weight. Field speculated that the fetus might be compensating for the depressed mother's inactivity by a heightened activity level of its own.

There are a number of possible mechanisms by which the mother's depression might influence the fetus's development, including genetic similarity. Field proposed that the mother's activity level, her heart rate, and intrauterine hormones may all play a role. As we see in Chapter 9 ("Brain and Body"), the stress hormone, cortisol, plays a central role in depression. Field and colleagues[127] found elevated cortisol levels in the depressed pregnant women they studied and proposed that this may increase fetal cortisol levels and, in turn, account for adverse effects on fetal development. Another factor potentially contributing to problems in fetal development is the depressed mother's impaired care of her own physical health (e.g., poorer eating and sleeping patterns, cigarette smoking) as well as her engaging in less frequent and less adequate prenatal care.[128]

This research is in its early stages, and the impact of prenatal stress on subsequent development is just beginning to be studied. One group of researchers found that mothers' anxiety (but not depression) in the prenatal period was associated with children's behavioral and emotional problems at 4 years of age.[129] Yet the effects were relatively mild in degree, because a host of other developmental factors come into play postnatally. Like genetic makeup or any other single factor, prenatal stress does not cast your fate in stone. However, these findings underscore the importance of coping with stress during pregnancy as well as seeking treatment when necessary.

TEMPERAMENT

Many adults who struggle with depression feel as if they were "born depressed"—they have felt depressed for as long as they can remember. The research on prenatal development might suggest a grain of truth to this possibility, and I have more to say about infant depression in Chapter 6 ("Childhood Adversity"). Of course, depression can also begin in early childhood, as it does in adulthood, from a combination of genetic vulnerability and stress. However, the feeling of having been depressed as long as one can remember also could be based on a temperamental disposition to depression.

We tend to think of a "temperamental" person as being moody. Technically, *temperament* refers to a broad range of *biologically based personality characteristics*, all partly rooted in genetic makeup. For example, some children are naturally more active, more impulsive, or more sociable than others; such temperamental differences are also evident in primates and other mammals.[130]

ANXIOUS TEMPERAMENT AND NEUROTICISM

One of the best-researched temperaments is anxiety proneness—depression's close companion. Developmental psychologist Jerome Kagan[131] observed that about 20% of children show an inhibited (anxious) profile, whereas about 40% show an uninhibited profile. When exposed to unfamiliar people, situations, objects, or events, inhibited children show avoidance, distress, or subdued emotion. For example, when introduced into a group of other children, the inhibited toddler is likely to sit alone and observe, whereas the uninhibited toddler will plunge eagerly into play.

Temperament is not destiny. Temperament and environment interact such that temperamentally inhibited children who are exposed to stressful environments are likely to *remain* that way rather than grow away from it. Under more favorable circumstances, temperamentally inhibited children can become less inhibited. Yet temperament constrains development: inhibited infants can move into the middle range, but they don't go all the way over to the uninhibited end of the spectrum.

Neuroticism—proneness to distress—might be construed as an adult extension of anxious temperament (see Chapter 1, "Depression"). Neuroticism has a partly genetic basis, and a neurotic disposition significantly increases susceptibility to depression, especially in the context of high levels of stress.[5,132]

DEPRESSIVE TEMPERAMENT

German psychiatrist Emil Kraepelin[53] proposed that "depressive temperament is characterized by a permanent gloomy emotional stress in all the experiences of life" (p. 118). Contemporary psychiatrist Hagop Akiskal[133] elaborated the concept of affective (emotional) temperaments, linking them to fundamental biological processes. Akiskal[134] characterized temperamentally depressive persons as somber, humorless, skeptical, gloomy, brooding, suffering, self-critical, guilt-prone, preoccupied with inadequacy and failure, nonassertive, self-sacrificing, introverted, critical, and complaining. Yet depressive temperament has its advantages: Akiskal observed that persons with depressive temperament are likely to be reliable and devoted; they're hard workers.

Depressive temperament is not a psychiatric diagnosis, nor is it as carefully defined or well researched as anxious temperament. Moreover, depressive temperament has fuzzy boundaries: in childhood, depressive temperament shades into persistent childhood depression, and later in life, depressive temperament shades into depressive personality disorder. I mention depressive temperament merely to emphasize the role of genetic and other biological factors in the development of depression.

CHEERFUL TEMPERAMENT

Recall from Chapter 1 ("Depression") that we can construe persons with depressed mood as being low on the spectrum of positive emotionality. Positive emotionality is another facet of temperament[4] and, for many persons, socializing is a prominent source of positive emotion.[135] To reiterate, a hallmark of cheerful temperament is *extraversion*, a central personality characteristic influenced partly by genetic makeup. Akiskal[134] formulated the opposite end of the spectrum from depression as being *hyperthymic* temperament. He characterized hyperthymic persons as being cheerful, optimistic, extroverted, talkative, confident, energetic, and uninhibited. He also proposed a *cyclothymic* temperament as involving an alternation between depressive and hyperthymic states.

TEMPERAMENT WARS

Persons who are temperamentally depressive tend to be put off by entreaties from more characteristically cheerful souls to "Buck up!" or the like. William James[136] drew a contrast between "morbid-minded" and "healthy-minded" persons, observing that "there are men who seem to have started life with a bottle or two of champagne inscribed to their credit; whilst others seem to have been born close to the pain-threshold, which the slightest irritants fatally send them over" (p. 152).

Citing the truism that good and bad are essential aspects of existence, James noted that the healthy-minded are characteristically attentive to the former, the morbid-minded oriented to the latter. The morbid-minded person's ruminations engender a "joy-destroying chill" that elicits this kind of healthy-minded response: "Stuff and nonsense, get out into the open air!" and "Cheer up." But James—himself prone to depression—averred, "Our troubles lie indeed too deep for *that* cure" (p. 157).

Persons of a temperamentally depressive bent are in good company. James weighed in this way:

> What are we to say of this quarrel? It seems to me that we are bound to say that morbid-mindedness ranges over the wider scale of experience, and that its survey is the one that overlaps. The method of averting one's attention from evil, and living simply in the light of good is splendid as long as it will work. It will work with many persons; it will work far more generally than most of us are ready to suppose; and within the sphere of its successful op-

eration there is nothing to be said against it.... But it breaks down impotently as soon as melancholy comes; and even though one be quite free from melancholy one's self, there is no doubt that healthy-mindedness is inadequate as a philosophical doctrine, because the evil facts which it refuses positively to account for are a genuine portion of reality; and they may after all be the best key to life's significance, and possibly the only openers of our eyes to the deepest levels of truth.[136] (p. 182)

One could object to the process of solidifying a depressed mood into a philosophy; no doubt, those with a depressive bent risk becoming mired in existential despair. With this prospect in mind, philosopher Simon Blackburn[137] commented, "It is sad when we become like that...we need a tonic more than an argument. The only good argument is, in a famous phrase of [philosopher] David Hume's, that it is no way to make yourself useful or agreeable to yourself or others" (pp. 80–81). Blackburn has science on his side, and James was right to use the term "healthy-minded"; extensive psychological research demonstrates the health benefits of optimism.[138]

GENDER

Depression is twice as prevalent among women as men, but this gender difference does not emerge until puberty. Boys are as likely as girls—if not somewhat more likely—to be depressed. Yet the prevalence of depression in boys remains stable, whereas the prevalence of depression in girls begins to rise at the onset of puberty and continues to increase until late adolescence, at which point the prevalence among girls has doubled that among boys. This gender difference persists throughout life.

These gender differences result from a combination of biological, psychological, interpersonal, and cultural factors. The following summary relies heavily on psychologist Susan Nolen-Hoeksema's[139] masterful integration of the complex research findings.

BIOLOGICAL CONTRIBUTIONS

Depression's associations with puberty, menses, the postpartum period, and menopause raise questions about a distinct hormonal contribution to depression for women. The divergence between females and males in prevalence of depression at the onset of puberty is particularly striking. In addition, a significant minority of women show symptoms of heightened emotional distress in conjunction with menses; this syndrome has been termed *premenstrual dysphoric disorder* and affects somewhere between 3%

and 8% of women. *Postpartum depression* refers to a major depressive episode in the first few weeks after giving birth; it affects between 10% and 15% of women. Women at highest risk for postpartum depression are those with a family history or personal history of depression, the latter including depression during pregnancy. Research has not consistently shown increased risk of depression in conjunction with menopause.

Hormonal contributions to depression are well demonstrated, for example, in thyroid disease. Yet women in general do not appear to be at greater risk for mood changes in conjunction with these gender-related periods of hormonal changes. Rather, these hormonal changes interact with genetic vulnerability and stress, such that the *combination* of all these factors could render some women particularly susceptible to depression at times of hormonal changes.[139]

PSYCHOLOGICAL, INTERPERSONAL, AND CULTURAL CONTRIBUTIONS

A multitude of psychological and social factors contribute to gender differences in depression; I review several here: negative body image, exposure to stress and trauma, social inequalities, and coping strategies conducive to depression. None of these factors is exclusive to women, but they are more prominent among women.

Physical changes associated with puberty go well beyond hormones, and they have a major impact on development. Body image is a major component of self-esteem for members of both sexes.[140] Yet the physical changes of puberty, whereas typically welcomed by males, are often unwelcome by females—particularly in the context of early onset of puberty.[139] Negative body image, associated eating disturbances, and their impact on self-esteem all play an important part in depression among adolescent girls.[141,142] Moreover, likely in conjunction with concerns about self-image, dating is more stressful for adolescent girls than adolescent boys.[139]

These observations of the role of stress in the early development of gender differences raise broader questions: First, are women more often exposed to stressful events than men? Second, when exposed to stressful events, are women more likely than men to respond with depression? Recent research suggests that similarities outweigh differences, although women and men are responsive to different *kinds* of stressors. One study, for example, found women to be more prone to depression in the face of interpersonal stress and men to be more prone to depression in the face of occupational stress.[143] Notably, however, men were more prone to depression in response to separation and divorce, perhaps because men are more likely than women to be lacking in social support. Although differential sensitivity to stress in general remains an open question, one study found that women were more likely than men to become depressed at lower levels of stress, whereas women and men were equally likely to become depressed in response to higher levels of stress.[5]

Although there may be more similarities than differences between men and women in overall exposure to stress, there is one glaring exception: women are far more likely to be exposed to sexual trauma than men. Such trauma includes childhood sexual abuse and sexual assaults at any age. In addition, women are more vulnerable to battering in adult attachment relationships, which may include sexual, physical, and psychological abuse as well as psychological neglect. Moreover, women are vulnerable to sexual harassment in a number of contexts. All these traumatic experiences confer a high risk for depression in women.[144] Of course, as is becoming more widely appreciated, boys are also vulnerable to childhood sexual abuse, and they are also at risk for posttraumatic depression in the aftermath of such abuse.

Short of such blatantly traumatic stressors, women experience other noteworthy adversities, including inequities in relationships with men. In intimate relationships with men, women may have less power over decisions and they may take on a greater share of the workload. In the workplace, women are likely to be more poorly paid, restricted from activities, or devalued. Yet higher-level professional women are not immune. Research in the 1970s revealed that 46% of women physicians had experienced depression; among the small sample of women psychiatrists, the rate was 73%. Among multiple possible explanations for this finding, the authors proposed that high pressure under adverse conditions of prejudice may have played a role.[145]

Poverty is a notorious risk factor for a wide range of psychiatric disorders, and the fact that women are more likely to live in poverty than men is yet another factor that has been proposed to account for gender differences in depression.[146] A classic study of stress and depression in women conducted in London by George Brown and colleagues[93] highlighted the impact of poverty. Single mothers raising young children in conditions of poverty were at exceptionally high risk for depression.

Finally, gender differences in ways of coping with stress may contribute to vulnerability to depression. As I discuss in Chapter 12 ("Flexible Thinking"), a tendency to ruminate—recycling worries and negative thoughts—contributes to the downward spiral of depression, perpetuates depressed mood, and interferes with productive problem solving.[147] Compared with men, who tend to be more action oriented, women are more prone to ruminating, and this propensity also contributes to their risk of depression.[139]

INFLUENCING FATE

This chapter addresses several constitutional factors that potentially contribute to the risk of developing depression. None of these factors causes depression; as you have begun to glimpse, the developmental pathways to depression are exceedingly complex, with biological, psychological, and environmental contributions all entangled at every step. I've construed these constitutional factors as constraints, and they leave ample elbow room for agency: how you live your life, how much stress you encounter, and how you cope are partly up to you. Although many risk factors are beyond your control, you play an active role in your fate.

Understandably, if you have children, you might worry that you have passed on some of the vulnerabilities I've just discussed. However, the same logic applies: these potential risk factors do not mean that your children are destined to become depressed. Knowing about risks can alert you to signs of developing problems, and knowing about coping and treatment options can help you intervene promptly and effectively should signs of illness appear.

• C h a p t e r 5 •

ATTACHMENT

Author Andrew Solomon[114] characterized depression as a fatal flaw in love: "To be creatures who love, we must be creatures who can despair at what we lose, and depression is the mechanism of that despair" (p. 15). Solomon was echoing Freud:[148] "We are never so defenceless against suffering as when we love, never so helplessly unhappy as when we have lost our loved object or its love" (p. 33). Freud thus identified the two pervading themes in depression: *loss* and *failure*. We experience losses through separations and deaths. However, Freud also recognized that we suffer from *loss of love*; the love object's disapproval and rejection spawn depressive feelings of inadequacy and failure.

Just as stressful attachment relationships play a major role in vulnerability to depression, comforting attachment relationships are a pathway to healing. Accordingly, attachment relationships remain a central concern throughout this book. This chapter lays the foundation by reviewing basic attachment concepts and describing the benefits of secure attachment relationships. Although the next chapter addresses various forms of childhood adversity in greater detail, I begin addressing childhood origins of depression in this chapter by drawing a parallel between two different patterns of insecure attachment and the two major themes in depression, loss and failure. The chapter concludes by highlighting the flexibility of attachment over the lifetime; we count on the capacity for growth in promoting recovery from depression and decreasing vulnerability to further episodes.

THE BENEFITS OF SECURE ATTACHMENTS

British psychiatrist John Bowlby[149] began developing attachment theory in the 1950s from observing children's reactions to separation and loss. Bowlby conducted extensive observations of children's responses to temporary separations during hospitalization. At that time, children who were dropped off at the hospital or placed in residential nursery care did not see their parents again until they were picked up—days, weeks, or even months later. Bowlby was struck by the sheer intensity of the distress and misery these children experienced during the separation as well as by the potentially enduring disturbance in attachment relationships evident after they returned home. His work contributed to public awareness of the potential harm done by such policies. Fortunately, we now take it for granted that parents can stay with their hospitalized children continuously if they so choose.

Through observing the impact of separations, Bowlby came to appreciate the significance of *emotional bonds*. In his words, it is essential for mental health that "the infant and young child should experience a warm, intimate and continuous relationship with his mother (or permanent mother-substitute) in which both find satisfaction and enjoyment"[149] (pp. xi–xii). This close emotional bond is the core of a secure attachment relationship.

Although he was concerned primarily with mental health, Bowlby came to believe that attachment served a biological function; our capacity for attachment is part of our biological constitution. Because we are social beings, attachment is as essential to our survival as air, water, and food. Attachment is fundamentally a mammalian adaptation, although it is also evident in some ground-nesting birds.[149] From the standpoint of evolutionary biology, Bowlby contended that the primary function of attachment is protection: proximity to the attachment figure protects offspring from predators. Without the protection afforded by attachment, offspring would not survive and mammalian species would not have evolved. Early in life, offspring must stay close to stay safe. We can recognize the emotional legacy of this evolutionary process: throughout life, when we are frightened, we want to be close to an attachment figure.

Secure attachment is an ideal; yet, as Bowlby's initial observations of the effects of separation revealed, insecurity in attachment relationships is not uncommon. Bowlby's collaborator, Mary Ainsworth, brought different attachment patterns into bold relief by developing a clever laboratory procedure, the Strange Situation, to study infants' and mothers' reactions to separation and reunion.[150] First, an experimenter brings the mother and infant into a playroom. Next, a stranger enters, and then the mother is asked to leave the infant alone with the stranger. The mother eventually comes back into the room, allowing the infant to respond to her return. Then the mother and stranger leave the infant all alone, after which the mother returns for a second reunion. Thousands of parent–infant pairs have been studied in this laboratory situation, and different patterns of infant behavior during the reunions have been identified.

Most infants studied in this laboratory situation show the pattern of *secure attachment*. These infants are keenly aware of their mother's presence and absence. Depending on their temperament, securely attached infants may be more or less distressed by the separation. Regardless of their reaction to the separation, they seek closeness with their mother when she returns, making eye contact or approaching and greeting her. They may be hugged or picked up and held. The attachment works: the reunion quells whatever distress the infant experienced from the separation. With the feeling of security reestablished through contact with their mother, securely attached infants confidently return to playing and exploring their environment.

Ainsworth's research demonstrates secure attachment in its archetypal form. As Bowlby[151] stated, secure attachment is not just essential for infant development; attachment needs are "characteristic of human nature throughout our lives 'from the cradle to the grave'" (p. 82). Over the course of development, secure attachment serves several functions beyond providing physical protection: it provides us with a safe haven and a secure base; it promotes our ability to regulate our physiological arousal; and—introducing an unfamiliar word—it fosters our ability to *mentalize*, that is, to understand ourselves and each other as persons with minds.

A SAFE HAVEN

Bowlby's concept of the safe haven captures our intuitive sense of attachment as an emotional bond that provides comfort in times of distress. As Bowlby[149] stated, along with physical protection, attachment provides us humans with a *feeling of security*. We need more than physical safety, although we certainly need that; we need to feel emotionally secure. When we are suffering—ill or injured, physically or emotionally—we desire contact with an attachment figure. Secure attachments entail trust, the hallmark of which is confidence that the attachment figure will be available and emotionally responsive in times of need.

A SECURE BASE

Bowlby[151] proposed that the safe haven of an attachment relationship also provides a *secure base* for exploring the world. He made no bones about the significance of this idea: "No concept within the attachment framework is more central to developmental psychiatry than that of the secure base" (pp. 163–164). Imagine a toddler confidently exploring the playground while keeping tabs on his mother, occasionally checking back to make sure that she's nearby. Confident in his mother's availability, he toddles off on his own. Growing older, we toddle farther away for longer periods of time, but we continue to need a secure base in attachment—as Bowlby stated, from the cradle to the grave.

The concepts of a safe haven and a secure base form an elegant partnership; secure attachment not only provides a feeling of emotional connection but also promotes individual autonomy by encouraging exploration of the wider world. Of course, secure attachment doesn't just foster playful exploration; it also enables us to explore possible solutions to serious problems.[152] Keep in mind that much of our exploration is social exploration, which ultimately allows us to form a range of supportive relationships and to avail ourselves of help when we need it.

REGULATING PHYSIOLOGICAL AROUSAL

In times of distress, reunion with the attachment figure calms distress and dampens excess physiological arousal. Moreover, repeated experiences of soothing contact are crucial in promoting healthy development of the nervous system and other organ systems.[153,154] In a secure attachment relationship, mothers and their infants are in sync not just emotionally but also physiologically: their schedules and rhythms become mutually adapted, for example, in sleep–wake cycles and feeding cycles.[155] Through a process of gradual learning, regulation of emotional and physiological arousal in attachment relationships promotes *self*-regulation, our ability to calm ourselves by ourselves. Loss of attachment connections at any point in life perturbs mind and body, but disruption in attachment early in life can interfere with the *development* of the capacity to regulate distress, thereby increasing vulnerability to depression. Conversely, secure attachments at any point in life provide a buffer against stress.

MENTALIZING

Following Bowlby, we tend to think of attachment in terms of physical proximity: the distressed child runs to the mother's arms, and this physical contact provides a feeling of security. Yet we get this feeling of security not only from touch but also through a *feeling of connection*—a meeting of minds. What makes this feeling of connection possible? Here I want to introduce a concept from contemporary attachment theory: *mentalizing*.[156] Mentalizing entails perceiving and interpreting behavior as based on mental states, such as desires, goals, emotions, and beliefs. For example, when you're empathizing with another person's distress, you're mentalizing. When you're trying to figure out why you did something, you're mentalizing. When you're thinking about feelings—your own or someone else's—you're mentalizing. Thus mentalizing provides the foundation for relationships with others as well as self-awareness.

Like speaking language, mentalizing is an innate capacity that takes time to develop. Like speaking, mentalizing develops in the context of relationships. British psychologist Peter Fonagy and his colleagues[157] have shown how mentalizing develops best in the context of a secure base in attachment. That is, secure attachment not only fosters the exploration of the outer world but also facilitates the exploration of the inner world, the world of the mind. In Fonagy's view, the essence of a secure attachment is this: each person has the other person's *mind in mind*. Likewise, self-awareness entails mentalizing, having your own mind in mind. A common form of mentalizing is talking about feelings. You can appreciate the importance of secure attachment to the development of mentalizing capacity when you consider how you are more inclined to talk about feelings—your own or the other person's—when you are in a trusting relationship.

A moment's reflection should convince you of the need to mentalize in coping with depression. You need to make sense of the difficulties in your own mind as well as those in your attachment relationships. I have written this book to assist you in this process, but there's no substitute for a secure attachment relationship to help you sort all this out. Catch-22: depression often stems from insecure attachment. Understanding the basis of insecurity can help you work toward more secure attachments.

INSECURE ATTACHMENTS AND DEPRESSION

At any time in life, secure attachment provides an antidote to stress, whereas insecure attachment is a prominent source of stress. Along with secure attachment, Ainsworth and colleagues[150] identified two prominent patterns of insecure attachment in infancy: ambivalent and avoidant. In the laboratory situation, infants who show the *ambivalent attachment* pattern are more focused on their mother than the toys in the playroom. They respond to separation with intense distress, and they are not easily comforted by the reunion with their mother. Their attachment behavior is infused with ambivalence, frustration, and anger: they may seek contact but angrily resist comforting, in effect, biting the hand that feeds them. In adulthood, this pattern of ambivalence is manifested in strong dependency needs coupled with a hypersensitivity to abandonment and resentment of the attachment figure's shortcomings. This combination of dependency and hostility can result in unstable and stormy relationships; in one of our educational groups, my colleague, psychologist Helen Stein, aptly dubbed ambivalent attachment the *kick-and-cling* pattern.

In contrast, infants who show the *avoidant attachment* pattern appear nonchalant in the laboratory situation, seemingly unaware of their mother's whereabouts and more interested in the toys. Ostensibly unperturbed by her departure, avoidant infants appear indifferent when their mother returns, perhaps wanting to be put down if picked up. Yet this outward appearance is misleading; avoidant infants show a pattern of elevated physiological arousal in response to the separation, and this arousal does not abate with the reunion.[158] In adulthood, this avoidant pattern is evident in a dismissing attitude toward attachment: "Who needs it? I'll take care of myself!" This stance works reasonably well, in childhood or in adulthood, as long as the distress remains at manageable levels. In the face of stress pileup, however, the sense of isolation coupled with the inability to rely on supportive attachment relationships contributes to the development of depression.

On the basis of a splendid career's worth of research, psychologist Sidney Blatt[159] distinguished two forms of depression anchored in insecure attachments: dependent and self-critical. These two forms reflect the two major themes in depression: loss and failure. In overview, dependent depression is associated with the theme of loss and the ambivalent attachment pattern; self-critical depression is associated with the theme of failure and the avoidant attachment pattern (see Table 5–1).

Before describing dependent and self-critical depression, I want to head off two possible misunderstandings. First, insecure attachment is not the only pathway to depression; it is one of many. Second, I don't want to imply that there is a straight path from infant attachment to adult attachment; that way of thinking would be a kind of "attachment determinism" akin to the idea of genetic determinism I took pains to dispel in Chapter 4 ("Constitution"). Like genetic makeup, early attachment history is one of myriad developmental factors that contribute to vulnerability to depression. Like genetics, early attachment may play a greater or lesser role. Finally, attachment patterns are not cast in stone;[160] on the contrary, even in infancy, the pattern of attachment will depend on the nature of the infant–parent interaction. An infant may be secure with her mother and insecure with her father or vice versa, depending on the quality of their emotional interactions.[161] If the quality of the interaction changes, the pattern of attachment

TABLE 5-1.   Two types of depression

	Dependent	Self-critical
Parental contribution	Depriving, inconsistent	Demanding, critical
Attachment pattern	Ambivalent	Avoidant
Interpersonal style	Neediness	Aloofness
Precipitating stressor	Separation and loss	Failure
Adaptive aspect	Seeking attachment	Striving for success

is likely to shift accordingly. For example, an infant who has been securely attached to her mother might shift to an avoidant pattern if her previously emotionally attuned mother subsequently became characteristically more irritable and rejecting as a result of marital stress.

In sum, attachment patterns reflect a balance of stability and change that parallels the stability and change in the pattern of interaction in attachment relationships. Based on these interactions, we develop what Bowlby[151] called *working models* of relationships. We tend to apply the models we have learned, but we can form different models with different persons, and we can update our models based on new experiences. We bank on this capacity for change in attachment relationships as a means of overcoming the vulnerability to depression associated with the insecure models I am about to describe.

DEPENDENT DEPRESSION

As the label implies, the dependent form of depression reflects sensitivity to separation and loss. Dependent relationships are characterized by what Blatt[159] calls *neediness*: an excessive desire for closeness, contact, comforting, soothing, nurturance, protection, and security. Sensitivity to separation and abandonment may be reflected in clinging behavior, coupled with manipulative and coercive efforts to prevent the attachment figure from leaving. Ironically, persons with this vulnerability become caught up in a vicious circle, because their pattern of neediness tends to drive the attachment figure away, thereby escalating the pattern of neediness.

In the dependent pattern, depressive episodes are precipitated by disruption in attachments—any potentially significant interruption in the sense of being cared for. The broken emotional bond leaves the individual feeling unwanted, unloved, unlovable, neglected, and abandoned. The ensuing depression is reflected in feelings of helplessness and loneliness.

The ambivalence in the attachment is characterized by the intermingling of dependency with feelings of frustration and hostility stemming from unmet needs. Yet feelings of frustration and anger associated with dependence are generally stifled for fear that expressing anger directly will further alienate the attachment figure and precipitate the dreaded loss. Typically, however, the resentment is expressed intermittently or indirectly.

Ambivalence can come into attachment relationships at any point in life as a consequence of disruptions—glaringly, for example, as a response to a spouse's affair. Yet a proclivity to ambivalence also can develop in childhood, stemming from parent–child relationships characterized by neglect, deprivation, or lack of emotional availability. The hallmark of attachment relationships that promote ambivalence is inconsistency: love and care may be used to control the child, for example, through overindulgence or withdrawal of love. Importantly, these relationships are characterized by episodic love and warmth, but they lack the dependability and stability of secure attachment relationships.

There is an advantage to the ambivalent pattern: the individual hasn't given up on seeking attachment. Keep in mind that being dependent is good;[108] a capacity for dependency is a cornerstone of secure attachment. The vulnerability to dependent depression stems from *excess* dependency.

> Doug entered the hospital at the insistence of his son. He had become progressively more depressed over a 2-year period and had spent the bulk of the time over the previous 3 months in bed with the curtains pulled shut and the lights turned off. He began psychotherapy feeling frustrated and despondent about his inability to pull himself out of his depression.
>
> Doug traced his depression back to a period of neglect in early adolescence after his parents' divorce. He recalled his mother as having been domineering and critical of both him and his father before the divorce. He had been close to his father and had relied on him for emotional support and comfort. Doug was devastated when, soon after the divorce, his father left the state to marry another woman. His mother then became depressed; Doug remembered a period of 2 years after the divorce when she hardly paid any attention to him, except to scold him occasionally. He felt alone and deprived; his only solace was to eat dinner occasionally at the home of his best friend, whose mother doted on Doug when he was there. By midadolescence, Doug's mother had pulled out of her depression, but he didn't feel he could depend on her. As he remembered it, every time he needed her help, she was "bossy and critical."
>
> Although frustrated with his mother, Doug remembered pulling out of his early adolescent "funk" and capitalizing on his strengths. In his senior year of high school, he began dating Harriett, a relatively shy girl who was fond of him and very accepting. He was able to confide in her and could see, in hindsight, that she had taken the role of his father.

Doug had worked throughout high school and put himself through community college. He obtained a stable job as a mechanic and married Harriett. He recalled the initial years of marriage as happy, but the marriage began to go downhill after they had children—three in close succession. Doug felt increasingly neglected as Harriett devoted more and more of her attention to the children. He dealt with his resentment by spending more time away from home, often at the bar with his drinking buddies. In turn, Harriet became resentful of having to take all the responsibilities for the home and the family. She was irritated about his drinking. She wanted him to be around more and to take more of an interest in her and the children. She complained that they were out of contact, and she wanted more communication. The more she tried to pull him back, the more he pushed away.

As Harriett became more critical and their relationship became more distant, Doug started becoming depressed. His drinking provided temporary relief but ultimately compounded his depression. Just before his slide into severe depression, he had learned—a few months after the fact—that Harriet had engaged in a brief affair with her boss. Doug was devastated and he was furious at her for betraying him—as his father had done. They made an effort at reconciliation and decided to stay together, but Doug's slide into depression was unstoppable. He was unable to work and, as he put it, withdrew into a cave.

Doug was fortunate that his son had insisted on hospitalization. He was forced to be up and around; he got back into a regular routine of activity, eating, and sleeping; and he found it helpful to have some social contact. Yet he remained seriously depressed despite intensive treatment that included antidepressant medication. He was tied in an emotional knot. He recognized that, despite the distance that had evolved in his marriage, he was desperately dependent on Harriett. Having been betrayed, he was fearful of allowing himself to depend on her again. He could not leave her, but neither could he allow himself to get close to her. In addition, he was afraid that if he let her know how angry he continued to be, she might leave him for good; he generally stifled his resentment but occasionally let loose and berated her.

Doug was difficult to help. Although he got along well with the other patients, he complained that the hospital staff never had enough time for him and that his psychiatrist wasn't giving him the proper medicine. Yet he was afraid to express his anger for fear that they would dislike him and help him even less. It became clear that his anger and frustration got in the way of getting help from any relationship in which he felt dependent. He was stuck.

Fortunately, Doug had a strong incentive to get better: he was suffering. He had a lot of determination, and he was very insightful. He was able to see how his early feelings of neglect and resentment had adversely influenced his marriage and his treatment relationships; inadvertently, he was playing an active role in his ongoing suffering. At one point he realized that he had been operating on the self-defeating principle that if he just suffered intensely or long enough, maybe someone would finally help him. He came to recognize that he needed to help himself more, and he was able to get past his resentment to communicate more openly with his wife and his therapists, thereby getting more emotional help from them as well.

SELF-CRITICAL DEPRESSION

The self-critical pattern of depression is associated with feelings of low self-worth and hopelessness. Self-critical individuals struggle with a sense of inadequacy, inferiority, or worthlessness, coupled with feelings of guilt and shame. They may compensate for feelings of inferiority by relentless striving for success—at the extreme, becoming perfectionistic. Yet any real success will feel hollow to the extent that the sense of worthlessness endures. A wide range of stressors might precipitate episodes of depression; any experience of failure will do. The failure may relate to lack of success at school or work or to rejection in close relationships.

The self-critical pattern is associated with a pervasive vulnerability to *disapproval*, not just from within but also from without. Because of low self-worth and anticipation of disapproval, close and secure relationships are difficult to maintain. Hence the attachment pattern is *avoidant*: dismissing of close relationships, the self-critical individual may appear stoic, aloof, or hostile. Moreover, to the extent that the criticism is also directed outward, it may evoke hostility from others, creating a vicious circle of self-criticism, criticism of others, rejection, and more self-criticism.

The self-critical pattern can take root in parent–child relationships characterized by excessive control coupled with a lack of warmth. Parents may be demanding, intrusive, deprecatory, punitive, hostile, and rejecting. The child's autonomy is thwarted, as he or she feels loved only for compliance or performance. In this context, the child develops an avoidant attachment pattern, but avoidant behavior does not solve the problem; parental criticism and rejection are internalized in a pattern of self-criticism—hostile attacks on the self by the self.

Elaine sought psychotherapy for the first time in her mid-40s after her anxiety and depression escalated to the point that—to her horror—she began thinking about suicide. She attributed her depression to the fact that she was a "fool" for allowing herself to have been "completely humiliated."

Exceptionally bright and hard working, Elaine had risen to the level of full professor in a prestigious liberal arts college. Although widely respected for her teaching and academic record, she felt she never really belonged, because she was generally perceived as critical and aloof. She agreed with this appraisal, characterizing herself as "not suffering fools lightly" and as being "driven," a "workaholic," and a "loner."

Elaine had been married for a brief time in her early 20s. She said that she had married impulsively and that she and her husband soon came to recognize their basic incompatibility. Not one to give up easily, Elaine was inclined to try to work out their problems. However, she ended the marriage abruptly after discovering that her husband had rekindled his relationship with a former girlfriend after feeling rebuffed by Elaine's "coldness." In turn, Elaine felt rejected and bitter, and she resolved never again to put herself in such a vulnerable position.

Elaine had dated on and off in the two decades after her divorce, but she was quick to find fault with any man who took a serious interest in her. She knew her life was out of balance; she was consumed by work, had little contact with her family, rarely saw her one close friend who had moved to a distant city, and only occasionally socialized with a few colleagues whom she described as "acquaintances." Reluctantly, she acknowledged that she had felt lonely at times.

In the months preceding her depression, however, Elaine had allowed herself to become attached to a charming and talented colleague, Jeff, who had recently joined the faculty in another department. In hindsight, she saw that—uncharacteristically—she had thrown caution to the wind, against her better judgment allowing herself to be vulnerable. Jeff appeared utterly enamored with her, and she was pleased by the boost to her self-esteem that the relationship provided. She had taken some satisfaction in her intellectual ability but never considered herself to be very attractive. Owing to Jeff's greater sociability, Elaine began to develop more of a social life. She actually felt proud to be seen with Jeff around the campus. Then, to her dismay, she heard through the grapevine that Jeff also was involved in a romantic relationship with one of his graduate students, a fact that had been known to others in this small academic community. Echoes of the past: she felt betrayed—and worse, utterly mortified.

Elaine's feeling of public humiliation was matched by ruthless self-attacks. She felt duped. She—of all persons—should have known better. Worse yet, she believed that she had "lost all credibility" among her colleagues and students, as if all her accomplishments were for naught. She was so distraught that she couldn't sleep for more than 2 or 3 hours a night, and she slept fitfully at best. Her teaching was going downhill, and she feared that she would be unable to fulfill a book contract. She considered resigning but began to feel like a "total failure" and doubted that she could find a comparable position elsewhere. She felt trapped.

Elaine wisely sought psychotherapy, although she did so only in desperation; priding herself on her independence and good judgment, she considered her need for professional help to be another humiliation, a further reflection of her failure. Clearly, in the midst of her depression, she had lost all perspective. Her longstanding pattern of isolation, coupled with her acute sense of shame, had made it impossible for her to confide in anyone, which might have helped her to regain a more objective view of her situation.

In the therapy process, Elaine's longstanding vulnerability to self-critical depression became apparent. She had grown up in a high-achieving academic family; she had survived on an emotional diet of sporadic praise for accomplishments intermingled with keen attention to flaws, leavened by little warmth or nurturance. She identified with her highly self-critical father, whom she also characterized as a workaholic. To compound matters, she recalled that her mother not only tended to be critical of her father but also consistently had disapproved of all the boys Elaine had dated in high school and college. She realized that much of her perception of the "incompatibility" in her first marriage was based on her *mother's* criticism of her husband. In retrospect, Elaine was disheartened to think that taking on her mother's disapproval might have contributed to the alienation that ultimately led to the dissolution of that relationship. Elaine's involvement in psychotherapy began a long process of self-exploration that gradually led to better balance in her life; she became more self-accepting and began developing a greater capacity for warm relationships.

I have reviewed Blatt's[159] distinction between dependent and self-critical forms of depression not only to highlight the pervasive themes of loss and failure in depression but also to emphasize how depression is commonly embedded in attachment relationships. Many persons find their depression bewildering; they give some reasons for their depression but protest: "That's no reason to be *this* depressed!" As a starting point in recovery, it's helpful to make sense of the depression. The depth of the developmental roots can be obscure. Blatt's distinction provides a helpful orientation to exploring the deeper meanings. I offer the distinction here in hope that it might help you clarify the basis of your own depression.

However, I do not want to overstate the distinction. Dependent and self-critical depression are not mutually exclusive; they can be intermingled. The loss of love entailed by disapproval and rejection is, after all, a *loss*—a severing of an emotional bond. When you feel abandoned, you're likely to feel you have failed. Whether you feel abandoned or you feel you have failed, you're likely to feel alone. Not infrequently, loss and failure seem to have equal weight in the creation of depression.

HEALING ATTACHMENTS

Recognizing that depression is embedded in attachment relationships offers hope, because attachment needs are enduring and attachment patterns are malleable. As with all other areas of development, attachment evolves over the lifetime. Initially tied to infant–caregiver interactions, attachment subsequently is shaped by relationships with nonparental caregivers, siblings, and members of the extended family. Beginning with the school years, attachment relationships expand to include peers, teachers, coaches, neighbors, and members of the clergy.[162] We also develop attachments to groups and institutions; the feeling of belonging potentially attained by affiliating with a group can be a significant source of attachment security for some persons.[163] Attachments to animals also can be powerful;[164] our mammalian kin have attachment capacities akin to ours,[165] and we can form affectionate bonds with them, especially when they are furry and provide comforting touch.

To reiterate, attachment relationships show both stability and change over the course of development.[160] Keep in mind that the infant is *biologically disposed to form a secure attachment*. I think of the need for secure attachment as a driving force in relationships throughout life. Fortunately, being adaptive, attachment is somewhat fluid: from infancy to adulthood, the opportunity to form a close relationship with a sensitively responsive attachment figure offers the possibility of change from insecure to secure attachment.[166] Accordingly, only rarely does a person to arrive at adulthood without *some* capacity to form a positive, close, and secure attachment—even in the face of a history of traumatic attachments.[167] We bank on the enduring quest for secure attachment in promoting recovery from depression; a network of supportive relationships is a good antidepressant.

Yet, in campaigning for attachment, I don't want to slight the importance of independence and achievement. Keep in mind that the safe haven and the secure base of attachment jointly promote both connection and autonomy. Blatt and Blass[168] highlighted two broad lines of development that are essential to well-being for all of us: relatedness and self-definition. Vulnerability to depression entails an imbalance in attachment: dependent depression is an indication of focusing on relatedness to the exclusion of self-definition; self-critical depression is an indication of focus in self-definition to the exclusion of relatedness.

Psychoanalyst Joseph Lichtenberg[163] neatly captured the balance of relatedness and self-definition in his conception of *self-dependence*, which he distinguished carefully from independence or avoidant attachment. To be self-dependent involves the capacity to depend on others as well as to depend on yourself when others are not available. *Self-dependence is the capacity to bridge the gap between separation and reunion.* What makes bridging the gap possible? A sense of connection that endures in periods of absence; the attachment figure becomes a benevolent mental presence.[169] As Lichtenberg summarized, "To be self-dependent is to be able to rely on the self—to evoke the other in a period of absence, to bridge the gap until reunion or restoration of the attachment" (p. 104). Plainly, a self-critical mental presence will undermine self-dependence, as will a fear that the attachment figure cannot be counted on in times of need. Secure attachment provides a pathway out of depression, not just in strengthening supportive relationships with others but also in improving your relationship with yourself (see Chapter 8, "Internal Stress").

I conclude this chapter by reminding you of the positive facets of attachment to brace you for the next chapter, which addresses the more severe forms of childhood adversity—trauma in attachment relationships at worst. I have emphasized the balance between stability and change. On the side of stability, we can carry forward patterns of insecure attachment from child-hood to adulthood or slip back into them in the face of severe stress. I have included this chapter and the next because we need to be aware of our vulnerability to these destructive patterns so as to stay out of them. History need not repeat itself, especially when you are aware of its influence.

Chapter 6

CHILDHOOD ADVERSITY

Understanding the childhood origins of vulnerability to depression serves two broad purposes: first, to make sense of adulthood depression, and second, to help prevent depression in future generations. I launched this discussion in the last chapter by describing how different patterns of insecure attachment relate to different forms of depression. This chapter continues in the same vein by focusing on three additional forms of adversity that contribute to insecurity in early attachment relationships: mother–infant depression, separation and loss, and attachment trauma. In addition, I consider the adversity associated with depression in childhood and adolescence. All these adverse experiences can contribute to stress pileup and vulnerability to depression later in life. I conclude the chapter with a counterweight, emphasizing that we must pay equal attention to developmental factors that promote resilience to stress; the whole point of coping with depression is to promote resilience in an ongoing way.

MOTHER–INFANT DEPRESSION

We all experience emotional contagion;[170] being around someone who is agitated makes us agitated. Fortunately, enjoyable emotions are also contagious; laughter is a prime example. Like other emotions—anxiety, irritability, and excitement—depression is contagious, even in infancy.

There's nothing magical about emotional contagion; it's based on patterns of interacting. We tend automatically and intuitively to mirror one another's behavior and emotional states; our capacity for empathy evolves from this tendency.[171] Our attachment relationships are especially subject to emotional contagion because of their emotional closeness and the sheer frequency and repetitiveness of the interactions. In infancy, our primary attachment relationships have a considerable impact on our emotional state.

We have particular reason to be concerned about the potential impact of maternal depression on infant development, because postpartum depression is so common. Thus I begin this section with a brief review of postpartum depression and then consider how maternal depression affects infants by virtue of the interactive dance inherent in the mother–infant relationship. Yet the extent to which postpartum depression affects infant development depends on many other factors, and clinicians have developed a range of effective interventions to prevent adverse consequences.

POSTPARTUM DEPRESSION

Postpartum depression is diagnosed when the episode begins within 4 weeks of childbirth.[8] Postpartum depression is distinguished from more transient *baby blues*, which are highly common during the first 10 days but do not interfere with the mother's functioning. Postpartum depression affects 10%–15% of women, and at worst, it can be potentially disabling, lasting a matter of months.[139] Symptoms may include dramatic mood fluctuations, preoccupation with the infant's well-being, fear of being alone with the infant, indifference to the infant, and a high level of anxiety.

By definition, postpartum depression coincides with childbirth and thereby is intertwined with that major life event. Yet childbearing per se does not increase the risk of depression, and postpartum depression is not a distinct form of depression.[172] Although the postpartum period is associated with substantial hormonal changes, the relation of these hormonal changes to the mood disturbance is unclear; perhaps the combination of a predisposition to depression—for example, from a family history, a personal history, or depression during pregnancy—in conjunction with the hormonal changes plays a role in triggering episodes.[139] Of course, childbirth is a life-changing event that reorganizes the network of attachment relationships.

I discuss the relationship between stressful life events and depression in the next chapter (Chapter 7, "Stressful Events"), and postpartum depression can be understood best in this context. Thus factors that increase risk for postpartum depression are stressful events during pregnancy and delivery, marital conflicts, and lack of social support.[172] Childbirth also can wreak havoc with schedules and routines—especially sleep—which also can increase the risk for depression in vulnerable persons (see Chapter 11, "Health"). Finally, doubts about one's competence as a mother—perhaps associated with a history of insecure attachment—also play a significant role in postpartum depression, potentially as a contributing factor to depression and as a consequence of depression.[173,174]

THE INTERACTIVE DANCE

We can best appreciate the impact of maternal depression on the mother–infant attachment relationship by considering the interactive dance between mother and child. The behavior of each partner contributes to the flow of this dance.[89] Infant researchers have focused their attention on *contingent responsiveness:*[175] for the interaction to proceed smoothly, the mother's behavior must be contingent on what the infant does and vice versa. Meticulous studies of videotaped interactions show the split-second coordination between mother's and infant's behavior in patterns of gazing, smiling, vocalizing, and touching.[176] This coordination develops early in infancy and characterizes our interactions with each other throughout life.[177] If the mother's behavior is out of sync with the infant's behavior, then the infant will become distressed. Although I focus here on the mother's behavior, keep in mind that the dance is a partnership, and the infant's capacity to dance also plays an important role in the interaction. A host of constitutional factors play a role in the infant's interactive style and responsiveness; some infants are inherently easier to engage and more responsive than others.

As psychologist Tiffany Field[126] and many other researchers[176,178,179] have observed, severely depressed mothers have difficulty engaging in an interactive dance with their infants. These mothers engage in less touching, looking, and talking; they are less animated in their face and voice. Researchers have identified two patterns of behavior common among depressed mothers: withdrawal and intrusiveness.[180,181] The *withdrawn* pattern entails less active engagement and responsiveness as well as failure to support the infant's activities, whereas the *intrusive* pattern includes such behaviors as interrupting the infant's behavior, poking, rough handling, aggressive teasing, and speaking in an angry tone of voice.

Infants of depressed mothers accommodate to their mother's interactive style and show a number of behavioral signs characteristic of depression: less activity, less vocalizing, fewer positive facial expressions, and a greater tendency to look away from the mother. These infants also show distress, and they protest; they are more likely to appear sad or angry and less likely to show expressions of interest. Interactively, depressed mothers and infants are dancing in an uncoordinated fashion; as Field[126] described it, "The face-to-face interactions of the depressed mothers and their infants were choppy, uncoordinated and unpleasant to observe" (p. 62). Consistent with the fact that depression is characterized by high levels of negative emotion and low levels of positive emotion (see Chapter 1, "Depression"), depressed mothers and their infants are less likely to show matching of positive emotions and more likely to show matching of negative emotions—less positive and more negative emotional dancing.

ADVERSE IMPACT

As I have just described, infants of depressed mothers show depressed behavior; they also show evidence of physiological distress that includes not only elevated heart rate and stress hormones but also changes in patterns of brain activity consistent with diminished positive emotionality and increased negative emotionality.[182] Such observations have led researchers to investigate a crucial question: does postpartum depression have long-term adverse effects on child development?

Developmental psychologists have been particularly concerned about the potential impact of postpartum depression on the quality of subsequent mother–infant attachment; some studies have found that postpartum depression is associated with greater risk of insecure attachment, whereas others have not.[183,184] Similarly, researchers have been concerned about the impact of postpartum depression on children's cognitive development, given that mother–infant interactions play an important role in shaping the infant's attention and capacities for learning as well as regulating emotional distress that would interfere with attention and learning.[174,185] Consistent with these concerns, some studies have shown that postpartum depression is associated with poorer performance on measures of ability in early childhood.[184]

Yet the extent to which postpartum depression adversely affects development depends on a host of other considerations.[185] It is the quality of the *mother–infant interaction* that affects development, not the mother's depression per se—although these are obviously related. But many mothers who have postpartum depression are able to interact effectively with their infants. As you might expect, the severity and duration of the postpartum depression is a crucial factor; relatively short-lived depressions will have a lesser impact. Moreover, not just the depression but also the extent of additional stress in the mother's life plays a significant role. Thus many possible contributors besides depressed mood may contribute to problematic parent–child interactions, including a history of childhood adversity in the parent.[181] The greatest adverse impact of postpartum depression is associated with generally high-risk situations, for example, adolescent mothers living in poverty with minimal social support. As this latter point implies, the nature of the infant's other relationships will be an important influence in development. For example, infants who show depressed behavior in interactions with their depressed mother perk up when they interact with their nondepressed father[186] or other caregivers.[187]

INTERVENTION

Given the potentially adverse impact of postpartum depression not only on the mother but also on the infant and family, it is important to keep in mind that something can be done about it.[188] Both pregnancy and breastfeeding are significant considerations—although certainly not absolute barriers—to taking antidepressant medication.[189] Given the impact of childbirth on relationships, interpersonal therapy can be helpful for depression at this time as well[190] (see Chapter 13, "Supportive Relationships").

Fortunately, a wide range of interventions have been developed not only to ameliorate postpartum depression but also to facilitate a more positive pattern of mother–infant interaction,[126,173,191,192] although brief interventions are more likely to have short-term rather than long-term benefits.[193,194] Not only counseling but also stress reduction techniques such as massage therapy and listening to music are helpful to depressed mothers. In addition, helping mothers to understand how problems in the relationship with their infant are associated with their own attachment history can be beneficial. Yet it is also important to focus directly on the problematic mother–infant interactive patterns. For example, when depressed adolescent mothers learn to massage their infants, the infants' mood improves and their levels of physiological stress decrease. In addition, coaching mothers to interact with their infants has proven to be helpful. For example, mothers who are relatively withdrawn are taught ways of getting their infant's attention so as to increase their level of engagement, whereas mothers who are more intrusive are taught to imitate their infants so as to increase their level of sensitivity.[192]

Starting at the ground floor of childhood adversity, I have focused this section on postpartum depression; of course, parental depression can influence child development at any time period.[195] Parental depression is associated with a range of emotional and behavioral problems in children and adolescents.[196] As is true in infancy, the adverse effects of parental depression will depend on a wide range of other factors, and older children and adolescents are subject to a wider array of influences beyond the family, for better or for worse. As much of the material reviewed in this book attests, parental depression is intertwined with many other factors—such as stress and other psychiatric disorders—that also will affect children and influence parent–child relationships. Psychologist Constance Hammen[197] summarized four broad factors that affect the children of depressed parents: parents' symptoms, chronic stressors such as marital problems that accompany parental depression, episodic stressors that impinge on parents, and other stressors in the child's life. There are many potential avenues of help, including treatment for the parents, treatment for the children, and family therapy.[188]

SEPARATION AND LOSS

In Bowlby's[198] words, "Loss of a loved person is one of the most intensely painful experiences any human being can suffer" (p. 7). Bowlby emphasized the similarities between children and adults in responses to loss and, in either case, he was critical of the "tendency to underestimate how intensely distressing and disabling loss usually is and for how long the distress, and often the disablement, commonly lasts" (p. 8). Bowlby also criticized the assumption that we should not only get over the loss quickly but also should get over it completely. In connection with this latter point, Bowlby[198] quoted a letter of consolation Freud wrote to a colleague whose son had died:

> Although we know that after such a loss the acute state of mourning will subside, we also know we shall remain inconsolable and will never find a substitute. No matter what may fill the gap, even if it be filled completely, it nevertheless remains something else. And actually this is how it should be. It is the only way of perpetuating that love which we do not want to relinquish. (p. 23)

CHILDREN'S RESPONSES TO SEPARATION

Bowlby[198] emphasized the similarities between children and adults in response to loss. He discovered a typical sequence of children's emotional responses to separation: protest, despair, and detachment. The initial *protest* reaction—angry crying, for example—expresses outwardly the intensity of distress and, at least initially, it is intended to forestall the separation. After a time, protest turns into quiet *despair*, which can be mistaken for diminished distress. Prolonged or repeated separations eventuate in *detachment*, the polar opposite of attachment; the child defensively blocks the natural desire for close emotional bonds to prevent the pain of future separations.

Such detachment is most strikingly evident upon reunion with the mother; the child might not even recognize her.

Here's how Bowlby[199] described the sequence:

> Whenever a young child who has had an opportunity to develop an attachment to a mother figure is separated from her unwillingly, he shows distress; and should he also be placed in a strange environment and cared for by a succession of strange people, such distress is likely to be intense. The way he behaves follows a typical sequence. At first he *protests* vigorously and tries by all the means available to him to recover his mother. Later he seems to *despair* of recovering her but nonetheless remains preoccupied with her and vigilant for her return. Later still, he seems to lose his interest in his mother and to become emotionally *detached* from her. Sooner or later after being reunited with his mother, his attachment to her emerges afresh. Thenceforward, for days or weeks, and sometimes for much longer, he insists on staying close to her. Furthermore, whenever he suspects he will lose her again he exhibits acute anxiety. (pp. 26–27)

We might readily identify depression with the despair phase, which Bowlby identified as showing increasing hopelessness. As he described,[149] the child "may cry monotonously or intermittently. He is withdrawn and inactive, makes no demands on people in the environment, and appears to be in a state of deep mourning" (p. 27). However, the other phases also play a role in depression. Bowlby's[199] observations on the protest phase highlight the role of anger and resentment in response to separation; these emotions play a powerful role in depression (see Chapter 8, "Internal Stress"). Bowlby noted that children naturally express anger at being left, and sometimes their anger indicates hope: their angry reproaches may serve as a deterrent, discouraging the parent from leaving again. In adults as well as children, such angry reproaches are coercive, attempting to cement the emotional bond. Yet intense and persistent anger, which may take the form of deep resentment, also can weaken the emotional bond, promoting detachment—a defensive giving up on attachment.

CHILDHOOD LOSS AND ADULTHOOD DEPRESSION

As I discuss in the next chapter, ample research shows that stressful events often precede depressive episodes; nevertheless, most persons who are exposed to stress do *not* become depressed. A landmark study of depression in women examined developmental factors that increased the risk of depression in response to stress and discovered that loss of mother through death before age 11 stood out.[93] In this study, neither later loss of mother nor loss of father at any age was associated with adulthood depression.

Yet subsequent research on the relation between childhood loss of a parent and risk of depression in adulthood has not yielded consistent findings, suggesting that the *context* of the loss also must be taken into account.[128] Bowlby[198] drew attention to the "enormous importance of a child's experience after the loss" (p. 312) and observed that children often experience inadequate care subsequent to the loss as well as being rebuked for their normal grieving. A child who has lost a parent will do best if the relationship with the parents was secure prior to the loss; if the child is well informed about what happened; if the child is included in the grieving rituals; and—most crucial from an attachment perspective—if the child "has the comforting presence of his surviving parent, or if that is not possible of a known and trusted substitute, and an assurance that the relationship will continue" (p. 276).

Unfortunately, as Bowlby recognized, he set forth stringent conditions for the well-being of the child in the aftermath of a loss. Sadly, such losses not infrequently expose children to additional stressors and adversities, including financial hardships, geographical moves, and—potentially most problematic—maltreatment. Confirming Bowlby's clinical experience, British psychologist Antonia Bifulco and colleagues[200] conducted research to explore further the context of attachment relationships following childhood loss and their relation to depression in adulthood. They found that vulnerability to depression in adulthood was associated with lack of maternal care prior to the loss, lack of paternal or substitute care after the loss, and the child's experience of helplessness in the aftermath of the loss. This brings us to the domain of childhood trauma as a vulnerability factor for adult depression.

ATTACHMENT TRAUMA

Exposure to traumatic stress at any point in life is a prominent contributor to the stress pileup that eventuates in depression.[95] *Trauma* refers to the lasting adverse effects of exposure to extremely stressful events. Depression is one among many such lasting effects. Potentially traumatic events have both objective and subjective aspects.[8] Objectively, such events pose a severe threat to the integrity of the person, such as death or serious injury. Subjectively, these events are experienced with feelings of helplessness and horror.[8] Of course, it is the subjective emotional experience of the stressful situation that is potentially traumatizing. I believe that the essence of traumatic events is feeling emotionally overwhelmed and *alone*. The traumatic impact of extremely stressful events can be ameliorated by the availability of a secure attachment relationship that restores the sense of security and safety as well as providing an opportunity to make sense of the traumatic experience.

There are innumerable forms of trauma, and I find it helpful to distinguish among them by the extent of interpersonal involvement.[144] All else being equal, it is worse to be traumatized by another person, especially when you depend on that person. Thus I distinguish three broad categories:

1. *Impersonal* trauma, such as an earthquake, tornado, tsunami, or dam collapse;
2. *Interpersonal* trauma, caused deliberately or negligently by another person, such as combat, terrorist attacks, assaults, or motor vehicle accidents stemming from drunk driving; and
3. *Attachment* trauma, inflicted in an attachment relationship, consisting of abuse and neglect.

Attachment trauma may occur in attachment relationships at any point in life, ranging from childhood maltreatment[201] to battering in marriages[202] to elder abuse.[203] Attachment trauma is particularly troubling because it promotes distrust in close relationships that interferes with the person's ability to form secure attachments, which are the most important means of healing.[144] Attachment trauma in childhood, our concern here, poses what my colleagues Peter Fonagy and Mary Target[204] call a *dual liability:* it not only provokes extreme stress but also undermines the *development* of the mental and interpersonal capacities to regulate that distress.

FORMS OF ATTACHMENT TRAUMA

In pursuing the childhood origins of vulnerability to depression in adulthood, Bifulco and her colleagues carefully distinguished several forms of maltreatment.[205,206] Broadly, maltreatment can be divided into abuse and neglect, and several forms of each can be distinguished.

Following others, Bifulco distinguished between physical abuse and sexual abuse. Going beyond others, she refined our understanding of "emotional abuse" by distinguishing between antipathy and psychological abuse. *Antipathy* refers to rejection, which may be either hot (e.g., cursing at the child) or cold (e.g., the silent treatment). *Psychological abuse* refers to cruelty and sadism directed toward the child, which may take many forms, including terrorizing (e.g., locking a child who's afraid of the dark in a closet), humiliating (e.g., shaming the child in front of her friends), depriving (withholding food or destroying valued belongings or pets), and corrupting the child (e.g., involving the child in pornographic or other illegal activities).

Bifulco discovered that all these forms of childhood abuse increase the risk of depression in adulthood,[207] and her findings have been confirmed by many other studies.[144] Not only does childhood maltreatment increase the likelihood of developing depression in adulthood but also it may contribute to the severity of the episode,[208] the likelihood of suicidal behavior,[209] and the likelihood of recurrence.[210] In some respects, however, psychological abuse (cruelty) potentially has the most devastating impact on development and relationships, and it bears the strongest relationship to depression in adulthood.[211] Yet psychological abuse is almost invariably intertwined with other forms of maltreatment, such as antipathy, neglect, and sexual and physical abuse; ultimately, it is the extent of pileup of the abuses that raises the risk of depression in adulthood.

In comparison with abuse, the impact of childhood neglect has been relatively ignored,[212] yet its adverse impact on development may equal or even exceed that of abuse.[213] Broadly, two forms of neglect can be distinguished. *Physical neglect* includes failure to provide for basic needs such as food, clothing, shelter, health care, and hygiene as well as lack of supervision, which compromises the child's safety (e.g., leaving the child in a dangerous environment).[214] *Psychosocial neglect*, a failure to support the child's psychosocial development,[206] includes emotional neglect (lack of responsiveness to the child's emotional states), cognitive neglect (failure to nurture and support cognitive and educational development), and social neglect (failure to encourage and support the development of peer relationships). Of course, all these forms of neglect may be intertwined as well as combined with various forms of abuse. For example, Bifulco and colleagues[215] found that neglect, physical abuse, and institutional stays were associated with higher risk of sexual abuse. As Bowlby recognized, this study exemplifies how one trauma—such as the loss of a parent—can lead to a whole cascade of other traumas.

CHILDHOOD AND ADOLESCENT DEPRESSION

Stress pileup can begin in the womb, and depressed behavior can be evident soon after birth. As in adulthood, childhood depression emerges in conjunction with biological vulnerability and environmental stress. Moreover, depression itself is stressful, and I am covering childhood and adolescent depression here because they can contribute to stress pileup and increase the risk for later depression.[216]

Depression in children and adolescents is not a distinct disorder from adult depression; the symptoms are similar throughout the lifespan.[47] There are two minor differences in diagnostic criteria:[8] first, children and adolescents may show irritable mood rather than depressed mood; second, dysthymic disorder is diagnosed on the basis of a 1-year duration of symptoms (as opposed to 2 years for adults). Like adults, children and adolescents can have double depression (major depressive episodes on top of dysthymia), and like adults, children and adolescents with depression often have additional psychiatric problems, including anxiety, conduct disturbance, attention-deficit disorder, and substance abuse.[216]

CHILDHOOD DEPRESSION

Although clinicians debate about whether a formal diagnosis of depression can be made in infants and toddlers,[216] there is no question about the existence of depressive behaviors from the beginning of life. One case series revealed serious depression in a small number of preschool children.[217] In addition to showing all the symptoms of depression seen in older individuals, all these children complained of physical symptoms, and two-thirds engaged in suicidal behavior. All these depressed preschoolers were from broken homes, and all had been abused or severely neglected.

The prevalence of depression gradually increases with age from the preschool years to adolescence.[47] As is true of adults, episodes of depression are likely to last several months in children, and they are also likely to be recurrent. Of great concern is emerging evidence that rates of depression in childhood as well as adolescence are increasing, perhaps in relation to social changes that include increasing family disruption, greater exposure to stress, and less availability of resources and supports.[45] Childhood depression interferes with functioning in school and in peer relationships; this interference hampers the development of academic and social skills, undermines the sense of self-worth, and places the child at increasing disadvantage.

Sadly, quite early in life, stress pileup can build in vicious circles. As psychologist Constance Hammen[47] put it, a cyclical process is activated, "proceeding from reduced competence to depressed affect to even more dysfunctional behavior, which then evokes negative consequences that perpetuate or exacerbate symptoms" (p. 177). Problematic family interactions are likely to be intertwined with the child's difficulties: parent–child interactions may be characterized by lack of emotional attunement, hostility, or frank maltreatment stemming from parents' psychological problems or substance abuse. Thus depressed children are likely to be hampered in developing secure attachments both inside and outside the family.

ADOLESCENT DEPRESSION

By adolescence, the prevalence of depression is comparable with that in adults. The fact that depression runs in families is evident in adolescence as well as adulthood; depression in either or both parents substantially increases the likelihood of depression in the adolescent.[218,219] Commonly, parents' and adolescents' problems fuel each other; for example, depressed parents tend to be more critical and their adolescents' disturbance may fuel the criticism.[220]

As in adulthood, episodes of adolescent major depression can be prolonged; in a large community (nonhospitalized) sample, for example, Lewinsohn and Essau[221] found that 25% recovered from the episode by 3 weeks, 50% by 2 months, and 75% by 6 months.[221] Of considerable concern, 40% experienced relapses within 1 year. Moreover, having an episode of depression in midadolescence substantially increases the likelihood of depression (as well as anxiety disorders) in later adolescence and young adulthood.[222]

Depression in adolescence is a serious problem in its own right, just as it is in adulthood. As it is with depression in childhood, however, the seriousness of the disorder is compounded by its potential impact on many facets of development. Consider these observations from Lewinsohn and Essau:[221]

> These formerly depressed young adults were less likely to have completed college, to more recently have been unemployed, to have a lower income level, to have higher rates of child bearing, to be smoking cigarettes, to have lower levels of social support from family and friends and smaller social networks, and to be experiencing some (i.e., subsyndromal) depressive symptoms, elevated stressful life events, low life satisfaction, low self-esteem, elevated mental health treatment, and poor physical health. It is important to note that the above-mentioned impairments were detectable even in participants who remained free of depression recurrence in young adulthood. (pp. 548–549)

How would an episode of depression from which the adolescent recovers have such a wide-ranging impact on subsequent development? Apparently, the adolescent loses developmental ground during the depression and has difficulty catching up.[223] In addition, adolescent depression can be both persistent and recurrent, and even if the adolescent recovers from the severe episode, residual depressive symptoms can have a significant impact on functioning. Moreover, not uncommonly, the adolescent's depressive episode is embedded in a wide range of stressful circumstances and impairments in functioning, such as family disturbance and trauma coupled with adolescent substance abuse and poor educational achievement. Like depression, these circumstances and impairments tend to be persistent in their own right.[222]

In Lewinsohn and Essau's research,[221] about 60% of depressed adolescents were receiving some kind of mental health treatment (although only 9% were receiving medication); this figure could be seen as a glass half-empty or half-full. Plainly, given its far-ranging consequences, identifying depression in adolescents and finding adequate treatment is extremely important. Yet given the impact of depression on many areas of functioning, ameliorating depression may be only the first step. Teaching depressed adolescents more positive ways of thinking and effective methods of problem solving is one promising strategy to promote healthy development.[224]

RESILIENCE

There are enormous individual differences in response to stress, even to such severe adversities as being raised in a highly depriving orphanage.[225] What enables some individuals to cope more effectively than others? There's no simple answer to this key question, because we all follow mind bogglingly complex developmental pathways influenced by a combination of environmental risk and protective factors as they interact with our individual vulnerabilities and strengths over the course of our lifetime.

I hope I've made it amply clear that no single risk factor—a particular gene, prenatal stress, or postpartum depression—exerts a great impact over development. I use the stress pileup concept because serious developmental problems like psychiatric disorders typically result from multiple adversities that interact with each other. Most problematic are negative *chain reactions* in which the individual's response to stress creates additional stress.[225] For example, an adolescent living in poverty who becomes depressed in relation to her parents' violent fights might turn to drugs, drop out of school, and become pregnant, further fueling her stress and depression.

However, we must attend to wellness as much as illness; fortunately, positive chain reactions also occur when strengths promote successes that afford opportunities for additional growth and for coping with challenges. On this positive side of the ledger, developmental psychologists have long been keenly interested in *resilience*, which

> refers to an ongoing process of garnering resources that enables the individual to negotiate current issues adaptively and provides a foundation for dealing with subsequent challenges, as well as for recovering from reversals of fortune. Resilience doesn't *cause* children to do well in the face of adversity. Rather, resilience reflects the developmental process by which children acquire the ability to use both internal and external resources to achieve positive adaptation despite prior or concomitant adversity.[226] (pp. 249–250)

As you reflect on your early development, it's worthwhile considering the positives. Unsurprisingly, a number of characteristics have been shown to promote children's effective functioning:[226–229] ability to regulate emotional distress, high intelligence and academic competence, positive self-esteem and self-efficacy, easygoing temperament and ability to elicit positive regard and warmth from caregivers, and social competence. Children of depressed parents are likely to cope best if they can distance themselves from the parent's depression, for example, by involvement in school or extracurricular activities.[228] They also benefit from mentalizing—that is, understanding their parent's depression as an illness rather than blaming themselves for problems in the relationship.

Yet we cannot bank on children's strengths alone to promote resilience. Although conveying "unambiguous respect for what children bring to their life successes," reviewers of the research[227] literature concluded that "the overarching message is simply that [children] cannot make themselves enduringly resilient, remaining robust despite relentless onslaughts from the environment" (p. 532). Furthermore, these reviewers concluded that "in large measure, *resilient adaptation rests on good relationships*" (p. 544). More specifically, a secure attachment relationship with a sensitive and responsive caregiver early in life is the foundation for the development of resilience.[226,227] Yet many developmental stressors that impinge on children also impinge on their parents, rendering it difficult for the parents to provide sensitive care. Parents may be beleaguered by the stresses of poverty, psychiatric disorders, martial conflict, or the challenges of single parenting or stepparenting. Thus, to promote children's resilience, it is often essential to promote their *parents'* resilience, for example, through the support of family and friends, community resources, and mental health services.[227]

As much as we might wish to do so, we cannot change the past. Yet we can aspire to decrease our risk and vulnerability and increase our resilience. In the next part, I discuss stress at greater length. Being aware of the stressors will help you find ways of minimizing them and learning to cope with them more effectively, thereby diminishing your risk and enhancing your resilience.

Part III

PRECIPITANTS

Chapter 7

STRESSFUL EVENTS

We can regard the depressed state as symptomatic of the brain's response to sustained stress.[230] The preceding part of this book ("Development") reviewed various forms of early life stress as well as constitutional factors that render persons more vulnerable to depression in the face of stress. This chapter and the next consider stressors in adulthood that precipitate depression; this chapter focuses on external stress (observable events), whereas the next focuses on internal stress (emotional conflicts), although these two realms of stress are inextricable.

A caveat: extensive research indicates that a large majority of depressed persons—80% in one series of studies—experience a severe adverse life event prior to the onset of depression.[231] Thus I have ample reason to be paying so much attention to stress. Yet there remains a group of individuals whose depression seems to come out of the blue; indeed, depression sometimes comes into "the lives of people who are not only stress-free, but often leading advantaged and apparently attractive existences"[232] (p. 327). As a clinician who is accustomed to working with patients who have become depressed in the face of blatantly obvious stress, I found the idea of out-of-the-blue depression to be incomprehensible until my colleague, psychiatrist Lauren Marangell, opened my eyes to this possibility: the *cumulative stresses of ordinary life* might be enough to trigger a depressive episode in individuals with sufficient biological vulnerability. One source of such vulnerability is prior episodes of depression. Further neurobiological research will clarify the nature of this vulnerability. Yet we must also keep in mind the need to determine if general medical conditions are causing or contributing to the biological vulnerability—whether or not obvious current life stress is involved (see Chapter 10, "Related Disorders").

A forewarning: I wrote Chapter 3 ("Agency and Elbow Room") partly with the present chapter in mind, striving to head off self-blame when considering the possibility of your active role in the stress you experience. Granted, as I discuss shortly, much stress that leads to depression is utterly unavoidable. Yet much other stress that leads to depression—most notably, stress in interpersonal relationships—is partly self-generated, albeit often unknowingly and unintentionally. Accordingly, as foreshadowed in Chapter 3, this chapter brings to the fore the need to juggle two perspectives on depression: on the one hand, depression is an *illness*; on the other hand, depression both stems from and contributes to *problems in living*.[233] You have *some* leverage over problems in living, and you need to make use of it so as to recover and remain well. Here's where you're challenged to work on self-awareness for the sake of change without lapsing into self-blame.

This chapter covers a lot of ground. First, I summarize a particularly informative research project conducted in London on the relation between stress and episodes of depression in adult women; this research underscores the joint role of acute and chronic stress in depression. Then I discuss the contrast between unavoidable and self-generated stress, the point at which agency comes into play. Next I tie this chapter back into the developmental perspective, highlighting some research that shows how adulthood stressors can evolve from a cascade of stress beginning earlier in life. I then point out that traumatic stress in adulthood contributes to depression, just as it does in childhood. Looking forward, I consider the impact of ongoing stress on the course of depression. Lastly, I attend to the challenges in minimizing stress, bringing agency back into consideration.

STRESSFUL LIFE EVENTS AND DIFFICULTIES

British sociologist George Brown and his colleague, Tirril Harris,[93] conducted landmark research on the social conditions that contribute to episodes of clinical depression in adult women. This research provided a foundation for our understanding the relation of stress to depression, because these investigators employed intensive interviews to assess meticulously the major stressors impinging on women, and they carefully determined the timing of the stressors in relation to onsets of depressive episodes.

In the majority of cases, depressive episodes were preceded by *provoking agents:* stressful life events and ongoing difficulties. Yet despite the fact that depression typically was preceded by stress, only a minority of women exposed to stress became depressed. Thus the authors sought to determine the vulnerability factors that placed this minority of women at risk for developing depression in response to stress. Importantly, this research highlights the importance of the *meaning* of the stressful events to the individual.

PROVOKING AGENTS

Importantly, Brown and Harris distinguished two types of provoking agents: stressful life events and ongoing difficulties. *Stressful life events* primarily revolve around losses and disappointments, and they often involve a feeling of failure. As discussed in Chapter 5 ("Attachment"), loss and failure are the main themes of depression. Examples of losses include separations or the threat of separation, a life-threatening illness in an attachment figure, significant material loss, and being forced to change residence. Also significant is the loss of a cherished idea or disillusionment as, for example, when a woman learns of her husband's infidelity.

Most research on depression has focused exclusively on acute stressors—discrete events, like the loss of a job or the breakup of a relationship. Yet ongoing or chronic stress may be even more important.[100] Wisely, Brown and Harris also investigated the role of ongoing *difficulties* in generating depression; these problems are associated with unremitting stress. Such difficulties include problems at work, inadequate housing, ill health, difficulties with children, marital conflict, and financial hardships. The researchers used a stringent criterion: to be considered severe, the difficulties must have gone on for at least 2 years; in fact, the severe difficulties they observed averaged 4 years' duration.

Both life events and difficulties were extremely common in the period preceding depressive episodes. The great majority of stressors took place within the 6-month period preceding the episode, and more than half took place in the several-week period preceding the episode. Consistent with the concept of stress pileup, the combination of ongoing difficulties and life events often precipitated depression, and life events directly linked to ongoing difficulties exerted the most powerful effect.[234] For example, ongoing marital conflict (difficulty) that eventuated in a separation (event) would be a powerful provoking agent. Naturally, stressful events related to major life goals and commitments, such as the loss of a treasured job or the breakup of a love relationship, were especially significant provoking agents.

MEANING

Brown and Harris[93] painstakingly assessed the severity of stressful life events and difficulties from an objective perspective; that is, they evaluated their likely impact on the average person. Yet they insisted that the *subjective* impact of stress—its meaning to the person and thereby its emotional impact—determines the risk of depression. Brown and colleagues[235] identified two prominent subjective responses to stress: feelings of humiliation and of entrapment. Humiliating events were associated with a feeling of being devalued, for example, being rejected or degraded by one's husband or children. Entrapment involved irresolvable ongoing difficulties including relationship conflicts, housing problems, employment problems, or health concerns. In general, only losses that involved humiliation and entrapment led to depression. There was one notable exception: death of a loved one; such a loss, by nature, has a significant long-term adverse impact.

The researchers proposed that depression stems from stressful events and difficulties that lead the person to feel hopeless. Humiliation, entrapment, and loss through death are particularly likely to lead to feelings of being defeated, powerless, and helpless; feeling defeated, the depressed person believes there is no escape and is unable to imagine a way forward. A sense of failure, low self-esteem, and lack of self-confidence also play an important role in the transition from stress to a sense of defeat and hopelessness. On the other hand, a close and supportive relationship can be a buffer for a person with low self-esteem. Such a relationship fosters hope because it offers the prospect of additional resources that will help the person cope; when you don't feel up to the challenge, having help makes all the difference.

In many respects, Brown's work supports psychiatrist Aaron Beck and colleagues'[236] cognitive theory of depression, because the individual's *interpretation* of stressful events is the key factor (see Chapter 12, "Flexible Thinking"). Like Brown, Beck and colleagues identified generalized hopelessness as a significant factor in depression. Yet they emphasized that depression stems from *distorted* interpretations of stressful situations, whereas Brown[237] challenged this view: "Psychological research on depression has tended to place particular emphasis on the inappropriateness of negative cognitive sets. By contrast, I would emphasize their appropriateness and how such cognitions may be fully understandable in light of the person's current milieu" (p. 367). No doubt distorted depressive thinking can make a bad situation seem worse, but Brown's research makes plain the level of real hardship that depressed persons typically face.

STRESS GENERATION

Throughout this book I have been emphasizing how depression stems from a pileup of stress rather than from a discrete stressful event. Moreover, as I emphasize throughout Part V ("Coping With Catch-22"), being depressed creates additional life stress. Thus researchers studying the relationship between life stress and depression have been challenged to sort out the chicken-and-egg problem: which came first, the stress or the depression?[238] A further complication: not only depression but also difficulties in maintaining stable relationships can contribute to what psychologist Constance Hammen[100,239] calls *stress generation:* playing an active—if unwitting—role in creating stress in your life, the problem I foreshadowed in Chapter 3 ("Agency and Elbow Room"). The chicken-and-egg problem arises because depression contributes to relationship conflicts and results from them; depression can be both cause and effect.

To disentangle cause and effect, a number of researchers have taken pains to distinguish between *fateful* stressors—those completely independent of the person's actions or beyond the person's control—and nonfateful stressors, what I call partly *self-generated stress,* that is, stressful events in which the person's actions and difficulties played a role. We must consider these latter stressors *partly* self-generated, because they always involve external factors (typically other persons), and the degree to which each individual plays a role will vary greatly from one event to another. This distinction between partly self-generated and fateful events has a great deal of practical importance because, to the extent that you can identify any active role you've played in the stress in your life, you have some leverage in reducing it. Agency comes in here, and as I emphasized in Chapter 3 ("Agency and Elbow Room"), we must aim for compassionate understanding rather than blame, self-condemnation, self-punishment, and further suffering.

We start with fateful stress. Uninfluenced by the characteristics or actions of the individual, fateful events can be regarded as bad luck. For example, one group of researchers identified a wide range of fateful events preceding major depressive episodes, carefully ensuring that the depressed person had played no part in their occurrence.[240] These events included loss of a family member or close friend, losing the home, being assaulted, employment problems, and inability to obtain treatment for illness and injury. They also determined the degree of disruptiveness of the events, that is, the extent to which the events had life-changing effects. The results were clear: the odds that persons with depression had experienced a disruptive fateful event were 2.5 times greater for depressed persons when compared with nondepressed persons in the community. Numerous other studies have confirmed the role of fateful stressors in depression.[231]

Psychiatrist Kenneth Kendler and colleagues systematically compared the contribution of fateful and partly self-generated stressful events to the onset of depression in women.[241] They focused on stressful events occurring within 1 month of the depressive episode, and they carefully determined the extent of long-term threat posed by each of the stressors. Both fateful and partly self-generated stressful events increased the risk of depression. Yet partly self-generated events were more problematic in three ways: first, they were slightly more frequent than fateful events; second, they were generally more severe in the sense of having more threatening long-term implications; and third, even apart from the level of threat, partly self-generated events were more likely than fateful events to precipitate an episode of depression.

As I have emphasized, the concept of stress generation applies primarily to interpersonal relationships,[100] and the developmental challenges covered in Chapters 5 ("Attachment") and 6 ("Childhood Adversity") predispose individuals to these potentially self-perpetuating cycles of stress and depression. A prime example: early loss and subsequent trauma can lead to a pattern of insecure attachment that endures into adolescence and adulthood and then contributes to conflict in intimate relationships. The risks are glaring: for both men and women, being in an unhappy marriage is associated with a 25-fold increase in risk for depression, although interpreting this finding poses the chicken-and-egg problem, namely, that the marital problems can contribute to depression and vice versa.[242] One study designed to disentangle the chicken from the egg assessed spouses who were *not* depressed at the initial interview and then followed up with them 1 year later.[243] This study found that dissatisfaction in the marriage rendered spouses three times more likely to develop a depressive episode, and nearly 30% of the episodes were related to marital dissatisfaction. To reiterate, as described in Chapter 5 ("Attachment"), stressful events and personality interact; persons who are more dependent are more likely to become depressed in response to problems in relationships.[244] Accordingly, working on problems in attachment relationships can be crucial in diminishing vulnerability to depression (see Chapter 13, "Supportive Relationships").

TRAUMATIC STRESS

As I described in Chapter 6 ("Childhood Adversity), childhood trauma in attachment relationships—maltreatment—is a significant factor in creating vulnerability to depression in adulthood. Here I merely want to draw attention to the fact that traumatic stress in adulthood also plays a significant role in depression.[144]

To reiterate, we can define *trauma* as the lasting negative effects of going through extremely stressful events.[95] Traumatic stressors entail a significant threat to your physical or psychological integrity and are experienced with a feeling of terror or helplessness.[8] Some traumatic events, such as tornadoes and car wrecks, are impersonal in origin. Other traumatic events are interpersonal in origin and involve some degree of culpability, ranging from recklessness (e.g., in accidents stemming from drunk driving) to deliberate intent to harm (e.g., assaults). Interpersonal stress can be particularly traumatic, because it engenders distrust, which is especially true in attachment trauma: being frightened, hurt, and betrayed in a relationship where you are depending on the other person for security can render closeness dangerous, and then you lose the foundation for healing—secure attachments.

A short list of potentially traumatic stressors includes natural disasters, accidents, combat, criminal assaults, rape, child abuse, witnessing violence, battering relationships, elder abuse, terrorism, and torture. Many of these potentially traumatic stressors—combat and abusive relationships—involve a combination of repeated stressful events and chronic stress, the worst of stress pileup. All such experiences can lead to posttraumatic stress disorder (PTSD), itself an extremely stressful illness (see Chapter 10, "Related Disorders"). With or without PTSD, depression is one of the main traumatic effects of these various forms of extreme stress.[95]

DEVELOPMENTAL CASCADES AND VULNERABILITY

As this chapter illustrates, stressful events play a prominent role in triggering episodes of depression. Brown's pioneering research highlighted the importance of taking the individual's immediate life context into account in evaluating the meaning of stress. Yet throughout this book, I have promoted the theme that we must consider the *whole life context* in vulnerability to depression. Exposure to stress is ubiquitous; many depressed patients point out that other persons they know seem to have experienced similar stressors but have not become depressed. They ask: why me?

Brown and his colleagues investigated factors that contribute to susceptibility to depression. Only about 20% of women exposed to severe life events and difficulties became depressed in their aftermath. What distinguished this vulnerable minority? The initial study[93] identified four risk factors: loss of mother prior to age 11, caring for a child under the age of 6, having three children under the age of 14 at home, and lacking an intimate confiding relationship. Having a job outside the home served as a protective factor, buffering the impact of stress. Notably, low self-esteem also proved to be a significant vulnerability factor, and self-esteem was linked to all four risk factors. Brown was especially interested in social conditions, and he found a strong relation between social class and depression: working-class women were more likely to have depression than middle-class women—not because social class per se relates to depression but rather because lower social class is associated with higher levels of adversity and stress.[232]

Subsequent research clarified the contributions of these various factors to vulnerability. Consistent with Bowlby's clinical work (see Chapter 6, "Childhood Adversity"), Brown found that loss of the mother early in life conferred vulnerability only when this loss was followed by lack of adequate care—either neglect or parental rejection.[245] Early inadequate care also contributes to low self-esteem, as does conflict in current close relationships. In turn, difficulties in close relationships are part and parcel of the context of another vulnerability factor: lack of social support. Having the support of a close relationship in the midst of a stressful crisis is a powerful buffering factor with respect to depression, and it is support in the trenches of the crisis that counts.[246] Women who became depressed were more likely either to lack support throughout the year preceding the depression or to have been *let down*: a previously supportive partner in whom the woman could confide her troubles—often a husband—did not provide support during the crisis, either because the crisis revolved around the relationship or because the partner was unsupportive (e.g., minimizing the significance of the problem or not wanting to deal with it). Single women who had a close relationship—typically with another woman, often a sister or mother—were far less likely to feel let down when seeking support in a crisis.

Extrapolating from Brown's research, we can easily imagine innumerable cascades into depression. For example, a girl who loses her mother in childhood is neglected in subsequent care. She develops low self-esteem and experiences significant conflicts in her relationships. Lacking close friends and not feeling worthy of love, she marries a troubled man who treats her poorly. She quickly becomes pregnant and soon is faced with the responsibility of caring for young children. Owing to marital conflict, her husband is unsupportive when she is faced with the crises of her father's dying and her youngest child's near-fatal injury. Feeling let down, she becomes clinically depressed.

Given the mind-boggling complexity of factors involved and all their possible combinations, researchers face a daunting task in trying to discover common patterns in the development of depression. Yet psychiatrist Kenneth Kendler and his colleagues took on this monumental challenge in their study of adult female twins.[247] Brace yourself for a pileup of information, which I present here only to underscore the developmental complexity of vulnerability to depression. Based on prior research, these researchers identified 18 factors that can play a role in susceptibility to depression, and they categorized these factors into five developmental periods:

1. Four *childhood* factors included genetic risk, disturbed family environment, childhood sexual abuse, and childhood parental loss;
2. Four *early adolescent* factors included neuroticism (proneness to emotional distress), low self-esteem, anxiety disorder, and conduct disorder (antisocial behavior);
3. Four *late adolescent* factors included low education, trauma, low social support, and substance abuse;
4. Two *adulthood* factors were history of divorce and past history of major depression; and
5. Four factors in the *preceding year* included marital problems, ongoing difficulties, fateful events, and partly self-generated stressful events.

As the sheer diversity of potential developmental factors implies, there are innumerable potential developmental pathways to depression, with genetic susceptibility, personality factors, and life experiences intertwined throughout. Employing statistical analyses to discern the forest from the trees, Kendler and colleagues identified three broad *developmental pathways* to depression, all intertwined with genetic contributions:

1. A genetic risk for depression was followed by early adolescent history of neuroticism, low self-esteem, and anxiety disorder; these in turn were followed by a history of major depression prior to the current episode.
2. Early adolescent conduct disorder and late adolescent substance abuse was followed by a previous history of depression, all of which culminated in the current episode.
3. Early childhood factors (disturbed family environment, sexual abuse, and parental loss) were followed by late adolescent factors (low education, trauma, and low social support) and adulthood factors (history of divorce and past history of depression), along with all forms of stress in the preceding year, to culminate in the current episode.

STRESS AND THE COURSE OF DEPRESSION

Thus far, I have focused on the role of stressful life events in precipitating episodes of depression. Yet we can continue the developmental perspective beyond the first episode to consider the role of ongoing stress in the subsequent course of depression. As you might imagine, ongoing stress plays a role not only in the speed of recovery but also in the generation of recurrent episodes.

RECOVERY

Not surprisingly, ongoing difficulties and stressful life events that occur during a depressive episode are likely to prolong the duration of the episode and to interfere with response to treatment, including treatment with antidepressant medication.[231,232] Conversely, Brown's research suggested that resolution of ongoing difficulties is associated with more rapid recovery.[248] In addition, Brown observed that a *fresh start*—a new relationship, new housing, a good employment opportunity—often heralded recovery. Sometimes fresh starts are the flip side of stressful events, such as when the breakup of a bad relationship provides opportunities for a better relationship. In addition, exposure to a potentially traumatic event—a brush with death—sometimes leads to a reassessment of priorities, greater agency in taking charge of one's life, and an improvement in mood.

RECURRENCE

Just as they play a role in the initial episode of depression, stressful events can play a role in recurrences—new episodes. Yet clinicians and researchers have taken a keen interest in a critical question: does stress play as significant a role in recurrences as it does in the initial episode? Psychiatrist Robert Post[249,250] presented extensive evidence that stressful life events play a greater role in initial episodes of depression than in recurrences of illness. He explained this observation on the basis of *sensitization*, namely, increased reactivity to stress as a consequence of repeated exposures to stress. Here we can make an analogy to bee stings: persons who are allergic can be sensitized such that each new sting has a more adverse effect than the last one. Important to the sensitization process is that depressive episodes are stressors in themselves. Thus Post proposed that, as part of the sensitization process, *episodes beget episodes*. The possibility that each episode confers increasing vulnerability to additional episodes underscores the need for vigorous intervention and exercise of agency in promoting recovery and wellness.

Post's concern about sensitization was a rallying cry for researchers, and the complex relation of stress to recurrence remains an active area of research.[100,232] For example, Brown and Harris[251] found that stress precipitated both initial episodes and recurrences, although there was a group of persons with particularly severe depression whose recurrences—not their initial episode—appeared *not* to be precipitated by stress. Subsequent research on the relative contribution of stress to early and late episodes had yielded contradictory results,[100] although some of the better designed studies confirm Post's concern that recurrences are less likely to be associated with obvious stressful events.[231]

Two studies of adolescent depression illustrate the potential role of stress in recurrences and underscore the adverse role of depression in development. The Oregon Adolescent Depression Project[252] found evidence for stress pileup in relation to initial episodes: adolescents experiencing three or more stressful events in a 1-year period were five times more likely to become depressed than those who experienced fewer events. Yet the number of stressful events experienced did *not* play a role in recurrences. Another study followed adolescent women over a 5-year period from the time of their high school graduation.[67] Alarmingly, 70% of participants who entered the study with a history of depression experienced a recurrence in the 5 years after high school graduation. This study found that episodic stress was a potent trigger for both onsets and recurrences of depression, whereas chronic stress triggered onsets but not recurrences. This study also showed that depressed adolescents go on to experience high levels of stress (partly self-generated) in interpersonal relationships, leaving them vulnerable to further episodes.

The complexity of research results is daunting, but we have ample reason to be concerned that stress and depression enter into self-perpetuating vicious circles such that your vulnerability to further episodes can increase over your lifetime—beginning in adolescence or earlier. To bring in further complexity, the relation between stress and recurrence of depression is affected by genetic risk. Kendler and colleagues'[253] study of adult women revealed two distinct pathways through which an individual could become sensitized. The *environmental* pathway pertains to persons with low genetic susceptibility: stressful life events play a greater role in triggering earlier episodes and a diminishing role in triggering later episodes (suggesting sensitization to stress over time). The *genetic* pathway, in contrast, pertains to persons with high genetic susceptibility: stressful life events play a lesser role in triggering both initial and subsequent episodes (suggesting a genetic sensitivity).

MINIMIZING STRESS

The prominent role of stress in depression poses two challenges: minimizing avoidable stress and learning to cope more effectively with stress of any origin. To recapitulate, a significant amount of stress that plays a role in triggering depression is fateful—unavoidable and out of your control. However, a prominent source of stress that contributes to depression is partly self-generated; this stress is avoidable—*in principle*, although not necessarily easily in practice. You can generate stress in your life in many ways, for example, by taking on more tasks, responsibilities, or commitments than you can manage; by engaging in risky activities; by abusing drugs or alcohol; or by neglecting your health—including failing to get enough sleep—and becoming unduly fatigued or ill. All these forms of stress generation attest to the importance of agency in recovering from depression and remaining well: you can exert some leverage here by making some lifestyle changes. I don't mean to imply that changing is easy; it can be extremely difficult, and it's a long-term project.

Yet lifestyle changes aren't the only daunting challenge. Problems in interpersonal relationships are the most significant source of partly self-generated stress that leads to depression.[100] Herein lies the greatest challenge in minimizing stress: developing more secure attachment relationships. However, identifying your participation in the creation and maintenance of stressful relationships is a crucial first step. For example, you might incautiously get into relationships too quickly and too deeply, thereby becoming attached to persons who are unreliable or who don't treat you well. Or you might pick persons whose troubles dovetail with your own, believing that you don't deserve better or imagining that you can reform these troubled souls. Or you might perpetuate patterns of insecure attachment from earlier relationships: an avoidant pattern will cause strain because it creates emotional distance; an ambivalent pattern will create friction and instability in the relationship.

More concretely, you might behave in various ways that fuel conflict: being critical, asking for reassurance only to reject it, being possessive or jealous, starting arguments, stonewalling, sulking, withholding affection, failing to ask directly for what you want and resenting not getting it, not following through with agreements, not communicating often enough or clearly enough, and so forth. All these are common human failings but, in sufficient measure, they can generate enough stress in relationships to create depression in predisposed persons. These problematic relationship patterns can be ingrained and hard to change—but you *can* change them with effort and with help, for example, with interpersonal psychotherapy and marital therapy (see Chapter 13, "Supportive Relationships").

This chapter has focused on external stress—stressful events and difficulties that can be observed by others, described objectively, and carefully researched. Yet I have also emphasized that, ultimately, it's the subjective experience of these events—what they mean to you—that creates the stress. In the next chapter, I focus on internal stress—the unobservable stress that goes on in the realm of your mind. Here too, we are dealing with partly self-generated stress, and here too, there's hope: you have some potential leverage over it.

Chapter 8

INTERNAL STRESS

We can describe stressful life events objectively, from the outside: your spouse died, you were divorced, you lost your job, or you were assaulted in a parking lot. Yet it's your *subjective emotional experience* of such events that renders them stressful, and your emotional response will be determined by what the events *mean* to you—how you believe they reflect upon you and what you anticipate their long-term consequences will be. In the face of extreme or relentless stress, you might come to feel humiliated, trapped, or hopeless. You might feel beleaguered by many painful emotions: anxiety, fear, shame, guilt, anger, and despair, to name a few. Whatever their source, it's these prolonged and painful emotional states that lead to depression—itself a prolonged and painful internal emotional state.

This chapter focuses on three forms of internal emotional stress that are common in depression: perfectionism; guilt and shame; and anger and resentment. The chapter concludes by linking all these forms of emotional stress to your relationship with yourself. As with some stressful life events discussed in the last chapter, the emotional stress I discuss here is self-generated, rooted in internal conflicts. If you can stay out of self-blame, there's a hopeful message here: you have *some* leverage over this internal stress. Yet I advocate an attitude of humility here: I don't believe you can fully control your emotions, but I do believe that you can influence them somewhat for the better.

PERFECTIONISM

Perfectionism is a prime example of self-generated stress that can provide continual mental fuel to stress pileup. Being perfectionistic, you are preoccupied with evaluation, criticism, and making mistakes.[254] You continually put yourself on trial, subject to disapproval from within and without. Perfectionism spawns an array of distressing emotions, including anxiety, frustration, shame, resentment, and depression. Perfectionism not only escalates negative emotion but also undermines positive emotion: being perfectionistic, you deprive yourself of pleasure and satisfaction by focusing all your attention on how you've fallen short rather than enjoying whatever success you've achieved. No matter how well you do, no matter how successful you may be, you can continue to raise the bar, fall short of your high aspirations, and feel like a failure. There's a vicious circle here too: to compensate for feelings of failure, you set your sights on increasingly unrealistic aspirations, only raising the likelihood of additional failure.[255]

Reading this, you might rightly object: perfectionism isn't all bad. *Positive perfectionism* involves holding high standards; it is associated with a high need for achievement and can contribute to healthy competitiveness.[256] Such perfectionism reflects *conscientiousness*, an adaptive personality trait. Positive perfectionism can be associated with high performance and a sense of personal satisfaction. Yet perfectionism can become oppressive when high standards are coupled with self-doubt, a pervasive sense of inadequacy, and unstable self-esteem. When you pursue perfection for the sake of overcoming feelings of insecurity or inferiority, you're likely to wind up in the vicious circle of a losing battle that fuels anxiety and depression.

TYPES OF PERFECTIONISM

Perfectionism covers a lot of territory, and different aspects of perfectionism lead to different problems. You might be perfectionistic in one or more different domains of life, for example, in work, school, writing, speaking, or physical appearance. Plainly, the more domains in which you seek perfection, the greater the emotional pressure and strain will be.

In addition, researchers distinguish among three types of perfectionism.[256] *Self-oriented* perfectionism involves *setting high standards for yourself*. When these standards are reasonable, self-oriented perfectionism is positive and adaptive. When your standards are unreasonable, self-oriented perfectionism will lead to self-criticism, anxiety, and feelings of inadequacy. *Socially prescribed* perfectionism involves believing unrealistically that *other persons are demanding perfection* from you; your parents, teachers, boss, or spouse expects you to do the impossible. Socially prescribed perfectionism leaves you vulnerable to feeling criticized and leads to a range of negative emotions that include not only anxiety but also resentment. Because it revolves around feeling negatively evaluated by others, socially prescribed perfectionism is particularly likely to be associated with painful feelings of guilt and shame. Socially prescribed perfectionism also contributes to stress in interpersonal relationships, owing to unrealistic beliefs about others' demands, expectations, and criticisms. Your anxiety and resentment are liable to lead to conflict in these relationships as well as contributing to distance and feelings of alienation. *Other-oriented* perfectionism involves your *demanding perfection from others*, for example, your children, students, employees, or spouse. Other-oriented perfectionism also contributes to interpersonal stress and conflict by alienating others, evoking feelings of anxiety, shame, and resentment in them—oppressing and depressing them as well.

Although they can be distinguished from one another, all three forms of perfectionism can feed into each other. For example, you might project your own perfectionism onto others and believe unrealistically that they are equally demanding of you. Alternatively, you may hold others to the same unrealistic standards you have for yourself. Accordingly, although it takes various forms, perfectionism potentially contributes to stress pileup in three ways: perfectionism creates internal emotional pressure, generates conflict in interpersonal relationships, and undermines social support. Moreover, perfectionism goes hand in hand with the kind of stressful lifestyle that compounds stress pileup, for example, being a workaholic.

DEVELOPMENT OF PERFECTIONISM

There are many developmental pathways to perfectionism, and it's important to consider not only the environmental contribution (e.g., in the family) but also the part the child plays.[257] On the environmental side, a child might identify with perfectionistic parents (self-oriented perfectionism), or a child may be driven toward socially prescribed perfectionism by other-oriented perfectionistic parents. Common in the family background of perfectionists are a high level parental demands coupled with a low level of warmth and affection.

Thus early attachment relationships can play a significant role in the development of perfectionism. As described in Chapter 5 ("Attachment"), psychologist Sidney Blatt[159] distinguished two major types of depression: dependent and self-critical. Maladaptive perfectionism exemplifies self-critical depression at the extreme. The harsh and punitive childhood relationships are internalized; the externally driven and pressured child becomes internally driven and pressured, a pattern that may continue into adulthood. As noted in Chapter 5, the feeling of rejection in childhood leads to an avoidant attachment style: relying on yourself rather than risking further rejection. Avoidance can continue into adulthood, and the sense of interpersonal isolation is further disrupted by the perfectionist's critical judgments of others.

By providing structure and organization, perfectionism also can be a child's way of coping with a chaotic and neglectful family environment. In addition, a child who is subject to parental abuse may cope by trying to be the perfect child, or the child may try to avoid the fate of an abused sibling by striving for perfection. Of course, the family isn't the only crucible for perfectionism; peers, teachers, and social norms also contribute. For example, current social conditions are notorious for providing pressure to have a perfect body, and eating disorders are one manifestation of perfectionism.[258]

Yet the environmental contribution to perfectionism is only one side of the coin. Some children may respond to perfectionistic parental models or demands for perfection by becoming rebellious—doing the opposite of what is expected. On the other hand, children with a conscientious temperament and an inclination to persist at problem solving are more likely to become perfectionistic. In addition, children with a fearful temperament are also more vulnerable to becoming perfectionistic; their fearfulness may be evident in concern about making mistakes, intolerance of criticism, sensitivity to punishment, and a high need for approval. Finally, having some area of ability or talent—for example in school, sports, or music—will also play a part by providing an avenue for perfectionistic strivings.

TAMING PERFECTIONISM

Cognitive-behavioral therapy, which addresses maladaptive beliefs (see Chapter 12, "Flexible Thinking"), has been applied to overcoming perfectionism; the book *When Perfect Isn't Good Enough*[259] provides systematic strategies. You need to lower your aspirations, which will entail reconsidering your goals, priorities, and values. To put it bluntly, you need to give up your grandiosity—being perfect—for humility—being human. However, lowering your expectations and giving up lofty goals may entail painful losses, and you will need to learn to tolerate the anxiety associated with falling short of perfectionistic standards, so that your anxiety can diminish over time. Some patients in my educational group advocated an end-run strategy: they find areas of activity in which they can set aside performance expectations—a time out from critical evaluation—to be a good way to start circumventing perfectionism. New hobbies or artistic pursuits are examples—provided you don't turn them into contests. By trying this end run, you might find that the feeling of freedom from criticism (whether from yourself or of others) is rewarding and can be generalized to other areas of your life.

I don't want to imply that perfectionism is easily given up. On the contrary, problems in early attachment relationships lead to powerful internal conflicts that are difficult to modify—especially when perfectionism alienates the person from close and affectionate relationships that might moderate the self-criticism. Hence catch-22: perfectionism has been found to be an obstacle to psychotherapy.[256] For starters, perfectionists are relatively unlikely to seek therapy, feeling as if they should be able to solve their problems without help. In addition, each form of perfectionism can contribute to problems in the therapeutic relationship, just as it may in other relationships. A self-oriented perfectionist may feel a need to be the perfect patient. A socially prescribed perfectionist may feel that the therapist is critical and demanding of unattainable perfection. An other-oriented perfectionist may demand perfection from the therapist and feel frustrated by the therapist's shortcomings.

Blatt and his colleagues[260] found that perfectionistic patients responded relatively poorly to brief treatment with psychotherapy and medication. Perfectionists had more difficulty forming a therapeutic alliance, that is, a trusting and productive working relationship with the therapist.[261] Yet perfectionists benefited greatly from more intensive long-term insight-oriented psychotherapy. This more intensive process allowed trust to develop gradually, enabling the patient to express and explore critical views of the self, others, and the therapist. Bringing the criticism out into the open set the stage for acceptance—by the therapist and oneself—to begin taking hold. Hence, given ample time to grapple with relationship conflicts, perfectionists can make good use of their conscientiousness and drive to derive substantial benefit from psychotherapy.

GUILT AND SHAME

Whether or not they are perfectionistic, depressed persons almost invariably struggle with feelings of failure. With a sense of failure come the emotions of guilt and shame; both are potentially painful and enduring. Both feelings also are embedded in relationships with others: they're *self-conscious emotions* that begin developing in the second year of life when children become both self-aware and sensitive to others' reactions to them.[262]

GUILT FEELINGS

Guilt feelings stem from having done harm to others, and guilt feelings are most painful when we feel we have done grievous harm to those we love. When we've done harm, guilt feelings can be adaptive: they can prompt us to right wrongs and to avoid repeating them. Yet severely depressed persons often feel unreasonably guilty in the sense that their guilt *feelings* far exceed whatever harm they have actually done to others. Feelings of guilt are so prominent in depression that they are included among the diagnostic criteria.[8] Of course, to the extent that we have actually done harm to others, we all must find ways of living with some guilt feelings.

Adding insult to injury, depression itself tends to escalate guilt feelings. For example, if you're prone to depressive rumination, you're likely to go over and over the events you feel guilty about. In addition, you might feel guilty owing to the *effects* of your depression. You might feel that you've let others down by virtue of being unable to carry on with your usual responsibilities. You might recognize that others are burdened by your depression—at the very least worried and perhaps resentful as well. Bear in mind that, although it's likely that others will be burdened, it's also likely that you're exaggerating the extent of that burden as a result of your depressed mood.

SHAME

In contrast to guilt feelings, which focus on the effects of specific actions, shame relates to your basic sense of self-worth. At worst, shame can reflect a pervasive feeling of defectiveness, a sense that your core self is bad. As contemporary philosopher Martha Nussbaum[263] put it, shame can "sully the entirety of one's being" (p. 216). Shame comes with feeling damaged, worthless, and inadequate. Of course, guilt and shame can overlap; when you've hurt or let someone down and you feel guilty, you might also feel ashamed, attributing the hurtful actions to your core badness.

Like guilt feelings, shame can gnaw on you as well as come in painful bursts. Shame can be an excruciatingly painful emotion—searing in intensity. Both shame and guilt feelings are stressful and wearing, and shame contributes to depression not only because of the emotional strain but also because it's isolating.[264] The basic impulse associated with shame is withdrawal—covering your face and hiding.[265]

Shame plays an especially powerful role for persons who show the self-critical pattern of depression.[266] As we have seen in the context of perfectionism, self-critical individuals not only view themselves as deficient and unworthy; they also view persons with whom they interact as critical, demanding, and disapproving. In effect, shame comes from the inside and the outside, and it goes hand in hand with feeling alienated, an outcast. In contrast, persons showing the dependent pattern of depression are somewhat protected from alienation and shame because they are more likely to reach out for support.

OVERCOMING FEELINGS OF GUILT AND SHAME

Frank, a man in his early 60s who had reached the height of success in his career as an attorney, suddenly quit work in the firm and plummeted into a profound depression. He spent weeks in bed, being completely unable to function. His depressive retreat mystified others who had viewed him as exceptionally competent, as well as kind and caring. In his depressed state, his view of himself was completely at odds with that of others; he felt utterly incompetent, useless, and worthless. Although he had amassed considerable financial resources as well as acquiring exceptional professional skills, he was convinced that he would no longer be able to support his wife and two daughters—indeed, that his family would ultimately wind up living in poverty. He felt extremely guilty that he had let his family down, and he could not stop ruminating about all the dire consequences of his inability to work, continually adding fuel to his guilt feelings.

Throughout Frank's career, outward appearances and internal experience had been at variance. Although he was very talented, Frank had pushed himself hard and had chronic anxiety that he successfully concealed from others. In the months preceding his depressive episode, changes at the firm escalated his anxiety. He had had a longstanding aversion to computers, and a new computerized billing system was implemented that he could not avoid learning. He felt unable to ask for help and thereby trapped. These new demands came on top of changes in the business climate, because the firm was threatened by new competition. When he got wind of plans to downsize, he was convinced he would be the first to be let go—notwithstanding that he was one of the most experienced, highly valued, and well-liked attorneys in the firm.

This was Frank's first experience with depression, and he had never had any form of psychiatric treatment before. Although he had struggled with anxiety for a long time, he had never considered the basis for it. His depression forced him to explore the psychological basis of his feelings for the first time. Plainly, he fit the prototype of self-critical depression, which had origins in his childhood. His mother was the dominant figure in the household; she was not unaffectionate, but she had extremely high expectations for him as the oldest son. She was disappointed that her husband was not more successful, and she resented the financial strains this imposed. She was determined that her oldest son would not follow in his father's footsteps, a determination that was abetted by Frank's obvious abilities. He became the star of the family, but not without internal strain.

Having achieved the pinnacle of success, Frank foresaw that he was about to fall off the pedestal, given the changes at the firm. He was certain that his income would plummet; he felt trapped, humiliated, and hopeless. Even though he had stable and loving relationships with his wife and daughters, he withdrew into virtually total isolation, taking to bed. Being unable to function, he had no recourse but to seek hospital treatment. Hospitalization only added to his guilt feelings, because it further eroded the family finances. It also added to his feelings of shame and humiliation; he could not tolerate the feeling of being a "mental patient." Moreover, he had little hope that the treatment would help.

Feeling ashamed and inadequate, Frank found the hospital setting to be extremely challenging. He was expected not only to become socially engaged with other patients in a range of informal activities but also to attend a number of group treatment meetings. In psychotherapy, he was expected to talk about his painful feelings. He wanted to retreat and to hide. Quiet as he was, patients and staff members found him to have an appealing manner, and they reached out to him. As he became more engaged, his mood gradually improved. He began to see that his fears of poverty were unfounded; he could retire if need be, although not without financial sacrifice. To his own amazement, he occasionally began imagining that he could return to work. He began to consider options.

The act of seeking treatment played a significant role in Frank's recovery. He had been severely handicapped by his inability to reach out for practical help and emotional support. He came to feel trapped and doomed. He could see how he had been driving himself relentlessly and that he could find a middle ground—not needing to make a fortune. He also could consider reaching out to colleagues for help rather than floundering alone with respect to the new computer technology. As his mood improved, he became keenly aware of how his depression had skewed his view of reality and his view of himself.

Guilt feelings and shame—feeling blameworthy and worthless—seem to come with the territory of depression. These feelings are often fueled by unreasonable views of the self, and they drive the depressed person away from potential sources of support. The isolation from others promotes rumination, and the depressive spiral only deepens. Somehow, the process of painful self-denigration must be reversed. The first step—perhaps the hardest—is going against the grain and reaching out to others. Isolation is a depressant; social engagement is an antidepressant. As Frank's experience exemplifies, talking with others who can be more objective—and feeling accepted by them—can begin reversing the feelings of guilt and shame.

ANGER AND RESENTMENT

As a burst of emotion, anger is adaptive and often essential. With its cousin, fear, anger is part of the fight-or-flight response that evolved for the sake of self-protection. Natural anger can be a source of energy and power, for example, motivating you to stand up for yourself or to engage in a needed confrontation. Thus, effectively expressed—which is not easy to do—anger can play a helpful role in resolving interpersonal conflicts. Of course, at extremely intense levels, such as in explosive rage, anger can be highly damaging to relationships.

Here I focus on two ways in which anger relates to depression: when it's self-directed and when it's stifled and turns into chronic resentment.

SELF-DIRECTED ANGER

You might have heard the idea that depression is anger turned inward. This is blatantly true, for example, when you're angry with yourself and berate yourself. Anger turned inward is a common reflection of self-critical depression, and we have seen that self-critical depression can have origins in early attachment relationships. Freud's insights about depression have been pivotal in this understanding.

Freud asked a simple question with a complex answer: in the wake of a loss, why are some persons able to mourn successfully, whereas others develop prolonged depression?[267] He took his cue from the central difference between normal grief and melancholia; in the latter, the person reacts to the loss with violent self-reproach. Freud believed that the question's answer lay in the *ambivalence* of the relationship—love intermingled with hate—although the hate was often unconscious, out of awareness. Reproaches against the person who was loved and lost turn into *self*-reproaches. The tendency to identify with the person you've lost plays an important role: you hang on to the relationship by incorporating the person into your self, but then your anger becomes self-directed. Freud also observed that this process of anger directed toward the self is not limited to loss through death but also may follow a wide range of situations in which you have felt hurt, wounded, let down, disappointed, or neglected. Blatt's[159] concept of self-critical depression is a further development of Freud's insight about the relationship of ambivalent attachments to depression.

RESENTMENT

It is the chronic stress imposed by enduring emotions like anxiety, guilt feelings, and shame that is most likely to contribute to the wear and tear that eventuates in depression. I am convinced that resentment—as an enduring source of strain from chronic anger—plays a paramount role in depression for many persons. I think of resentment as stifled anger; both the resentment and the stifling impose chronic strain. As I described in Chapter 5 ("Attachment"), resentment is prominent in both types of depression related to problems in early attachment relationships. Persons who are vulnerable to dependent depression are highly sensitive to separations and losses, yet they are in a bind: they fear that expressing their resentment will alienate the person on whom they depend, and they stifle it, suffering the chronic emotional strain in the process. Persons with self-critical depression—perfectionism in the extreme—are likely not only to berate themselves for their shortcomings but also to carry resentment toward those (past and present) for whom they feel they are not measuring up.

Why is resentment depressing? To be sure, resentment is stressful; it's one form of chronic emotional strain. Yet I think resentment is also depressing because it's taking a one-down, subordinate position. Resentment is associated with feeling oppressed, and oppression is depressing: you feel trapped, squelched, and stifled. I have presented ample evidence that people don't become depressed without reason, although the reasons are sometimes obscure, particularly when they date back to early attachment relationships. In my view, depressed persons typically have reason to feel angry and resentful. Many also feel guilty about their anger and resentment, because these feelings clash with love, gratitude, and loyalty. The natural impulse associated with anger and resentment is to hurt back or take revenge,[268] and you might feel guilty about your resentful inclinations, even if you haven't actually carried them out and hurt anyone. In addition, you might feel ashamed of your anger and resentment—as though these feelings make you a bad person at the core. Thus, already tied in the emotional knot of resentment, you can tie yourself in a double-knot of guilt and shame regarding your resentment. Untying this emotional double-knot requires facing and accepting the feelings of anger and resentment and acknowledging the reasons for them. Although the feelings may be out of proportion—as childhood holdovers—they are not likely to be without basis.

The solution to resentment requires nothing less than resolving problems in attachment relationships. Often enough, these problems go back to relationships with parents and other caregivers, and it may not be possible to resolve them in the present. Then you must come to terms with these conflicts in your own mind. I believe that these old resentments are often fueled by parallel conflicts in current relationships, and addressing these current conflicts can take much of the steam out of resentment from the past.

> Greta, a woman in her 40s, sought inpatient treatment for an episode of depression that had gone on for 2 years. She first became depressed in childhood in conjunction with repeated battles between her parents. She described her father as aloof and irascible, at best coldly putting her mother

down and, at worst, violently berating her. Her mother was chronically depressed, and Greta resented her for not standing up to her father or divorcing him. Greta also resented her mother's squelching her, urging her to be quiet and well behaved so as to avoid antagonizing her father. Greta felt that her mother was so concerned with maintaining the peace—a futile endeavor—that her mother had no interest in her. Greta felt emotionally neglected and resentful about that as well.

Determined not to repeat the past, Greta married Joe, an even-tempered man who treated her with affection and respect. Yet over the course of having three children, their relationship gradually deteriorated. Joe took a job that involved a great deal of traveling, leaving Greta to care for the children, one of whom was particularly demanding owing to hyperactivity and another of whom had a chronic illness. Greta felt unsupported and began to resent Joe. When he was home, she was irritable and distant, subtly critical for what she perceived as his inadequate efforts to help with the children as well as with household tasks. Greta and Joe drifted into a vicious circle of mutual resentment, in which Joe spent more and more time traveling and was more withdrawn when he was at home. Greta came to resent his emotional neglect, paralleling her experience with both parents in childhood. She, too, withdrew—into depression.

When she entered treatment, Greta just felt depressed; she was not aware of feeling angry. Yet her critical comments about Joe had an irritable edge that was evident to her fellow patients as well as her therapist. Greta seemed to seize on any minor shortcomings in Joe, such as his failure to call exactly on time, adding to her stockpile of resentment. At first she was defensive when this pattern was brought to her attention; she viewed anger and resentment as sinful. Over the course of therapy, when she reviewed the ample basis for anger in childhood as well as its current basis in her marriage, Greta became more accepting of her feelings. She was also able to see how her lingering resentment from the past was amplifying the resentment from her marriage.

As Greta became more accepting of her anger, she was freed up to address her conflicts with Joe more forthrightly. Joe was willing to make some adjustments in his travel schedule, and Greta also was able to find other sources of support.

FORGIVENESS

I believe that the most straightforward antidote to resentment is resolving problems in current relationships that perpetuate and amplify it. Yet there is another important antidote: forgiveness. Acknowledging resentment and working with it are crucial, because the obsessive preoccupation with having been wronged is a major source of emotional stress as well as conflict in relationships.[269]

Forgiveness is a hard-won achievement, and the extent to which one should aspire to forgive is debatable. Although I am not championing resentment, it is worth noting that some arguments have been made in favor of it. Philosopher Jeffrie Murphy[270] proposes that resentment in response to wrongdoing can serve positive functions: maintaining self-respect, promoting self-protection, and reinforcing respect for the moral order. He argued that forgiveness should be given cautiously, and it's not easy to do. Moreover, as philosopher Claudia Card described,[271] forgiveness is not an all-or-nothing matter, because it includes renouncing hostility, accepting contrition, forgoing opportunities to punish, and reconciling. In many instances, partial forgiveness makes sense (e.g., renouncing hostility without renewing the hurtful relationship).

Self-forgiveness comes into play in relation to guilt feelings—when these feelings are proportionate to actual harm done. Forgiving yourself is no less complex than forgiving others, and to the extent that you've done harm, you're bound to contend with guilt feelings. It's not the feelings of resentment or guilt that are problematic—these are natural feelings, and they have an adaptive function. It's being mired in these feelings continuously, as opposed to contending with periodic bursts, that creates the chronic emotional strain associated with depression. You can learn to tolerate periodic bursts of these feelings, acknowledging and accepting them, and learn to understand their basis. This brings us to the pivotal matter, your relationship with yourself.

RELATING TO YOURSELF

In the previous chapter, I argued that problems in interpersonal relationships are a pervasive source of the stress that eventuates in depression. In this chapter, I have argued that it's the *internal* experience of these problems—the emotional wear and tear—that leads to depression. I believe that it's helpful to view this internal emotional stress from the perspective of your relationship with yourself. We are accustomed to thinking about problems with self-esteem and self-worth, but I also find it helpful to think in more active terms about what you are *doing:* how you are relating to yourself—valuing or devaluing yourself, for example. I'll start with self-worth and then take the perspective of your interactions with yourself, concluding with the proposal that you have an attachment relationship with yourself, for better or for worse.

SELF-WORTH

One of the most durable research findings is the association of depression with low self-worth; "feelings of worthlessness" is among the diagnostic criteria for depression.[8] Yet the relationship between self-worth and depression is complex, and self-worth itself has many facets.

Based on her research on the development of self-worth in childhood and adolescence, psychologist Susan Harter[140] proposed that global self-worth is determined conjointly by perceived competence in various domains of importance and the extent of approval from persons in valued relationships. Individuals differ in domains of competence that they value, for example, academic success, athletic performance, likeability, and physical appearance. Strikingly, physical appearance is the largest determinant of global self-worth across age groups, sexes, and nationalities. In addition, individuals differ in what relationships contribute most to self-worth; for example, some persons put more weight on acceptance from peers than parents, others the reverse.

Self-worth is both a relatively stable personality trait and a somewhat changeable state of mind; thus Harter distinguishes between baseline and barometric self-worth. Both facets relate to depression. Relatively enduring, low *baseline* self-worth contributes to vulnerability to depression. This cognitive vulnerability to depression appears to be consolidated by adolescence.[272]

However, the relationship goes both ways: the experience of depression lowers *barometric* self-worth; when you feel depressed, you focus your attention on all your failings. Furthermore, going through episodes of depression can have a lasting adverse impact on self-worth that extends beyond the resolution of the depressive episode.[273] For example, although you have recovered from the episode, you might lack confidence in proceeding with career plans or developing relationships for fear of becoming depressed again.

In principle, the sheer complexity of self-concept and self-worth should be a protective factor against depression in the face of adverse experiences. If you experience a setback at school or at work, for example, a supportive relationship that helps you feel good about yourself might serve as a buffer. Conversely, in the face of disruptions in a key relationship, other domains of success might buffer your mood. The barometer might dip but not plummet. Unfortunately, one of the hallmarks of depression is *global* negative thinking;[236] as the diagnostic criteria attest, a failure in any one domain can lead to generalized feelings of worthlessness.

We face another chicken-and-egg debate: does low self-worth precede depression (i.e., as a vulnerability) or does depression lower self-worth (in a kind of scarring process)?[274] As I have already implied, both are true. Harter found individual differences among adolescents in this respect. For some, a fall in self-worth precedes depression, for example, when a failure in school leads to self-hate and then depression. For others, depressed mood precedes a drop in self-worth, for example, when a social rejection and the ensuing depression leads to self-critical thinking.

Rather than debating the chicken versus the egg, we might best think of the relationship between depression and self-worth as a spiraling process, for example, as when stressful life events lead to depressive ruminations about all your shortcomings and failures, and then your thinking and your mood fuel each other in a vicious circle. As psychologist Rick Ingram and colleagues[275] pointed out in this context, a diagnosis of major depression requires 2 weeks of symptoms; depression does not develop overnight but rather requires a stabilizing process; it takes some time to dig yourself deep into the hole with negative thinking. As we will see in Chapter 12 ("Flexible Thinking"), learning to interrupt and block this stabilizing process is crucial in coping with depression.

INTERACTING WITH YOURSELF

Even allowing for barometric changes, the concepts of self-esteem and self-worth imply something static; you have it, at one level or another. I've been advocating the perspective of agency, focusing not just on your characteristics but rather on what you're doing so you can *do something about it*. We're looking for leverage. Thus I encourage you to think of your self-esteem and self-worth as a reflection of how you're relating to yourself.

The concept of a relationship with yourself may seem a bit odd, but I think it's profoundly important. We humans can form a relationship with ourselves, because we have two forms of consciousness.[276] First, like many other nonhuman animals, we have basic awareness. Asleep, we are unconscious; when we wake up, the switch goes on, and we are conscious. Second, to a degree far surpassing other animals, we are self-conscious, conscious of being conscious. We humans are not only self-aware; having language, we talk with ourselves continually.

Naturally, the way you relate to yourself will be influenced significantly by the quality of the relationships with others, especially early attachment relationships. As you learn to talk with others, you learn to talk with yourself. The way in which you talk to yourself about yourself will reflect the ways your attachment figures have talked to you about yourself. These early conversations can be enduring in the mind, lasting from childhood into adulthood; we often refer to this process as "playing old tapes" from the past.

Consider all the ways you relate to yourself. You think about yourself. You talk to yourself. In the process, you are often making emotional judgments about yourself. You evaluate yourself. You think *and feel* about yourself, relating to yourself emotionally. Just as in any other close relationship, your emotional relationship with yourself will have positive and negative tones. On the positive side, you can encourage, praise, reassure, and comfort yourself. On the negative side, you can discourage, criticize, berate, and torment yourself—as you are especially likely to do when you're depressed, thus depressing yourself further in a spiraling process.

You can think of shame and guilt feelings as stemming from the way you relate to yourself. Recall that these are self-conscious emotions; you can feel guilty and ashamed under the gaze of another person, and you can do so under your own gaze as well. You can relate to yourself in a guilt-inducing and shaming way, thereby diminishing your self-worth. Relating in this way to yourself can be provocative and frustrating, inducing anger and resentment, just as being in such a relationship with another person would do. Thus you can resent yourself—and perhaps you do, to the extent that you mistreat yourself. But all this is depressing.

The sheer pervasiveness of your relationship with yourself bears emphasis. You're with yourself all the time, although you can neglect yourself or obliterate your self-awareness with drugs or alcohol. Depending on the way you relate to yourself, the pervasiveness of this relationship could be a blessing or a curse.

BONDING WITH YOURSELF

To take this line of reasoning one step further, you can think of your relationship with yourself as an attachment relationship. New Zealand philosopher Christine Swanton[277] ingeniously referred to the process of *bonding* with yourself. Mirroring other attachment relationships, you might have a relatively secure or insecure relationship with yourself, being more or less able to count on yourself to be there for yourself in a supportive and emotionally attuned way. To be attuned, you must mentalize, having your own mind in mind—in effect, empathizing with yourself.

Swanton described bonding with oneself in the context of *self-love*; she viewed the bond as providing a sense of strength, vitality, and energy, just as a loving bond in any other attachment relationship would do. When you relate to yourself in a benevolent, loving, and compassionate way, you cultivate a more positive sense of self-worth. In the context of a benevolent relationship with yourself, you will be more accepting of constructive criticism from yourself, just as you would be from another person who has goodwill toward you. The alternative, relating to yourself in a threatening or self-denigrating way, can make you ill with depression.

• Part IV •

ILLNESS

• Chapter 9 •

BRAIN AND BODY

We are naturally active agents, intensely engaged with the world, exploring curiously, exerting our influence, and responding flexibly to events. We are purposeful, intelligent, and creative agents: we plan, draw on past knowledge, deliberate, generate options, and take action. We are social agents: we invest in attachments, and many of our projects involve collaboration with others. Thus we are mentalizing agents: we make sense of others as we aspire to influence them and to be receptive to their influence.

All this agency requires enormous bodily energy and brainpower that we ordinarily take for granted. In Chapter 3 ("Agency and Elbow Room"), I addressed a fundamental manifestation of catch-22: you need agency to recover from depression, and the illness constrains your agency. Depression limits your energy and capacity for creative thinking, including your capacity to relate to other persons. Thus, to reiterate a main point from Chapter 3: being ill, you cannot recover by a mere act of will. If you need biological evidence for that point, this chapter provides it.

Be forewarned: this chapter is relatively technical, and readers without any background in biology or neuroscience will find it challenging. You need not grasp all the biological details, but I believe you'll benefit from making some connections between your experience of depression and some of the biological changes that neuroscientists have identified. Be reassured that I intend to keep your mind in mind and to avoid losing you in your brain.

I begin with a primer on brain organization. This unavoidably dense material provides essential background for you to grasp the import of research showing how different areas of the brain are affected by depression. In this section on brain organization, you might pay particular attention to the part on "Agency in the Prefrontal Cortex," the main theme of this chapter. I next discuss how feeling ill when you're depressed relates to elevated stress hormones. While we're in the realm of chemistry, I discuss the key neurotransmitters involved in depression and its treatment—and challenge the oversimplified notion of a chemical imbalance. Then I come back to the theme of agency in addressing how altered patterns of brain activity undercut motivation and diminish your capacity for goal-directed activity, including social interactions. If you are inclined to skip the difficult bits, don't miss the two parts on reversibility ("Reversibility and a Hero: Brain-Derived Neurotrophic Factor" and "Reversibility With Treatment"), lest you infer that you're permanently stuck with a malfunctioning brain. Continuing the reversibility theme, I conclude the chapter by noting that catch-22 is not insurmountable.

BRAIN ORGANIZATION: A PRIMER

All of us who are not neuroscientists face a daunting problem: we know relatively little about the brain, yet the findings of biological psychiatry are becoming increasingly crucial to understanding depression and its treatment. There is only one solution: learning.

The sheer complexity of the brain humbles neuroscientists. The human brain is by far the most complex object in the known universe. The cerebral cortex, the outer covering of the brain, is estimated to contain 30 billion neurons (brain cells) and one million billion connections.[276] For over a century, neuroscientists have been striving to identify discrete areas of the brain and their relation to mental, emotional, and behavioral functions— areas related to speech, vision, fear, and movement, for example. Yet identifying discrete functional areas is only part of the challenge; their patterns of interconnectivity are equally important. For example, more than 30 areas of the visual cortex have been distinguished;[278] these areas are connected not only with each other but also with other areas of the cortex as well as subcortical structures (beneath the cortex). All brain areas and the neurons that compose them work in concert, analogous to a symphony orchestra.[279] The quality of the symphony will depend on the functioning of the individual instruments as well as the capacity of the different groupings to play harmoniously in continually changing patterns.

In the long run, you need not know your hypothalamus from your hippocampus, but you should appreciate that depression relates to alterations in brain functioning. This primer provides an overview of neuroanatomy to prepare you to understand how the psychological symptoms of depression are associated with changes in brain activity. I start with a brief description of the individual cells of the nervous system. Then I give an overview of brain organization by distinguishing the left side from the right, the front from the back, and the outside from the inside, noting some specific regions relevant to depression along the way. I conclude with a description of the prefrontal cortex, because this area plays such an important role in depression.

NEURONS

The prominent role of medication in the treatment of depression (see Chapter 14, "Integrating Treatment") has drawn our attention down to the finest level of detail, to the inner workings of the neurons (individual brain cells); this is the territory of molecular biology.[280] Like us, neurons are wonderfully adaptive, altering their functioning according to changes in the environment. Like us, their physical condition and functioning can be undermined by stress. Also like us, with proper care they can heal and thrive.

Neurons are highly social creatures, connected with each other in immensely complex networks. They secrete chemicals that act as signals; these chemicals bind to receptors on the receiving neuron, triggering an electrical current that leads the receiving neuron to secrete its own chemical signals, and so on. Neurons are interconnected by synapses, microscopic gaps that the chemicals cross to exert their influence on receiving neurons. It's a short trip across the gap; it takes about a millisecond.

Designed for communication, neurons have branches that extend outward from the cell body: *dendrites* on the receiving end and *axons* on the sending end. Axons of sending neurons make contact with dendrites of other neurons (as well as with their cell bodies and axons). Neurons are not like straight wires; they're more like intermingled trees and bushes. A single axon may have many branches and connect with dozens or even hundreds of targets. Similarly, a given neuron has many dendrites and may receive signals from hundreds or even thousands of sending cells. Thus, in making decisions about firing and secreting their chemical signals, neurons continuously integrate a wealth of information from other neurons.

The chemicals that neurons employ in signaling each other are called *neurotransmitters*, and there are dozens of them, a small number of which are the focus of current research on depression. I concentrate here on norepinephrine, dopamine, and serotonin. Performing any mental or physical activity requires that a subset of neurons spanning many brain areas fire synchronously at a given moment. All the instruments of the orchestra can't be playing loudly and at random at the same time. Thus the brain must always maintain a delicate balance of excitement and inhibition—too much excitement, for example, can result in a seizure—orchestral cacophony. Accordingly, some neurotransmitters, such as glutamate, are excitatory, increasing the likelihood that the receiving neurons will send their own signal; others, such as gamma-aminobutyric acid (GABA) are inhibitory, decreasing the likelihood that the receiving neurons will signal.

Like the groupings of orchestral instruments—strings, woodwinds, brass, and percussion—different areas of the brain specialize, playing different parts in the symphony. Unlike the orchestra, however, all areas of the brain are active at all times, although the relative prominence of different areas shifts continually depending on the task at hand. Unlike the orchestra, brain organization is fantastically complex. Brain organization can be approached from different vantage points, and I highlight a few of these: left-right, front-back, and outer-inner.

LEFT-RIGHT ORGANIZATION

You might be familiar with the popular idea of "left brain" versus "right brain" activities, stemming from the brain's division into two cerebral hemispheres. Although there is a great deal of overlap in functions, and the two hemispheres are connected point-to-point by a massive bundle of fibers (the corpus callosum), there is also considerable specialization between hemispheres.

Broadly speaking, the left (dominant) hemisphere analyzes details and organizes them into sequences, whereas the right hemisphere grasps the big picture.[281] The left hemisphere handles routines; the right grapples with novelty.[116] Accordingly, the left hemisphere is specialized for language, the right for emotion.[282] Owing to their tight interconnections, the two hemispheres work in concert. For example, when we listen to speech, we not only hear the words but also the music behind the words (in the tone of voice). The left hemisphere decodes the grammar and semantic meaning while the right hemisphere decodes the emotional import.

FRONT-BACK ORGANIZATION

The central fissure divides the brain into a front (anterior) portion specialized for movement and a back (posterior) portion specialized for perception. Combining front-back and left-right divisions, we can identify four quadrants. For example, whereas the left hemisphere as a whole is specialized for language, the anterior portion (Broca's area) specializes in speech production and the posterior portion (Wernicke's area) specializes in speech perception.

More specifically, each hemisphere of the cortex is divided into four lobes (see Figure 9–1). The anterior half is the frontal lobe, and the posterior half is divided into three lobes: the occipital lobes, at the very back, support visual perception; the temporal lobes, at the sides by the temples, support auditory perception; and the parietal lobes, the remaining portion, support spatial and body perception.

Although considered one lobe, the frontal portion of the cortex represents a large area with many subdivisions. Just anterior to the central fissure is the motor cortex, which organizes and generates movement. The anterior-most portion of the frontal lobe (behind the forehead) is called the prefrontal cortex, broadly construed as the brain's executive.[116] The dorsolateral prefrontal cortex, on the outer side, enables us to keep track of what we're doing in the outer world. The ventral prefrontal cortex, on the underside, enables us to monitor and regulate emotional experience. More about the prefrontal cortex shortly.

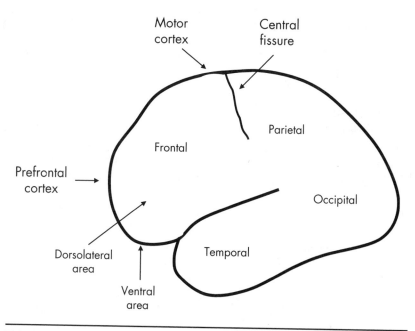

FIGURE 9–1.   Lateral view of the cerebral cortex (left hemisphere).

OUTER-INNER ORGANIZATION

Thus far I have concentrated on the outer surface of the brain, the cerebral cortex and its broad divisions. The cerebral cortex is most distinctly advanced in us humans (and other primates). It's highly folded and convoluted to allow a vast amount of tissue (30 billion cells) to be packed into the limited area of the skull. Stretched out flat, the human neocortex would have the size and thickness of a large table napkin.[276] Yet this evolutionarily advanced cortex sits atop subcortical brain structures we share with other animals.

Viewing brain organization from an evolutionary perspective, neuroscientist Paul MacLean[165] proposed that we have a *triune brain*—three brains that, although richly interconnected, operate somewhat independently. These three brains sit on top of what he called the *neural chassis*, the brain stem and spinal cord. The brainstem atop the spinal cord contains cell groups that secrete the neurotransmitters that regulate the level of arousal of the cortex. MacLean likened the neural chassis, by itself, to a vehicle without a driver.

The three drivers, inside to outside, are the reptilian brain, the paleomammalian (ancient mammal) brain, and the neomammalian (new mammal) brain. Thus far, I have been focusing on the neomammalian brain, the cerebral cortex. I only mention the innermost reptilian brain in passing; it governs basic habits, daily routines, and some of the basic expressions for social communication. However, we need to consider the paleomammalian brain, commonly called the *limbic system*, in some detail; it plays a central role in emotion, memory, and attachment—all of which we humans share with our more ancient mammalian kin. In depressed states, the limbic system gains the upper hand over the neocortex; the old mammalian equipment trumps the new.

Five structures within the limbic system play a significant role in depression (see Figure 9–2):

1. The *cingulate cortex* lies behind and beneath the frontal cortex, surrounding the corpus callosum that connects the two cerebral hemispheres. The anterior portion of the cingulate cortex, contiguous with the prefrontal cortex, plays a central role in emotion and attention, both of which are crucial in depression. The anterior cingulate is divided into a ventral (lower-most) area involved in emotion, a dorsal (top-most) area involved in attention, and a rostral (front-most) area that coordinates the ventral and dorsal areas.[283] If we think of the cerebral cortex as engaged with the outer world (environment) and the innermost por-

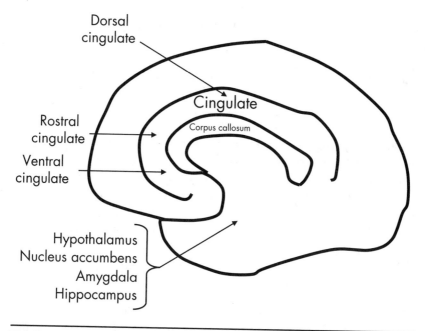

Dorsal cingulate

Cingulate

Rostral cingulate

Corpus callosum

Ventral cingulate

Hypothalamus
Nucleus accumbens
Amygdala
Hippocampus

FIGURE 9–2. Medial view of the limbic system (right hemisphere).

tions of the limbic system as engaged with the inner world (viscera), the cingulate cortex is an interface between the two. Yet within the anterior cingulate cortex, the dorsal area relates more closely to the outer world and the ventral area more closely to the inner world.

2. The *hypothalamus* integrates the nervous and endocrine systems, secreting hormones to regulate homeostasis. For example, the hypothalamus plays a central role in regulating basic survival functions, including temperature, appetite, thirst, and sexual responsiveness. The hypothalamus orchestrates the autonomic (involuntary) components of the stress response. That is, the hypothalamus adjusts the functioning of the internal organs, such as the heart and lungs, to behavioral demands, for example, raising your blood pressure when you're under stress.

3. The *hippocampus* plays a significant role in emotion and memory, creating episodic memories of personal experiences and converting short-term memories into long-term memories. In addition, the hippocampus regulates the secretion of stress hormones by the hypothalamus.

4. The *amygdala* is most noteworthy for its role in fear: it detects danger in a small fraction of a second (e.g., responding to a threatening face),

orchestrates the fear response (physiology and behavioral expression), and supports fear conditioning (learning to associate certain stimuli with danger).

5. The *nucleus accumbens*, rich in dopamine receptors, plays a significant role in pleasure and reward—experiences that, by their absence, are central to depression.

To summarize, the neomammalian brain, the neocortex, supports perception, language, abstract reasoning, and complex problem-solving, including the capacity to anticipate the future and plan our actions accordingly. Yet we must be attuned to the inner world as we navigate the outer world, because the inner world continuously assigns value to the outer world, steering us toward reward and away from harm. In depression, the cortical-limbic balance shifts, evidenced by a painful preoccupation with the inner world.

AGENCY IN THE PREFRONTAL CORTEX

Of all the areas of the brain, the prefrontal cortex plays a preeminent role in agency. Neuroscientist Elkhonon Goldberg[116] characterized the prefrontal cortex as the executive brain, likening its role to the orchestra conductor. As the seat of agency, the prefrontal cortex organizes and sustains goal-oriented behavior. As Goldberg put it,

> The prefrontal cortex plays the central role in forming goals and objectives and then in devising plans of action required to attain these goals. It selects the cognitive skills required to implement the plans, coordinates these skills, and applies them in a correct order. Finally, the prefrontal cortex is responsible for evaluating our actions as success or failure relative to our intentions. (p. 24)

The prefrontal cortex maintains a dynamic balance between persistence and flexibility in action.[284] Prefrontal activity is essential to creating mental representations, such as generating images of what you want to happen, and in keeping these representations in mind in the face of interferences and distractions. You use your prefrontal cortex to form and hold onto priorities and thus to override strong impulses or habits that don't fit your present situation or intention. You also use your prefrontal cortex to organize your actions in proper sequences, for example, your morning routine. In short, your prefrontal cortex keeps you on track. Without prefrontal organization, your behavior will be haphazard. You know your prefrontal cortex has abandoned you when you walk from your living room to your kitchen to get something and, by the time you've arrived in your kitchen, you've forgotten why you went in there.

Yet, counterbalancing the ability to keep you on course, your prefrontal cortex also enables you to change direction when the situation demands. You can respond adaptively to interruptions, novelty, and changing demands. Without prefrontal control, you perseverate: when you look over and over again in the same spot for something you've misplaced, your prefrontal cortex has gone missing too.

Neuroscientist Joaquin Fuster characterized the prefrontal cortex as the organ of creativity.[285] In effect, the prefrontal cortex flexibly draws upon information as needed from many other brain areas. Most generally, in organizing action, the prefrontal cortex integrates information from the outer world with information from the inner world. Your prefrontal cortex monitors and regulates emotional activity in the limbic system.[286] Thus your prefrontal cortex enables you to be guided by gut feelings in the course of planning actions and pursuing goals.[287] Well-coordinated prefrontal and limbic activity makes for emotional intelligence, the integration of emotion and reason.[288]

Emotional intelligence overlaps with social intelligence, the ability to read and relate to other people, our mentalizing capacity. Here too, the prefrontal cortex takes center stage. As Goldberg[116] put it, "The prefrontal cortex is the closest there is to the neural substrate of social being" (p. 111). Although we often take our ability to interact with each other for granted (when our prefrontal cortex is working properly), it's the most complex thing we do. Goldberg captured the challenge well: "In the earlier description of the essential executive functions I emphasized their sequential, planning, temporal ordering aspect. Now imagine that you have to plan and sequentially organize *your* actions in coordination with a group of other individuals and institutions engaged in the planning and sequential organization of *their* actions" (p. 107).

In this primer, I've merely hinted at the staggering complexity of brain organization, putting the prefrontal cortex at the apex as the conductor, the head agent that coordinates intellectual, emotional, and social activity. You won't be surprised to learn that depression is associated with impairment in the functioning of the prefrontal cortex, which I discuss later in this chapter.

With this overview of brain organization in mind, we are now in a position to consider key neurobiological changes in depression. We proceed on the chemical level, considering hormonal aspects of depression and neurotransmitter alterations before returning to our primary concern, changes in patterns of brain-mind activity.

ILL HEALTH AND ELEVATED STRESS HORMONES

Our intricate stress response evolved to adapt to acute stressors, but it's not well designed for chronic stress.[289] Neuroscientist Robert Sapolsky[290] neatly captured this human design flaw in his book title, *Why Zebras Don't Get Ulcers:* zebras just flee from the lion and don't obsess about the next encounter. With chronic stress, adaptation turns into illness. To put it bluntly, stress can make you sick—as you well know when you're depressed. You don't have much energy, you don't feel like eating, you can't sleep well, and you have little interest in sex. This state of physical ill health further erodes your agency by undercutting your energy, motivation, and mental functioning.

Stress hormones play a key part in these adverse bodily changes. As described earlier in this chapter, neurotransmitters rapidly exert their influence by neuron-to-neuron transmission across microscopic synapses. Yet neurons secrete hormones as well as neurotransmitters; hence we also need to consider the neuroendocrine response. Hormones exert their influence through circulation in the bloodstream, more slowly influencing the functioning of a range of organ systems, including the brain. To complicate matters, the brain also uses hormones as transmitters.

THE HYPOTHALAMIC-PITUITARY-ADRENAL AXIS AND CORTISOL

When we think of acute stress, we are most likely to focus on the fight-or-flight response. This sympathetic nervous system response is triggered by the neurotransmitter norepinephrine (a form of adrenaline), which is secreted by a group of cells in the brainstem, the locus coeruleus. The fight-or-flight response is an immediate emergency reaction to stress that is fine-tuned by the slower neuroendocrine stress response.

The heart of the neuroendocrine response is the hypothalamic-pituitary-adrenal (HPA) axis (see the circuit diagram in Figure 9–3). In response to stress, the hypothalamus secretes corticotropin-releasing factor (CRF), stimulating the pituitary to secrete adrenocorticotropic hormone (ACTH), in turn stimulating the adrenal cortex to secrete *cortisol*, a key stress hormone. Cortisol secretion has numerous short-term adaptive functions together with an array of long-term maladaptive functions.[289] Among its many functions, cortisol helps provide energy by regulating glucose availability. In acute stress, cortisol provides energy to the brain by increasing neurons' uptake of glucose; in addition, cortisol increases the neurons' level of excitability.

Yet a critical part of cortisol's adaptive function is *terminating* the stress response; thus cortisol also has been dubbed an *antistress* hormone.[291] The

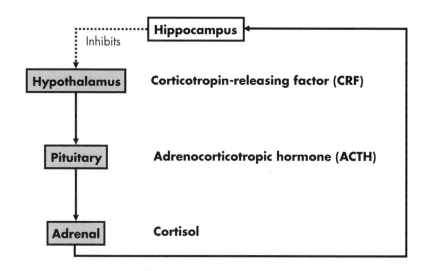

FIGURE 9–3. Overview of the HPA axis.

Source. Reprinted from Allen J: "Illness," in *Coping With Trauma: Hope Through Understanding.* Washington, DC, American Psychiatric Publishing, 2005, p. 143. Used with permission. Copyright 2005 American Psychiatric Publishing.

hippocampus is rich in cortisol receptors, and stimulation of these receptors leads the hippocampus to lessen further secretion of CRF by the hypothalamus, dampening the HPA axis. Yet excess levels of cortisol can damage neurons in the hippocampus, causing them to atrophy (shrink) and, at worst, to die. By adversely affecting the functioning of the hippocampus, elevated cortisol levels ultimately interfere with the containment of the stress response, increasing cortisol levels in a vicious circle. Unfortunately, such cell damage is not limited to the hippocampus but also is evident in the prefrontal cortex.[292]

A VILLAIN IN THE HPA AXIS: CORTICOTROPIN-RELEASING FACTOR

Consistent with the fact that depression is a high-stress state, a substantial minority of depressed outpatients and a majority of depressed inpatients show signs of excess cortisol secretion.[230] As psychiatrist Charles Nemeroff[293] put it, "Perhaps the most venerable finding in all of biological psychiatry is the increase in [HPA] axis activity in drug-free depressed patients. There is considerable consensus that this 'endocrinopathy' is due in part, and perhaps largely, to hypersecretion of CRF" (p. 523).[293] The role CRF plays in stress and depression goes beyond its pivotal place in HPA-axis activity. CRF is secreted by neurons in many areas of the brain, including the cerebral cortex, amygdala, and locus coeruleus.[293] CRF secretion enhances locus coeruleus-norepinephrine activity and vice versa, such that the fight-or-flight and HPA-axis responses can escalate each other.[294]

I have come to see CRF as a major villain in depression. As Nemeroff[295] and others[296] have discussed, CRF secretion, abetted by norepinephrine, induces anxiety along with a range of physiological effects that include increased heart rate and blood pressure, increased startle reflex, restlessness, and increased withdrawal to novel stimuli. Moreover, CRF plays a significant role in the generalized ill health associated with depression, interfering with appetite and sleep as well as sex drive and reproductive activity. In short, excess CRF secretion can make you ill.

DEVELOPMENTAL VULNERABILITY

Repeated exposure to manageable stress can increase your resilience as you become *desensitized:* as you encounter a stressor like public speaking, you gradually master it, being better able to cope and less emotionally reactive. Conversely, exposure to excessive or chronic stress can undermine your capacity to cope with subsequent stress; you can become *sensitized*, more reactive to stress rather than less so.[249] Neurobiological research, much of it conducted with animals, has demonstrated consistently that stressful experience early in life can induce a sensitization process that increases vulnerability to depression in response to stress later in life.[297] Our villain, CRF, plays a significant role in this process, although myriad chemical components of the stress response are all intertwined in sensitization.

Early life stress, such as maternal deprivation, not only increases CRF production but also increases CRF gene expression—that is, turning on neurons' CRF genes and increasing the rate of CRF synthesis.[295] Owing to sensitization, these early influences have persistent effects, enhancing CRF secretion and the HPA axis response to stress in later life.[296] As discussed in Chapter 4 ("Constitution"), biological vulnerability to stress and depression potentially begins prenatally in conjunction with maternal stress and depression; given that CRF production begins in the human fetus around the end of the first trimester, prenatal HPA axis disturbance might play a significant role in persistent vulnerability to stress and depression.[298,299]

As neurobiologists recognize,[296] these findings underscore what clinicians have long known: adult depression has significant origins in stressful childhood relationships.[144] This knowledge reinforces the need for early prevention and intervention. Treating maternal depression during pregnancy and after delivery should be a high priority. Yet the implications are far broader, highlighting the need to prevent childhood maltreatment and ameliorating other social ills such as poverty and its profoundly stressful and oppressing consequences.[300]

REVERSIBILITY AND A HERO: BRAIN-DERIVED NEUROTROPHIC FACTOR

Research on HPA-axis disturbance associated with early stress presents a grim picture. Thus it is crucial to keep agency in mind: you can do something about your vulnerability. Anything that reduces stress, including psychotherapy addressed to resolving internal conflicts, is likely to help.[301]

The knowledge that stress and depression are associated with neuronal atrophy and even cell death is especially alarming. Thus it's important to keep in mind the enormous plasticity of our neurons.[280] Atrophy of neurons in the hippocampus may reflect the cells' self-protective response, because it diminishes their exposure to the potentially toxic effects of excess neurochemicals.[302] Moreover, the hippocampus is capable of generating new neurons; thus the effects of cell death may not be irreversible.

Fortunately, counteracting the effects of the molecular villains, neurobiologists have identified a hero: brain-derived neurotrophic factor (BDNF).[294,297,303] BDNF is a brain-nurturing chemical;[118] it contributes to the differentiation and growth of neurons during brain development and continues to promote the generation, growth, and health of neurons in the mature brain. Furthermore, BDNF enhances neurotransmission. Although stress decreases BDNF expression, BDNF availability also protects neurons against the toxic effects of stress.

Here's the punch line: antidepressant treatment promotes BDNF production and, thereby, neuronal healing and health.[303,304] Thus molecular biology is illuminating intracellular processes that not only contribute to our understanding of depression but also point to the means by which treatments restore neuronal functioning and thereby normalize brain activity. Most importantly, this line of research promises to facilitate the development of increasingly refined and effective antidepressant interventions.

BEYOND THE CHEMICAL IMBALANCE

The advent of antidepressant medication has drawn widespread attention to the idea that depression stems from a chemical imbalance and that antidepressants restore the balance. I like one facet of this idea: it has infused the popular culture with the belief that depression is a real physical illness. Yet I dislike the inference that there's a special form of chemical-imbalance depression that has nothing to do with your mind or your life. The idea of a chemical imbalance doesn't explain anything; it calls for an explanation. What causes the chemical imbalance? Much of this book has been addressed to that question. I find the idea of a chemical imbalance to be mindless: we can't relate the *experience* of depression to a chemical imbalance. Rather, we must relate the experience of depression to broader changes in patterns of brain activity, as I discuss shortly. Nonetheless, brain activity runs on neurochemistry, and medication intervenes at this level; hence understanding depression and its treatment requires consideration of the chemicals—neurotransmitters.

Three neurotransmitters of central interest in the treatment of depression are norepinephrine, dopamine, and serotonin. These transmitters are produced by groups of neurons in the brain stem, and they are secreted into the upper levels of the brain, including the cerebral cortex. They are also called *neuromodulators* because, owing to their widespread pattern of secretion, they influence the responsiveness of large groups of cortical neurons. For example, the presence of neuromodulators affects neurons' responsiveness to glutamate excitation and GABA inhibition. Thus the levels of these neuromodulators exert broad effects on patterns of brain activity and thereby influence arousal and mood.

NOREPINEPHRINE AND AROUSAL

As I noted earlier, norepinephrine plays a central role in organizing the fight-or-flight response. Norepinephrine secretion puts the cerebral cortex into high gear, and the adrenal medulla activates the corresponding physiology in the body by secreting adrenaline (epinephrine) into the bloodstream, preparing for vigorous action, for example, by elevating heart rate and blood pressure.

More broadly, norepinephrine initiates and maintains arousal in the cerebral cortex, producing a state of alertness.[230,305] For example, in response to novel stimuli, such as a sudden noise, the norepinephrine system activates the cortex, orienting you and focusing your attention. Thus, when the norepinephrine system is working optimally, it facilitates attention, concentration, learning, and memory. With insufficient arousal, your thinking would be sluggish; with excess arousal, you would be agitated and distractible, unable to focus.

The findings regarding changes in norepinephrine levels associated with depression are inconsistent; some depressed persons show decreased levels, whereas others show increased levels.[230] There is consensus, however, that sustained stress can impair the functioning of the norepinephrine system, resulting in a compromised response to stress and challenge. Although norepinephrine abnormalities are likely to be secondary to the depressed state rather than a primary cause, the norepinephrine system appears to play an important role in recovering from depression.[305] The most commonly employed antidepressant medications (e.g., Prozac) target the serotonin system rather than the norepinephrine system, but some medications target the norepinephrine system primarily, and others target both systems. Keep in mind, however, that the major neuromodulators interact with one another; medications that directly influence any one of them influence the others indirectly (see Chapter 14, "Integrating Treatment").

DOPAMINE AND REWARD

Like norepinephrine, dopamine has an activating effect. Dopamine plays a central role in movement and, consistent with its role in action, dopamine activity is associated with brain systems involved in motivation. Dopamine activity in the limbic system (nucleus accumbens) is associated with a wide range of rewards, such as food, sex, and drugs of abuse. Animal research suggests that dopamine also plays a role in the rewarding experience of social behavior.[306] Amphetamines increase dopamine release, and cocaine blocks the reuptake of dopamine into secreting cells; thus both stimulants make more dopamine available in the brain.

Neuroimaging research on the effects of amphetamines has shown that subjective feelings of euphoria are associated with the magnitude of dopamine release in the vicinity of the nucleus accumbens.[307] It's tempting to regard dopamine as the "cerebral joy juice" that psychologist Paul Meehl[6] inferred was lacking in depressed persons. Yet we need to keep in mind that it's not the levels of chemicals in the brain that count but rather the activity of complex brain circuits; the brain circuitry associated with dopamine activity is complex indeed, involving widespread brain areas beyond the limbic system, including the prefrontal cortex.

Neuroscientists have proposed a number of hypotheses about the role of dopamine in the experience of pleasure and reward.[308] Dopamine activity appears most closely tied to the perception of *incentive value*, the power of a potentially rewarding stimulus to motivate behavior. Thus dopamine activity is more closely tied to the excitement about a forthcoming reward than to the enjoyment of it, more to wanting than liking. For example, dopamine activity relates more strongly to the craving for drugs than to the rush. Neuroscientist Jaak Panksepp[7] aptly described this dopamine-related brain circuitry as a *seeking* system; it's active when you're seeking something interesting, exciting, or rewarding. In his words, the seeking system "leads organisms to eagerly pursue the fruits of their environment—from nuts to knowledge" (p. 145). The seeking system is the motivational core of agency.

It's tempting to speculate that something is amiss with the dopamine system in depression, of which a cardinal symptom is lack of interest in formerly pleasurable activities. The seeking system is turned down, agency diminished. Stimulant drugs that produce euphoria (amphetamines and cocaine) activate this system. You might think that antidepressant drugs would target this system; some do, but most don't—at least not directly. Recall, however, that affecting one neuromodulator affects all; hence, a number of antidepressants could contribute to normalizing dopamine function.[230]

SEROTONIN, SELF-CONTROL, AND SOCIAL ENGAGEMENT

Serotonin-related brain circuitry plays a role in myriad functions and activities, ranging from circadian rhythms and appetite to social behavior. Serotonin plays a significant role in modulating the stress response[230] and in enhancing impulse control.[309] Sitting between the other two neuromodulator systems, the serotonin system can dampen the effects of norepinephrine-based arousal and regulate the dopamine-based propensity to action.[118] Given its role in regulating emotional arousal and behavior, it's not surprising that serotonin plays an important role in social functioning. Optimal serotonin function is associated with effective social engagement, whereas impaired serotonin function is associated with social anxiety and loss of social rank.[310]

Extensive research now demonstrates that depression is associated with alterations in serotonin function.[293] The most widely employed class of antidepressants, selective serotonin reuptake inhibitors (SSRIs such as Prozac) have the immediate effect of blocking the transport of serotonin from the synapses back into the secreting neurons. Yet merely increasing serotonin levels in synapses doesn't have an antidepressant effect, as the delayed therapeutic response to taking antidepressant medication attests.[118] Rather, increasing synaptic levels leads to a cascade of changes in the functioning of the neurons, for example, including changes in gene activity and alterations in levels of receptors.[311] Moreover, because the neuromodulators influence each other, as well as the effects of excitatory and inhibitory neurotransmitters, altering levels of serotonin also normalizes the functioning of the norepinephrine and dopamine systems.[230]

The importance of serotonin function in exerting control underscores the role of unregulated stress in depression. I have emphasized throughout this book how depression typically includes a combination of high levels of negative emotion and low levels of positive emotion, a point also to be elaborated in the next section of this chapter. It's noteworthy that SSRIs have therapeutic effects not only for depression but also for anxiety disorders, including panic disorder, social phobia, obsessive-compulsive disorder, and posttraumatic stress disorder; hence, these antidepressant medications also could be called antinervousness agents.[312] Yet patterns of brain activity, not levels of neurotransmitters, tie most directly to emotional experience.

ALTERED BRAIN ACTIVITY

In *Darkness Visible*, Styron[2] likened depression to a howling tempest in the brain. Here's how he related his knowledge of the altered brain chemistry to his personal experience:

> With all of this upheaval in the brain tissues, the alternate drenching and deprivation, it is no wonder that the mind begins to feel aggrieved, stricken, and the muddied thought processes register the distress of an organ in convulsion. Sometimes, though not very often, such a disturbed mind will turn to violent thoughts regarding others. But with their minds turned agonizingly inward, people with depression are usually dangerous only to themselves. The madness of depression is, generally speaking, the antithesis of violence. It is a storm indeed, but a storm of murk. (p. 47)

Albeit in metaphor, Styron was going in the right direction, aspiring to fathom how changes in brain chemistry might relate to changes in brain activity and linking them to his emotional experience. Neuroimaging technology now allows researchers to study the brain in action, for example, by measuring changes in blood flow, oxygenation, and glucose utilization in different areas while participants engage in various tasks. Although ignorance still abounds, we now know a great deal about how different brain areas relate to different psychological functions. Thus, if a particular area of the brain is damaged or improperly functioning, we can predict what abilities will be disrupted.

For example, knowing that the ability to interpret speech is mediated by the left temporal lobe, we can predict that damage to this area will impair speech perception. Correspondingly, neuroimaging research shows that when individuals are engaged in interpreting speech, brain activity increases in the left temporal lobe.[313] Accordingly, by identifying areas of the brain that show altered activity in depression, we can sharpen our understanding of the symptoms of depression. Most important, by studying how therapeutic interventions—not only medications but also psychotherapy—influence brain activity in these impaired areas, we can refine our treatment approaches.

SOME CAVEATS

Beware that I'm about to summarize a relatively new area of research; we have a combination of well-replicated findings and new frontiers. Readers unfamiliar with this territory should keep in mind several caveats:

- Individual brains differ from one another in physical structure and patterns of connection, owing to each individual's unique history. Research necessarily glosses over these individual differences by examining groups of individuals to look for general patterns.
- Beyond individual differences, neurobiological findings are influenced by sex and age differences as well as by differences in history of medication treatment.
- Depression is heterogeneous, varying in degree of severity and pattern of symptoms. Research indicates that different subgroups of depressed persons show different patterns of brain changes.
- Brain research focuses on major depression, and its implications for brain changes in other forms of depression, such as dysthymia, are unclear.
- Researchers are challenged to identify what brain changes reflect the current *state* of depression and what changes are indicative of a more longstanding *trait* that indicates an enduring vulnerability to depressive states.
- Different neuroimaging techniques yield different findings, and all neuroimaging technology faces limitations in the precision with which brain areas can be identified, as well as in the slice of time in which changes in activity take place. New refinements in technology will lead to far greater precision in future research.
- Finally, although it might not be obvious to the uninitiated, I am presenting the findings at a global level, glossing over innumerable details. Comparing the research I'm discussing to a mountain range with a highly variegated landscape, I'm taking a panoramic perspective, looking at a few conspicuous peaks from a great distance.

You're not reading this book for the purpose of learning neuroanatomy but rather to understand depression more fully. Thus I have organized this section according to psychological capacities and highlighted selected brain areas that relate to these capacities. You need not remember the specific brain areas involved; rather, you should appreciate that there *are* specific brain areas connected with the problems of depression.

EMOTIONAL IMBALANCE IN THE FRONTAL CORTEX

Although we prefer positive to negative emotion, we need both: negative emotion disengages us from things we need to avoid; positive emotion keeps us engaged with things we need for our well-being. As you know, depression brings imbalance: too much negative, too little positive.

Using electroencephalographic (EEG) recording of brain activity, psychologist Richard Davidson and his colleagues[314-316] linked this depressive imbalance to asymmetry in right-frontal versus left-frontal patterns of brain activity. As I noted earlier in this chapter, consistent with its holistic and novelty-oriented style of processing information, the right hemisphere is more specialized for emotion.[282] Yet Davidson's research refines this specialization. Activity in the right frontal cortex is elevated in the context of negative emotion, such as fearful withdrawal from a noxious stimulus. Conversely, activity in the left frontal cortex is elevated in the context of positive emotion, such as an inclination to approach a potentially rewarding situation.

Recall that your prefrontal cortex enables you to keep images and goals in mind; you need to have approach goals and avoidance goals, activation and inhibition. Keeping something you want to avoid in mind, you feel anxious, and your right frontal cortex is relatively active; keeping something you desire in mind—activating your seeking circuitry—you feel excited, and your left frontal cortex is relatively active.

Davidson also has discovered that more enduring emotional *styles*—being characteristically more cheerful or fearful—are associated with corresponding patterns of frontal imbalances.[314] That is, in childhood as well as adulthood, the resting level of electrical activity is elevated in the right frontal cortex for persons who are more prone to anxiety and elevated in the left frontal cortex for those who are more disposed toward positive emotion.

Depression is associated with diminished left-frontal activity, consistent with the cardinal symptoms of depression: decreased capacity for pleasure, decreased interest in potentially enjoyable activities, and a pervasive decline in goal-oriented motivation and activity.[317] Conversely, persons who characteristically show elevated left frontal activation also show a greater resilience in the sense that they are more able to use positive emotions to regulate and rebound from negative emotions.

These differences between cerebral hemispheres are evident early in life. For example, psychologist Tiffany Field and colleagues[127] found that depressed women and their newborns had elevated right frontal activation. As in adulthood, these patterns of activation relate to emotional behavior: infants who show elevated right hemisphere activation also show more sensitivity to separation from their mother, for example, being more prone to crying;[317] infants of nondepressed mothers show elevated left frontal activation when playing with their mothers, whereas infants of depressed mothers fail to show this pattern;[318] finally, for infants of depressed mothers, reduced left frontal activity is associated with lower levels of expressed affection toward the mother.[182]

EMOTIONAL IMBALANCE IN THE LIMBIC SYSTEM

Evidence of changes in amygdala activity demonstrates most directly how depression is a high-stress, high-anxiety state. As noted earlier, the amygdala rapidly responds to threatening situations and orchestrates fear responses.[319] Psychiatrist Wayne Drevets, who has conducted extensive neuroimaging research on depression, found elevated blood flow in the amygdala for depressed persons and, moreover, observed that the magnitude of the amygdala abnormality correlated directly with the severity of depression.[320] Furthermore, increased amygdala activity has been observed in depressed persons even during sleep.[321] The magnitude of abnormal amygdala activation in depression is substantial, roughly equivalent to the levels observed in animals who are exposed to fear-conditioned stimuli.[322] Fortunately, successful treatment normalizes amygdala activity, although persons who show persistently elevated amygdala activity despite treatment remain at risk for relapse.

Whereas the amygdala serves an alerting and arousing function, other areas of the limbic system participate in registering and regulating visceral activity, which we experience as gut feelings. Drevets[323] also observed abnormalities in the ventral part of the anterior cingulate cortex, which may be associated with the failure to regulate stress-related physiology.

Subcortical structures involved in pleasure and reward also have been studied in depression. As noted earlier, dopamine activation of the nucleus accumbens plays a significant role in responsiveness to potentially rewarding stimuli and goal-directed, appetitive behavior—seeking. Drevets[322] summarized research on depression indicating abnormalities in brain structure as well as dopamine function in the vicinity of the nucleus accumbens. Moreover, as we all know from experience, when we feel threatened—as we are likely to do with a hyperactive amygdala—we're less inclined to engage in rewarding activities.

To recap, at both the level of the cerebral cortex and the limbic system, abnormalities in brain structure and function are consistent with the experience of depression: it's a high-stress state, often associated with anxiety, accompanied by a reduced capacity for pleasure and a diminution of goal-directed activity.

IMPAIRED AGENCY AND PREFRONTAL FUNCTIONING

Numerous studies of depression have revealed widespread abnormalities in the prefrontal cortex. These studies have shown abnormalities in brain structure[292] as well as brain activity.[283,304,324,325] Thus, on top of decreased motivation, the impairment of prefrontal functioning further undermines the capacity to organize and maintain goal-directed action—the essence of agency.

Consistent with impaired executive functioning, depression notoriously undermines various aspects of cognitive functioning: attention, concentration, memory, and complex problem solving. One noteworthy neuroimaging study examined depressed and nondepressed persons while they were engaged in a complex problem-solving task.[326] Previous research had shown that successful performance of the task is associated with elevated prefrontal cortical activity and that the task is sensitive to cognitive impairments in depression. The task involves a combination of relatively easy and relatively difficult problems. When performing the difficult problems, depressed persons failed to show the expected activation of the prefrontal cortex. Not functioning optimally, the prefrontal cortex was unable to rise to the challenge. The depressed participants were unable to initiate and sustain the mental activity required to solve the problems, and they were unable to evaluate the adequacy of their responses.

As you think about the import of impairment in prefrontal functioning, keep in mind that interacting with others—mentalizing—is a cognitively and emotionally challenging endeavor that also depends substantially on the prefrontal cortex.[327–329] Like other forms of complex problem solving, social interactions require considerable brainpower. When you are depressed, you can find that it takes a great deal of effort to socialize. The sheer mental effort involved—when you're low on energy—is a major reason for depressed persons to withdraw from social encounters. Here catch-22 assumes major proportions, because social isolation is such a significant contributor to depression. Yet there's another important problem with isolation: owing to all the difficulties associated with prefrontal impairment—initiating activity, seeking pleasure, thinking flexibly, and solving difficult problems—you'll need to make use of help from other persons. All of us rely on each others' prefrontal cortexes; when you're depressed, you need to do so more extensively despite your inclination to withdraw from contact.

EMOTION AND REASON: COOPERATION AND COMPETITION

MacLean's notion of a neomammalian brain sitting on top of a paleomammalian brain is appealing in part because it captures the potential tug-of-war between emotion and reason that we all experience from time to time. Yet we should not be misled by either language or neuroanatomy into drawing a bright line between reason and emotion: we need emotion to guide our reasoning. Ideally, we reason emotionally, and coordinated prefrontal and limbic activity is the norm.[287] Yet, as we all know, powerful emotions can undo our reasoning and problem-solving capacities. There's an adaptive side to this: sometimes we need to quit thinking and go into the fight-or-flight mode. Thinking would just slow us down when we need to cope with a charging bear. Most often, however, we need reason and emotion working together.

As we've seen, the prefrontal cortex both interprets and regulates emotion; impairment of prefrontal functioning, in conjunction with hyperarousal in the limbic system, makes for a troublesome combination. Drevets[322] speculated that this dysfunctional pattern of the brain relates to a major problem in depression, obsessive rumination. Under the pressure of heightened emotional distress, and with diminished flexibility in thinking, you can spin your wheels in a rigid fashion, recycling depressing thoughts. This vicious circle fuels the spiral into depression and maintains the depressed state (see Chapter 12, "Flexible Thinking").

Catch-22 has lodged in the brain. Depression draws your attention inward. As Drevets spelled out, coping entails pulling yourself out of depressive ruminations by distracting yourself, engaging your mind in some productive activity.[330] You need to shift your attention from the inner world of distress onto the outer world of emotionally neutral—or positive—territory. However, you know this shift isn't easy, and your brain is organized so as to make it especially difficult when you're depressed. The brain areas implicated in depressed states (amygdala, ventral prefrontal cortex, and ventral anterior cingulate cortex) are reciprocal with those involved in productive cognitive activity (dorsolateral prefrontal cortex and dorsal anterior cingulate cortex); their reciprocity means that activating one region deactivates the other.

Deactivating the brain areas maintaining depression requires *active* engagement with the outer world, such as holding a conversation; passive attention, such as watching television, is insufficient. You need to shift gears, in effect, reorganizing your pattern of brain activity. This challenge goes against the grain of the brain. Knowing the brain circuitry might help you to appreciate why it's such an effort to disengage from depressive ruminations and to focus your attention outward. Often, you'll need the help of others to do it. Two prefrontal cortexes are better than one.

REVERSIBILITY WITH TREATMENT

Documenting changes in brain activity associated with depression attests to the seriousness of the illness. This knowledge can be both reassuring and alarming: reassuring in underscoring that there's reason for the difficulty you're having, but alarming in implying that your brain is damaged. You can temper your alarm with two considerations: first, the brain is highly plastic, otherwise we couldn't develop or learn anything; second, the brain changes associated with depression are at least partly reversible, otherwise no one would ever recover. Although the extent to which adverse brain changes are reversible is an area of ongoing investigation, two kinds of brain changes are associated with recovery: normalization of functioning, in which patterns of brain activity return to the predepressed state, and compensatory processes, in which new patterns compensate for remaining impairments.

Psychiatrist Helen Mayberg and colleagues' research exemplifies current efforts to investigate how patterns of brain activity change with treatment.[331] Consistent with the challenge of integrating emotion and reasoning, these authors emphasized the significance of altered *interactions* among different brain regions in depression:

> It is now generally understood that depression is unlikely to be the result of a single brain region or neurotransmitter system. Instead, it can be conceptualized as a multidimensional, systems-level disorder affecting discrete, but functionally integrated, pathways. Moreover, depression is not simply the result of dysfunction in one or more of these elements, but also involves failure of the remaining system to maintain homeostatic emotional control in times of increased cognitive or somatic stress. (p. 194)

To reiterate, the balance between limbic activation and cortical regulation shifts in depression. Mayberg and colleagues[332,333] observed that experimentally induced sadness and clinical depression increase limbic activity (in the ventral anterior cingulate) and decrease cortical activity (in the dorsolateral prefrontal cortex). Again, these findings demonstrate reciprocity between limbic and cortical functioning: when we're sad or depressed, emotion occupies our attention, and we focus inward as limbic-system activity predominates; our capacity for effective engagement with the outer world is diminished as cortical activity (particularly the dorsolateral prefrontal area) decreases.

Conversely, successful treatment with antidepressant medication suppresses limbic system activity below the normal level (a compensatory process) and increases prefrontal functioning (a normalizing process). The findings associating treatment interventions with changes in brain activity vary considerably from one study to another, depending on the patients treated and the specific treatment interventions. Yet the normalization of prefrontal functioning is the most consistently replicated finding.[333] This normalization is essential; both overactivity and underactivity are disruptive, as Mayberg[331] notes:

> Frontal hyperactivity is now viewed as an exaggerated or maladaptive compensatory process resulting in psychomotor agitation and rumination, serving to override a persistent negative mood generated by abnormal chronic activity of limbic-subcortical structures. In contrast, frontal hypometabolism seen with increasing depression severity is the failure to initiate or maintain such a compensatory state, with resulting apathy, psychomotor slowness and impaired executive functioning. (p. 197)

To reiterate, normal prefrontal functioning enables us to regulate emotional distress effectively, as well as to direct our attention flexibly to the outer world so as to distract ourselves from distress. As Mayberg[331] reviewed, a wide range of treatments—not only antidepressant medications but also electroconvulsive therapy, vagus nerve stimulation, and surgical procedures—dampen excess limbic-system activity and thereby enhance prefrontal functioning. Notably, when they are effective, placebos (neurochemically inert substances) also are associated with brain changes paralleling those with antidepressants, although to a lesser extent than active medication treatment.[334]

Of course, we routinely alter our pattern of brain activity by exerting mental control, for example, when we regulate our emotions by thinking realistically or engaging in a distracting activity. Naturally, we're better able to exert control when we're not depressed and our prefrontal cortex is fully functioning. Accordingly, as Mayberg reviewed,[331] cognitive therapy (see Chapter 12, "Flexible Thinking") is associated with changes in brain activity. Preliminary studies also suggest that interpersonal therapy (see Chapter 13, "Supportive Relationships") is associated with changes in brain activity.[335,336]

Although these treatment findings are encouraging, a great deal more work has been done on identifying adverse brain changes associated with depression than on the beneficial impact of treatments on brain functioning. In addition, far more work has been done on the effects of antidepressant medication than on psychotherapeutic approaches. The effects of all these treatments are by no means identical; as I warned at the beginning of the chapter, I've been glossing over differences.

Psychiatry has not reached the point of being able to employ neuroimaging to diagnose depression, much less to predict which individual will respond best to which form of treatment. Yet we can be hopeful that neuroimaging methods will inform clinical practice in the future. Mayberg and her colleagues, for example, are investigating how particular patterns of brain activity predict an individual's capacity to benefit from a particular form of treatment.[115] For example, based on different patterns of interaction among seven brain regions, these investigators were able to identify differences between patients who responded better to cognitive-behavioral therapy and those who responded better to antidepressant medication.

As psychologists Anthony Roth and Peter Fonagy[17] have proposed, the question is not what treatments work—they all do to varying degrees. Rather, what works best for whom? Psychologists have been chipping away at this question for decades, and now we can look forward to some help from neuroscience—perhaps in the not-too-distant future, given the pace and creativity of current research.

BRAIN, MIND, AND CATCH-22

All these neurobiological findings are consistent with viewing depression as a brain disease. Yet there's plenty of psychology behind the development of the physical illness. Viewing depression as the brain's response to sustained stress,[230] we should keep in mind that the stress is psychological and interpersonal. Ultimately, it's the *meaning* of stressful events and the *subjective emotional experience* that translates into sustained stress in the brain and body.

We can now begin to understand how brain and mind conspire in eroding agency and squeezing your elbow room. Catch-22: to cope with depression, you need to be able to think flexibly, to interact with others effectively, and to mentalize—be attuned to yourself and others. With your limbic system in overdrive and your prefrontal functioning compromised, all these tasks are difficult. To reiterate Styron's[2] apt phrase, you may be dealing with a "storm of murk." Remember that catch-22 makes recovery difficult, not impossible. You are not dealing with an all-or-nothing situation: no one has found a complete cessation of brain activity associated with depression! The findings show *altered* activity, increases and decreases. You'd best cut yourself some slack as you exert leverage over yourself with your remaining elbow room: it's not impossible to do the things you need to do, but it's much harder than it would be if you weren't depressed.

Fortunately, the mind-brain relation goes both ways. Antidepressant medication can help normalize brain functioning and, thereby, your physical health and mental well-being. Conversely, positive behavioral, psychological, and interpersonal changes can help reverse the changes in brain functioning. The interplay of physiology and psychology is the reason that the best treatment of depression often involves a combination of medication and psychotherapy (see Chapter 14, "Integrating Treatment"). Knowing what we do about the reversibility of brain changes in depression, it's clear that you can do something about it, but bear in mind that you can do it more easily with help from others.

Chapter 10

RELATED DISORDERS

Unfortunately, having one illness does not prevent you from having another; being diabetic doesn't preclude having hypertension. So it is with psychiatric disorders. Depression commonly occurs in conjunction with other psychiatric disorders, and this co-occurrence complicates the treatment of depression, just as depression can complicate the treatment of other psychiatric disorders or general medical conditions. A common example: alcohol abuse can worsen depression, and depression can promote alcohol abuse.

Accordingly, as you're aspiring to recover from depression and to remain well, you need to consider related psychiatric problems that should be addressed concurrently. Depression could be associated with many psychiatric disorders, and there's no room here for a mini-textbook of psychiatry. I highlight a few prominent disorders that are often intertwined with depression: bipolar disorder, anxiety disorders, substance abuse, and personality disorders. I also alert you to the potential role of general medical conditions in depression. Although they are not psychiatric disorders, I conclude with a discussion of suicidal states, because these are such a problematic aspect of severe depression.

BIPOLAR DISORDER

For most of its history, bipolar disorder has been called *manic-depressive* illness, because this disorder involves cycling between episodes of mania and depression. The term *bipolar* indicates that mood can swing in two opposite directions, one pole being manic, the other depressed.

POSITIVE EMOTIONALITY IN EXCESS

The concept of a spectrum of positive emotion helps pinpoint the distinction between mania and depression.[4] I've emphasized that depressed mood entails a low level of positive emotion: an inability to experience interest, excitement, pleasure, and joy. When you're depressed, you lack the incentive to do anything; nothing seems rewarding. In contrast, positive emotion facilitates behavioral activation, approach behavior, and responsiveness to reward—what Panksepp[7] aptly dubbed *seeking*. Thus, in a manic state, you are apt to be engaged in a wide variety of rewarding activities, being overly responsive to a range of incentives—everything seems appealing. The seeking system goes into overdrive, fueled by a feeling of boundless energy. Manic activities potentially include a high level of sociability, ranging from excessive talkativeness to indiscriminate sexual encounters; spending sprees, including gambling; imprudent business ventures, including risky investments; and, more generally, taking on an unmanageable number of commitments and becoming involved in unwieldy conglomerations of projects.

Although mood swings are the core of bipolar disorder, like depression, mania involves more than mood disturbance: changes in thought patterns, behavior, activity, and relationships also occur. Thus the diagnostic criteria for a manic episode include elevated mood and many other symptoms.[8] The mood criterion involves a period of at least 1 week of abnormally elevated, expansive, or irritable mood. Other symptoms include inflated self-esteem, decreased need for sleep, talkativeness, racing thoughts, distractibility, and an increase in goal-directed activity. Irritability and aggressiveness relate to the enhanced power of potential rewards: persons in a manic state are easily frustrated when their pursuit of incentives is thwarted. They are also liable to be dominating and controlling—at worst, steamrolling others into going along with their ill-considered plans.

Some of these polar contrasts between depression and mania are illustrated in Table 10–1. As the broad diagnostic criteria indicate, these polar opposites revolve around not just pleasure but also tempo, energy, activity, self-concept, and sociability. Note that sleeping and eating too little often

TABLE 10-1. The bipolar spectrum

Depression	Mania
Deficient pleasure	Excess pleasure
Slow tempo	Fast tempo
Low energy	High energy
Inactivity	Hyperactivity
Worthlessness	Grandiosity
Social withdrawal	Social intrusiveness

accompany mania, which is also true of depression, but there's a difference: in mania, you may feel *little need* to sleep or to eat, whereas in depression, you're likely to feel *unable* to sleep (due to insomnia) or eat (due to lack of appetite).

DEGREES OF MANIA

Like depression, mania occurs in degrees: mania is more severe than *hypomania* (*hypo* meaning beneath or below). Although hypomania involves a distinct change in mood, it doesn't lead to significant impairment in functioning. Indeed, many persons value hypomanic states not only because their mood is elevated but also because they feel energetic and can be highly productive.

Three levels of bipolar disorder are distinguished, based on the severity of the mania and depression.[8] *Bipolar I* disorder entails cycling between mania and major depression; *bipolar II* disorder entails cycling between hypomania and major depression. These two forms of bipolar disorder are fairly stable over time, such that bipolar II doesn't typically evolve into bipolar I.[337] The third (least severe) form of bipolar disorder is *cyclothymia*, which entails cycling between hypomanic and depressive symptoms. In cyclothymia, the depression falls short of major depression in severity.

Thus we can distinguish between bipolar depression (major depression in the context of bipolar I or bipolar II disorder) and unipolar depression (major depression with no history of mania or hypomania). Unipolar and bipolar *depression* are similar in symptom patterns and thought patterns (negative thinking and low self-esteem) as well as in the precipitating stressors (stressful life events).[338] In addition, bipolar and unipolar depression are likely to respond to the same forms of psychotherapeutic treatment, such as cognitive therapy or interpersonal therapy, although the pharmacological treatment will be different given the risk that treatment of bipolar depression with antidepressant medication alone might precipitate mania[189] (see Chapter 14, "Integrating Treatment").

STRESS AND MANIC EPISODES

Bipolar disorder is often regarded as being relatively biological, because genetic determinants are more strongly associated with bipolar disorder than with unipolar depression.[339] Yet the biological aspects of mania should not blind us to psychological factors any more than they should do so in relation to depression.

Stressful life events, for example, have been found to be predictive of mood episodes in persons with bipolar disorder, just as they have been for persons with unipolar depression.[340] Yet the *kind* of stressful events that trigger mania differ from those that trigger depression (including bipolar depression). Specifically, two kinds of stressful events have been shown to precipitate mania: social rhythm disruption and goal attainment.

Stressors that are disruptive to daily schedules, routines, and rhythms are particularly likely to trigger a manic episode.[341,342] Especially problematic are stressful events that disrupt sleep schedules. Social routines that lead to stable patterns of sleeping, eating, and exercise entrain circadian (24-hour) rhythms. Events that disrupt these rhythms have been found to trigger manic episodes. Common examples would be going to the emergency room in the middle of the night, traveling overseas, and doing shift work. However, breakups in primary relationships also can throw daily routines and schedules off kilter. Thus these psychological stressors have a disruptive biological effect by disorganizing body rhythms.

In stark contrast to depression, positive life events can trigger manic episodes.[343] Yet positive events in general do not trigger mania; the attainment of goals is the crucial factor. Examples are attaining a promotion, being accepted into college or graduate school, or starting a new romance. Why would attaining a goal trigger mania? Ordinarily, a person who has worked hard to attain a major goal will experience a letdown after achieving the goal. Having enjoyed the success, the person may coast for a while and take it easy. Persons with mania, on the other hand, can have the opposite reaction: they're hypersensitive to rewarding experiences. In a person predisposed to manic episodes, the pleasure-approach-reward system is easily revved up. Given a bit of a reward, the person goes into overdrive. Thus success could trigger a spiral of increasing goal-oriented or reward-seeking activity. Thus receiving an accolade could stimulate the person to launch a series of new projects with the hope of more accolades. Success whets the appetite for more.

Bipolar disorder fits right into the stress pileup model. First, although the *type* of stress differs, stress can precipitate a manic episode, just as it may precipitate a depressive episode. Second, as with depression, manic episodes have stressful consequences. Indeed, the consequences of manic episodes can be particularly devastating. One of the most significant problems with manic states is the impairment of judgment. Judgment involves two facets: anticipating the consequences of your actions and conforming your actions to those anticipations.[344] Thus reckless and impulsive behavior characteristic of manic episodes often leads to major life stress—relationship problems, debts, legal problems, and so forth. Hence part of the vulnerability to depression following mania is the further accumulation of stressful life events and the associated erosion of self-esteem.

INTERMINGLING OF MANIA AND DEPRESSION

The bipolar concept makes intuitive sense, because it's easy to identify manic-depressive opposites. Yet the bipolar stereotype obscures important clinical characteristics of mood disorder. Persons who have a manic episode and no history of depression are diagnosed as bipolar on the anticipation that they will ultimately cycle into a depressive episode. Yet a sizeable minority of persons—a fifth to a third—who experience a manic episode do *not* go on to develop depression.[338] Of course, the first manifestation of bipolar disorder might be a depressive episode; a 15-year follow-up study of persons hospitalized for major depression revealed that 19% subsequently developed mania and 27% developed hypomania.[345]

More puzzling than mania without depression is that a substantial minority of persons with bipolar disorder—roughly 30%–40%—experience *mixed states*.[346] In such states, depressive symptoms may alternate with manic symptoms from day to day or hour to hour.[347] These mixed states also may involve a more complex intermingling of manic symptoms not only with depression but also with anxiety and aggressiveness, a condition termed *dysphoric mania*.[348]

Given that depression and mania—not to mention anxiety and aggressiveness—occur in varying degrees of severity, the possible mixtures are endless. Moreover, these mixed symptoms may either exist simultaneously or fluctuate very rapidly. Furthermore, for a person with bipolar disorder, the process of recovering from one pole may entail an intrusion of symptoms from the other pole: in the course of recovering from mania, depressive symptoms may begin to intrude; alternatively, in the course of recovering from depression, manic symptoms may begin to intrude. Not to be confused with mixed states[349] is the phenomenon of *rapid cycling*, which involves a minimum of four distinct episodes of mood disturbance (including switches from one pole to the other) in a 12-month period.[8]

TREATMENT IMPLICATIONS

Problematically, many persons in the midst of a manic state are prone to deny difficulty and to resist involvement in treatment. Because manic states are pleasurable up to a point, mania is seductive and can be hard to give up. If persons in manic states will accept treatment, medication can be employed to facilitate recovery from manic episodes as well as in preventing relapse and recurrence.[350]

Notably, psychological interventions may be especially helpful in *preventing* manic episodes. As has been observed in depressive episodes, negative cognitive styles—an inclination to interpret stressful events in a self-referential and self-critical fashion—increase the likelihood of manic reactions to stressful events.[351] Accordingly, cognitive-behavioral therapy can be helpful in prolonging recovery and preventing recurrence. Moreover, research is helpful in having pinpointed the kind of stressors that trigger manic episodes. To the extent possible, persons who are predisposed to mania will do best to avoid disrupted schedules that interfere with sleep. Although it would be self-defeating to avoid attaining goals, predisposed persons can be attentive at such times to slowing down rather than revving up. In addition, disruption and conflict in close relationships plays a significant role in manic episodes,[352] so treatment that fosters the capacity to maintain stable and secure relationships is highly pertinent to bipolar disorder.

ANXIETY DISORDERS

I have emphasized throughout this book how depression and anxiety intertwine; hence many persons with depression meet criteria for an anxiety disorder.[353] Yet anxiety disorders are a heterogeneous lot, including generalized anxiety disorder, phobias, panic disorder, obsessive-compulsive disorder, and posttraumatic stress disorder (PTSD). All these disorders are associated with an elevated risk of depression. Most often, although not always, *symptoms* of anxiety precede depression. Similarly, most often, anxiety *disorders* precede depressive disorders.[353]

This sequencing of symptoms and disorders reflects an important difference between anxiety and depression: anxiety links to anticipated danger and a sense of uncertainty associated with feelings of *helplessness*; depression links to failure and loss associated with feelings of *hopelessness*. A period of uncertainty and anxiety typically precedes a conclusion that the feared outcome is unavoidable or has occurred. This sequence of helplessness and hopelessness is consistent with Bowlby's[198] observations on loss of an attachment relationship: agitation and anxiety are associated with the initial protest reaction which, over time, evolves into despair.

Diagnosing and treating anxiety disorders co-occurring with depression is essential, because the presence of an anxiety disorder on top of depression is associated with multiple adverse consequences: a prolonged time to recovery, a higher likelihood of chronicity and relapse, more impaired functioning, and a greater risk of suicidal states.[353] Although psychotherapeutic and medication treatment are effective for the combination of depression and anxiety disorders, it's crucial to tailor the treatment to the specific anxiety disorder.[354]

In this section, I focus on two anxiety disorders that frequently occur along with depression: generalized anxiety disorder (GAD) and PTSD. The diagnostic overlap between depression and GAD helps clarify the intertwining of anxiety and depression I've noted throughout this book, and the overlap between depression and PTSD underscores the role of traumatic stress in depression.

GENERALIZED ANXIETY DISORDER

Of all the anxiety disorders, GAD overlaps most prominently with depression.[353] The hallmark of GAD is excessive and uncontrollable anxiety and worry about a wide range of concerns, accompanied by symptoms such as restlessness, fatigue, concentration problems, irritability, muscle tension, and sleep disturbance.[8] These symptoms reflect a high level of negative emotionality; here the overlap between anxiety and depression is most conspicuous. Consistent with this overlap, genetic predisposition is shared between major depression and GAD, and this predisposition is evident in the personality trait of neuroticism (proneness to emotional distress) that, in turn, predisposes individuals to both disorders.[353]

To reiterate, although depression (low positive emotionality) and anxiety (high negative emotionality) are partly distinct from each other, they also show substantial overlap.[4,353] Rarely are persons with major depression free of negative emotionality; more commonly, persons with anxiety maintain their capacity for positive emotion, in which case they're not depressed—despite their anxiety. The hallmark of anxiety as distinct from depression is the physiological hyperarousal characteristic of sympathetic nervous system activation; symptoms include dizziness, heart racing, difficulty breathing, and feeling wobbly in the legs.[355]

POSTTRAUMATIC STRESS DISORDER (PTSD)

I have emphasized the central role of stress in the development of depression throughout this book, and I have highlighted trauma in childhood and adulthood as playing a significant part in stress pileup over the lifetime. Thus depression is a common trauma-related disorder.[144] *Trauma* refers to the lasting negative effects of exposure to extremely stressful events.[95] PTSD is one form trauma may take, and it's a particularly cruel illness: having gone through terrifying events, persons with PTSD continue to relive these events in their mind afterward, sometimes for months or even years.[8] These reexperiencing symptoms take the form of intrusive memories and powerful emotional upheavals, the hallmark of which is flashbacks, a feeling of reliving the trauma in the present. Sadly, sleep doesn't necessarily provide respite; traumatic events also can be reexperienced in the form of nightmares. Understandably, persons with PTSD have avoidance symptoms, for example, trying not to think or talk about the trauma as well as avoiding any situations that might evoke traumatic memories. At worst, such avoidance can lead to profound withdrawal and social isolation.

Darwin[33] prophetically observed that fear is the most depressing of the emotions, and persons with PTSD not only have gone through extremely frightening experiences but also remain afraid of the eruption of their symptoms—the reason for their avoidance behavior. Consistent with Darwin's view, a substantial proportion of persons with PTSD also have major depression.[144] As with other anxiety disorders, PTSD more often precedes depression than the converse.[356] Yet preexisting depression also increases vulnerability to developing PTSD in the aftermath of traumatic stress. Moreover, a history of depression puts individuals at a higher risk for exposure to traumatic stress perhaps, for example, by impairing their judgment or increasing the likelihood of interpersonal conflicts.[357]

Considering the potential role of trauma and PTSD in depression is essential, because PTSD complicates the treatment of depression, and interventions addressing trauma are essential when these two disorders co-occur.[144]

SUBSTANCE ABUSE

Substance abuse fits hand-in-glove with the stress pileup view of depression. As I've now belabored, most persons struggling with depression also must contend with anxiety. Both depression and anxiety are based on psychological stress coupled with altered patterns of brain functioning. Depression and anxiety are hard problems. Reducing depression and anxiety by improving psychological coping and interpersonal relationships is a major undertaking. It's little wonder that many depressed and anxious persons resort to altering their brain functioning directly by chemical intervention. The effects are powerful and immediate. Alcohol, for example, potently decreases negative emotion and increases positive emotion; hence depression and alcoholism often occur together. One study found that 30% of persons with a diagnosis of depression also had a diagnosis of alcoholism, and 40% of alcoholics also had a diagnosis of depression.[358]

The discovery that drugs alter mood is ancient. We humans cleverly have discovered and synthesized a wide range of substances that mimic our intrinsic brain chemistry,[359] serving as adjuncts to endogenous neurotransmitters and neuromodulators that play a role in arousal and mood.[360] Many of us use caffeine, alcohol, or nicotine routinely to alter our state of mind. Moderate use of substances like caffeine and alcohol can be beneficial,[361] but many of us are not so adept at regulating their use. We share with other mammals a proclivity to engage in compulsive self-administration of many substances. Like other mammals, our vulnerability to addiction is based on our genetic makeup and our history of stress. Unique among mammals, we've refined cultural tools for mood alteration over the ages and passed them on to future generations for ready use. Modern methods of manufacturing and distribution have rapidly increased the diversity, potency, and availability of addictive substances.

True, addictive substances dramatically relieve anxiety and depression, and they're readily accessible. Yet substance abuse also may serve as a *catalyst* for more severe depression, speeding up the process of becoming depressed by contributing to stress pileup (see Table 10–2). Alcohol is a prime example. Many persons use alcohol to avoid or escape distressing emotions, a proclivity dubbed *drinking to cope*.[362] We can view the pattern of drinking to cope as a red flag. A 10-year follow-up study showed that persons who drank to cope showed relatively high consumption and problem drinking; as you might expect, these individuals also were especially likely to increase their alcohol consumption during depressive episodes. Drinking while anxious and depressed is blatantly counterproductive: given stress pileup, abusing alcohol accelerates the slide into severe depression and prolongs your stay there. Author Andrew Solomon[114] speaks from experience:

> My experience is that alcohol is not particularly tempting when you are experiencing pure depression, but that it is very tempting when you are experiencing anxiety. The problem is that the same alcohol that takes the edge off anxiety tends to exacerbate depression, so that you go from feeling tense and frightened to feeling desolate and worthless. This is not an improvement. I've gone for the bottle under these circumstances and have survived to tell the truth: it doesn't help. (p. 226)

TABLE 10–2. How substance abuse contributes to stress pileup

Areas of stress	Examples
Stressful life events	Arrests, job loss
Interpersonal stress	Arguments, separations
Internal stress	Guilt feelings, shame
Stressful lifestyle	Time devoted to obtaining and using substances
Impaired coping	Impaired problem solving and emotion regulation
Illness	Exacerbates depression and other physical illnesses

A DEVELOPMENTAL PERSPECTIVE

The developmental pathways to depression and substance abuse are exceedingly complex, because there are innumerable possible routes to each of these disorders. Moreover, depression and substance abuse may influence each other in various ways over the course of development.

For many individuals, adolescence is a pivotal time for the development of both disorders. Just as in adulthood, depression and substance abuse are likely to compound each other in adolescence. A study of more than 1,000 high school students[363] distinguished those who had problems with depression or heavy drinking from those who had both problems. This mixed depression-alcohol group showed the highest levels of early childhood problems, stressful life events, poor coping, delinquent behavior, and substance abuse, as well as feeling they had poorer family support and performing most poorly academically. Notably, both the depression-only group and the mixed depression-alcohol group reported using alcohol to cope with their high levels of stress.

The Virginia Twin Registry study[247] illustrates how a number of developmental factors may cascade into substance abuse in adolescence then on to depression in adulthood. Two childhood risk factors were found to contribute to substance abuse in late adolescence: genetic vulnerability and childhood sexual abuse. Two additional risk factors in early adolescence also contributed to substance abuse in later adolescence: anxiety disorder and conduct disorder (antisocial behavior). Three stressors evident in late adolescence also fed into substance abuse during that period: low education, a history of trauma, and low social support. Contributing to stress pileup, substance abuse in late adolescence increased the likelihood of two important risk factors for depression in adulthood: being divorced and experiencing stressful life events.

PHYSIOLOGICAL CATALYSTS

A wide range of substances—opiates, nicotine, amphetamines, cocaine, alcohol, and cannabis—stimulate the brain reward system. Repeated use brings about long-term adaptive changes in the neurons, such that withdrawal results in the depression of this reward system. Thus failure to self-regulate drug use sets up a spiraling distress-addiction cycle.[360]

The fact that substance abuse may serve as a physiological catalyst for mood disorders is captured by the psychiatric diagnosis of *substance-induced mood disorder*. This diagnosis is made when a depressive or manic episode is precipitated by the *direct physiological effects* of a substance.[8] Substances that may trigger mood episodes include alcohol, amphetamines, cocaine, narcotics, and hallucinogens as well as a wide range of prescribed medications.

To warrant the diagnosis of substance-induced mood disorder, the mood disturbance must begin around the time of intoxication or withdrawal and persist beyond the typical period of intoxication or withdrawal. For example, a person who develops a clinically significant depression during withdrawal from cocaine and whose depression persists beyond 1 month after withdrawal is complete would be diagnosed as having cocaine-induced mood disorder with depressive features and onset during withdrawal. Notably, substance abuse also may trigger persistent symptoms of anxiety, which are diagnosed as substance-induced anxiety disorder.

DEPRESSANTS

The effects of central nervous system depressants, such as alcohol, barbiturates, and narcotics, illustrate how substances can be used in an effort to control depression and anxiety as well as how substance abuse may backfire. You can generally count on these substances to reduce anxiety dramatically—they inhibit neural excitement and dampen the anxiety circuits in the brain.[364] A careful study of the daily relationship between mood and drinking in moderate alcohol users showed that, over the course of a day, feelings of nervousness increased alcohol consumption, and drinking then decreased the feelings of nervousness.[365] This effect was particularly strong for men, for persons with a generally high level of anxiety, and for those with a family history of alcoholism. On the other hand, alcohol was less effective for reducing nervousness in persons with high levels of depression and those who were more prone to problem drinking. Importantly, pleasant moods also were associated with increased alcohol consumption, but depression and boredom were not. Although not shown in this particular study, for some persons depressants such as alcohol may temporarily reduce depression by producing a feeling of pleasure or euphoria. Even the relief from anxiety can produce pleasure.

The anxiety-relieving property of these central nervous system depressants, however, is just one side of the story. Withdrawing from them can produce rebound anxiety. Take away the anxiety-reducing agent, and the anxiety bounces back. The experience of withdrawal—or even the *anticipation* of withdrawal—contributes to the cycle of abuse and then to addiction. However, the most important point is the most obvious one: being central nervous system depressants, substances like alcohol and narcotics may ultimately make your depression worse.

STIMULANTS

Stimulants like amphetamines and cocaine have a direct effect on the pleasure circuits in the brain. Given that lack of pleasure is the core of depressed mood, stimulants are a direct intervention in depression. Yet high doses of stimulants can produce dysphoria—unpleasant moods—as well as paranoid anxiety. When you withdraw from stimulants, you may plummet into a state of depression. In addition, given that they activate brain circuits involved in excitement and pleasure, stimulants may trigger manic episodes in persons who are predisposed to bipolar disorder.

Moreover, whereas depressants dampen excitability in the nervous system, stimulants increase it. By increasing arousal, stimulants can activate the brain circuits that produce anxiety. This activation is especially risky for persons with a history of trauma who have PTSD. From the point of view of your nervous system, taking stimulants or withdrawing from depressants is akin to another blast of psychological stress[366,367] that further sensitizes your nervous system. Thus you may sensitize yourself to stress unwittingly by abusing stimulants or withdrawing from depressants. In addition, intoxication is a common contributor to traumatic events such as assaults and automobile crashes. Thus substance abuse, exposure to trauma, and a sensitized nervous system can be linked in a vicious circle.[144]

Abuse of depressants and stimulants entails using them erratically, in high doses and in various combinations, along with withdrawing from them. This erratic pattern is like having your nervous system on a yo-yo. The chemical intervention that briefly relieves anxiety and depression also undermines the stability of your brain functioning in a way that perpetuates anxiety and depression. No wonder people become addicted when more of the substance is needed to reduce its own adverse effects.

PSYCHOLOGICAL CATALYSTS

However, substance abuse is not just a physiological catalyst for depression. The psychological and interpersonal problems stemming from substance abuse contribute powerfully to stress pileup. The contribution of intoxication to traumatic events is just one glaring example. Consider also the internal pressure associated with substance abuse: quite often, persons who abuse substances feel preoccupied with the substance as well as ashamed and guilty. Also consider the external stress pileup: substance abuse undermines your ability to function, for example, producing restlessness, problems in concentration and memory, and malaise; then your impaired functioning may lead to further stress, for example, due to difficulties in maintaining a household or performing at work or school. Most important, substance abuse typically enflames interpersonal conflicts and thus provokes disruption in relationships. Such interpersonal stressors are the most common precipitant for depressive episodes, and they also impede recovery and provoke recurrences. Consider the flip side: social support is a prominent protective factor in relation to depression, and substance abuse commonly undermines that support.

Even without considering what's going on in your brain and the rest of your body, it's easy to see how substance abuse can be a catalyst in the stress pileup model. For example, you are at odds with your spouse, your drinking gets out of hand, your performance at work deteriorates, you lose your job, your spouse files for divorce, and you slide into major depression accompanied by alcohol dependence. The number of similar scenarios is endless.

SUBSTANCE ABUSE AND THE COURSE OF DEPRESSION

Substance abuse is problematic not only because it may speed the slide into depression but also because it interferes with the process of recovery from depression. One major research project tracked the relationship between alcoholism and recovery from depression over a 10-year period.[358] Compared with those who were not drinking, depressed patients with *active alcohol abuse* were *half as likely to recover* from their depression at any point in the 10-year period. Notably, those with a history of alcoholism who had stopped drinking were just as likely to recover as those with no history of alcoholism—regardless of the point during the 10 years they stopped drinking. It's never too late to stop.

Given that substance abuse can be a catalyst for depressive episodes and can interfere with recovery, we have ample reason to be concerned that substance abuse will increase the likelihood of recurrence after full recovery from depression. Stress plays a major role in initial episodes and in recurrent episodes of depression, and substance abuse contributes to physiological and psychological stress. Accordingly, a number of researchers[60,71] have identified substance abuse as one factor that contributes to relapse and recurrence of depression, although not all studies are consistent on this point. Surprisingly, the 10-year follow-up study just described did *not* find active alcoholism to be associated with recurrence of depression.[358] Yet a subsequent report of a 5-year follow-up of the patients in this study who showed both alcoholism and depression at admission found that remission in alcoholism did have a protective effect against recurrence of depression.[368] A study of more than 20,000 patients hospitalized for mood disorders in Denmark found that active alcoholism early in the course of depression significantly increased the risk of subsequent recurrence of depression, although alcoholism later in the course of the illness did not do so.[369]

No doubt, depressed persons should not drink when ill, nor should they resume drinking after they recover—not only because of the possibility of increasing the risk of relapse but also because drinking would interfere with recovery from future episodes if they were to occur.

DEPRESSION AND THE COURSE OF SUBSTANCE ABUSE

Two research projects illustrate how depression complicates recovery from substance abuse. One study of patients admitted to McLean Hospital for the treatment hospitalized for alcohol dependence distinguished those who had a diagnosis of major depression at admission from those who did not.[370] After discharge, patients who also had depression more quickly took their first drink and were faster to relapse back into alcohol abuse.

Another study of patients in a dual-diagnosis program[371] also showed that depression had an adverse impact on treatment of substance abuse (i.e., abuse of alcohol, heroin, and cocaine). Specifically, depression increased the likelihood of substance use after discharge from the hospital, and depression also decreased the likelihood of stable remission from substance dependence. Notably, patients who were depressed were three times as likely as those who were not depressed to relapse into substance dependence over the course of the 18-month follow-up period. The authors proposed that depression might contribute to recurrent problems with substance abuse in a number of ways: depression might interfere with the motivation or effort required to abstain from substance abuse; it might contribute to a pattern of negative thinking that would undermine abstinence; and it might contribute to self-medicating with substances.

TREATMENT IMPLICATIONS

Once depression and substance abuse become prominent, each must be treated in its own right. Even if depression clearly led to substance abuse, treating the depression and hoping that the substance abuse will take care of itself will *not* suffice. Conversely, even if substance abuse clearly led to a depressive episode that persists beyond the withdrawal phase, treating the substance abuse and assuming that depression will no longer be a problem will *not* suffice.

Substance dependence and major depression are inherently recurrent illnesses. Moreover, when you have both, the recurrence of either one will increase the chances of recurrence of the other. To reiterate, each must be treated in its own right, and each requires long-term self-care. In his book *Intoxicating Minds*, pharmacologist Ciaran Regan[372] concluded, "An addicted brain is distinctly different from a nonaddicted brain. Its metabolic activity, receptor sensitivity, and responsiveness to environmental cues are profoundly changed. Is addiction like other chronic relapsing illnesses, such as diabetes or hypertension?" (p. 75). Plainly, the answer is yes. A parallel argument could be made for depression, and both of these illnesses don't just produce changes in your brain; they also produce persistent changes in your *life*.

The treatment challenges are substantial, and you must take steps that extend beyond the period of acute recovery to maintain your health over the long-term. Ordinarily, treatment of severe depression will entail a combination of medication and psychotherapy. Treatment of substance abuse is similarly multifaceted,[373] and many persons benefit from 12-step programs in the process of recovery and in maintaining sobriety.[374] Yet persons with major depression have more difficulty becoming effectively engaged in 12-step programs,[375] attesting to the importance of treating depression in facilitating recovery from substance abuse.

Finally, in addition to proper treatment for each illness, positive lifestyle changes that enhance and maintain your general health and well-being will help prevent recurrence of both illnesses. As addiction specialist Avram Goldstein[359] maintained, the brain is a delicately regulated system that evolved over millions of years; he considered use of addictive drugs to be a "reckless chemical attack" on the brain and made the following analogy: "No prudent person would try to beef up the performance of a personal computer by jolting it with high voltage electric shocks" (pp. 68–69). Imagine instead manipulating your brain chemistry—turning up the reward system and turning down the anxiety system—with your mind, behavior, and relationships. Compared with abusing substances, this alternative is slow—

but sure. To reiterate, having both problems requires you to take care of your health over the long haul. There are worse fates.

PERSONALITY DISORDERS

I've emphasized several problems potentially linked to personality: the role of stress generation in interpersonal conflicts; attachment disturbance related to problems with dependency and self-criticism; and the trait of neuroticism. When such personality characteristics are associated with significant distress or impairment in functioning, personality disorders are diagnosed. Although personality disorders take many forms—as individual personalities do—they generally relate to persistent problems in interpersonal relationships.[376] The diagnostic manual[8] defines personality disorder more specifically as "an enduring patterns of inner experience and behavior that deviates markedly from the expectations of the individual's culture, is pervasive and inflexible, has an onset in adolescence or early adulthood, is stable over time, and leads to distress or impairment" (p. 685). Personality disorders are associated with stress generation and thereby linked to depression.

To a considerable extent, personality disorders reflect exaggerated personality traits. For example, a group of personality disorders characterized by anxiety and fearfulness includes *avoidant personality disorder*, reflecting social inhibition related to hypersensitivity to rejection; *dependent personality disorder*, reflecting submissive and clinging behavior associated with a need to be taken care of; and *obsessive-compulsive personality disorder*, reflecting a preoccupation with orderliness, perfectionism, and control. *Borderline personality disorder* is a more complex disorder, reflecting a pattern of emotional and interpersonal instability centered around attachment disturbance, namely, a fear of abandonment and aloneness.[377]

I have not picked these illustrative personality disorders at random; among all the personality disorders, they are most highly associated with depression.[378] The fact that the cluster of anxious personality disorders relates highly to depression is consistent with the general overlap between anxiety and depression. Borderline personality disorder is also characterized by a high level of anxiety and emotional distress[379] as well as highly stressful attachment relationships, in part owing to impairment in mentalizing capacities.[380]

In discussing variations in depression at the beginning of the book (see Chapter 1, "Depression"), I mentioned the provisional diagnosis of *depressive* personality disorder, a generalized pattern of unhappiness, pessimism, and feelings of inadequacy. Psychologist Theodore Millon[381] contrasted the symptoms in depressive personality disorder as being "less severe, more social in character, and more prolonged, if not lifelong, compared with those in the dysthymic diagnosis" (p. 289). Thus, in depressive personality, the focus is on interpersonal functioning, whereas in dysthymia the focus is on depressed mood. Nonetheless, there is considerable overlap, and the criteria for depressive personality disorder overlap considerably with neuroticism and negative emotionality; they include not only unhappiness but also worry, pessimism, and guilt feelings.

Given their overlap, disentangling depression, anxiety, and personality disorders is no small diagnostic feat. Yet diagnosing personality disorders is important, because they prolong the course of depression, increase the likelihood of relapse, and adversely affect treatment outcome.[72,382] Personality disorders are inherently stable and, as would be true of any habitual pattern of behavior, changing personality takes a great deal of time and effort. Yet given the entanglement of personality disorders with depression, the investment is justified. Fortunately, ample research shows that long-term psychotherapeutic treatment is effective for a wide range of personality disorders.[383–385]

GENERAL MEDICAL CONDITIONS

Innumerable general medical conditions can contribute to depression. Examples include endocrine disorders (e.g., thyroid disease), infections (e.g., HIV), degenerative diseases (e.g., Parkinson's disease), cardiovascular problems (e.g., stroke), and some forms of cancer.[8] Conversely, depression complicates the course and treatment of a wide range of general medical illnesses.[386]

Although it is far beyond the scope of this book to review this complex territory, I want to make one main point: you should obtain a thorough medical evaluation to investigate such possible causes of depression, even if the depression seems to have been brought on by a major stressor. If you're sufficiently imaginative, you can always come up with some possible psychological explanation for a depressive episode. Yet the fact that there is a bona fide psychological explanation by no means rules out the joint contribution of some general medical condition; psychology and biology conspire. If a medical condition is playing a role in your depression, it's crucial to diagnose and treat it.

More generally, your physical health plays a central role in your mood—and vice versa. Chronic stress, elevated cortisol, and depression are all intertwined. Stress can compromise immune function, contribute to type II diabetes, and promote heart disease.[289] Depression is associated with increased risk of heart attacks and strokes.[295,386] For such reasons, if you're grappling with depression, it's best to establish a relationship with a physician in which you receive periodic checkups to ensure that any pertinent medical conditions are diagnosed and treated. Conversely, maintaining your physical health plays a central role in improving your resilience to stress and depression.[387]

SUICIDAL STATES

The diagnostic criteria for depression include recurrent thoughts of death and suicide.[8] Some depressed persons long for respite through death without acting on that longing; others actively do something to bring about their death. As the diagnostic criteria imply, depression is the psychiatric condition most frequently associated with suicide.[388] The lifetime risk of suicide is reported to be in the vicinity of 15% of persons hospitalized for major depression;[64,389] the estimated risk is considerably lower—although still substantial—in depressed persons in the community. Of particular concern is the increasing rate of suicide among young persons,[390] which parallels the increasing prevalence of depression in this age group. Yet depression is only one of a wide range of psychiatric disorders associated with suicide; others include bipolar disorder, anxiety disorders, and substance abuse.[390] Moreover, as described earlier in this chapter, all these other conditions are often intertwined with depression.

Suicidal behavior is frequently confused with deliberate self-harm, namely, self-injurious behavior that does not involve an intent to die.[391] Examples are self-cutting without lethal intent, banging and burning oneself, and overdosing with pills for the sake of knocking oneself out for a while rather than dying. The primary purpose of such actions is to provide *temporary* escape from unbearably painful emotional states, whereas suicide is intended to provide *permanent* escape.[95] Of course, the line between deliberate self-harm and suicidal behavior can be blurry; in a distraught state, for example, a person might take a bottle of sleeping pills to knock herself out but be relatively indifferent to the possibility of death.

To complicate matters further, as Solomon[114] described, *thinking* about suicide can be a way of coping, also providing temporary respite to forestall permanent escape through action: "Knowing that if I get through this minute I could always kill myself in the next one makes it possible to get through this minute without being utterly overwhelmed. Suicidality may be a symptom of depression; it is also a mitigating factor. The thought of suicide makes it possible to get through depression" (p. 283).

I've worked with patients who have been continuously suicidal for months before they regained hope and wished to go on living. However, such prolonged suicidal states are rare. Far more commonly, a person with a vulnerability to suicidal behavior enters a relatively brief period of suicidal crisis. We need to understand what factors render some persons especially vulnerable to such crises so as to prevent suicidal actions during the crises as well as to decrease long-term vulnerability to suicidal states.

UNBEARABLE EMOTIONAL STATES

Many vulnerability factors increase the risk of a suicidal state. Not only are there genetic factors that predispose a person to depression but also there are genetic factors apart from depression associated with heightened suicide risk.[392] Other factors include a propensity to impulsive behavior, a history of aggression and violence, a family history of depression and suicidal behavior, and a history of substance abuse.[393,394] The most serious indication of suicide risk is a history of previous suicide attempts.[390]

What makes for a suicidal crisis? Quite often, as it is with depression more generally, a stressful life event—or series of events—brings on the acute suicidal state in a vulnerable person. Yet the *meaning* of the events to the individual is the crucial factor. Most crucial in the suicidal state is a feeling of being trapped and a conviction that the situation is hopeless.[395,396] However, the hopelessness in suicidal states relates specifically to the experience of being trapped in seemingly unending excruciating emotional pain. Often the events that trigger suicidal states involve an acute feeling of humiliation or shame.[393] Perfectionists are especially vulnerable to feeling mortified in the face of their ubiquitous feelings of failure; hence perfectionism is common in suicidal persons.[159] Accordingly, psychologist Roy Baumeister[397] emphasized *painful self-awareness* as the core of the suicidal state, and he viewed suicide as an *escape:* "The main appeal of suicide is that it offers oblivion" (p. 93).

INTERPERSONAL EFFECTS

We've seen that relationship problems play a central role in depression, and ruptures in attachment relationships—feeling let down, betrayed, humiliated, and abandoned—play a significant role in suicidal states. Yet deliberate self-harm and suicidal behaviors are extremely alarming to others and thus tend to escalate the very conflicts that precipitate them. For example, you might feel humiliated after being let down, then your suicidal reaction might drive a deeper wedge into the relationship by generating more fear and antagonism.

Quite often, other persons feel manipulated by self-injurious and suicidal behaviors, which they construe as attention-getting maneuvers. No doubt, some persons do employ suicidal threats manipulatively, for example, in an attempt to forestall abandonment—a maneuver that inevitably backfires. More often, however, as Baumeister[397] proposed, the intent is to escape from internal emotional pain; problematically, the suicidal person is *not* adequately considering the impact of their behavior on other persons.

Psychologist Mark Williams[396] made a useful point in construing deliberate self-harm and suicidal behavior as a *cry of pain* rather than a manipulative cry for help. He likened these cries to those of an animal caught in a trap and howling in pain. Although deliberate self-harm and suicidal behaviors are a means of escaping from pain, temporarily or permanently, they also serve as *expressions* of pain. Some persons feel that they cannot possibly express the depth of their emotional pain in words; only self-injurious actions will do. Yet these cries of pain evoke such alarming feelings that they often drive others away rather than reinstating the secure attachment ultimately needed to alleviate the emotional pain.

In her deservedly popular book on suicide, *Night Falls Fast*, Kay Redfield Jamison[390] poignantly addressed the impact of suicidal death on loved ones. Tragically, suicidal persons who are able to think beyond their personal pain to consider the impact of their death on loved ones get it backwards. As Jamison states, "However much it may be set in or set off by the outer world, the suicidal mind tends not to mull on the well-being and future of others. If it does, it conceives for them a brighter future due to the fact that their lives are rid of an ill, depressed, violent, or psychotic presence" (p. 292).

On the contrary, loved ones not only suffer from grief but also from traumatic loss—and potentially from depression. In the aftermath of a suicide, loved ones are likely to face horror, confusion, and—inevitably—guilt feelings, ruminating about what they might have done to prevent the suicide. By no means is depressive illness inevitable in survivors; yet active coping is essential to avert depression and other health problems. Sadly, the shame associated with suicide can undermine the process of obtaining social support when it is most needed. In this context, support groups can be especially helpful.

PREVENTION

We might liken suicidal states to a "perfect storm" in which many elements come together. I'd put emotional pain at the center of the storm. However, many other factors conspire. Anxiety or panic can add fuel to the suicidal fire. For a person who is in a suicidal state, intoxication with alcohol or drugs can be a primary catalyst for action, by virtue of clouding judgment and lowering inhibitions. Yet no one attempts or commits suicide without a method. Jamison[390] counseled:

> If someone is acutely or potentially suicidal, guns, razor blades, alcohol, knives, old bottles of medications, and poisons should be removed from the home. Medications that can be used to commit suicide should be prescribed in limited quantities or closely monitored, and alcohol use, which can worsen sleep, impair judgment, provoke mixed or agitated states, and undermine the effectiveness of psychiatric medications, should be discouraged. (pp. 258–259)

Tragically, persons in suicidal states believe that death is a *reasonable* way of coping with a hopeless situation. In the throes of deep emotional pain, they cannot see past their current plight. They cannot appreciate that their suicidal state is embedded in *illness*—as Jamison tersely put it, "Circumstances of life…dangerously ignite the brain's vulnerabilities" (p. 309). Having worked with a number of profoundly suicidal persons who have been glad to be alive years later, I'm convinced that suicide in depressed states is *un*reasonable. Looking back on her own nearly fatal suicide attempt, for example, Jamison declared simply: "I was fortunate enough to be given another chance at life" (p. 311).

Nowhere is the need for mentalizing more crucial, and nowhere is it more difficult than in a state of hopelessness in which all your mental energy is focused on escaping into oblivion. The first step toward mentalizing is the simple—but difficult—recognition that you are in a distressed *state*. I cannot overemphasize the importance of thinking in terms of a *state of mind*, particularly when you are in a suicidal state of mind. Here I want to emphasize the vast difference between *feeling* hopeless and *being* in a truly hopeless situation. You may *feel* hopeless when your situation is not hopeless. You may well be in a hopeless situation in the sense of finding it impossible to have something you treasure (e.g., after loss of a job, a death, or a divorce), yet you may slowly be able to find a way forward and not feel hopeless indefinitely (see Chapter 15, "Hope").

I can hardly think of a more difficult mental challenge than maintaining some sense of hope when you feel hopeless—a complex state of mind. Hence I keep emphasizing the fact that a suicidal crisis is a *state*. States change. Granted, an objectively brief suicidal state can seem like an eternity, given how painful and all-consuming the state can be. The ultimate mentalizing challenge: to be aware, when you're in the throes of suicidal despair, that your state of mind does not represent reality accurately. If you could only think "I'm in a state. How can I get myself out of it?" Catch-22 though it may be, you may need to reach out for help. At worst, if you feel completely without friends, you may need to seek public help, such as a suicide hotline or hospital emergency room. To the extent that your mentalizing capacity is limited, you need the objectivity that only another person can provide.

I realize that what I'm suggesting requires a huge mental feat: hoping when you feel hopeless and mentalizing when you want oblivion. Yet your capacity to mentalize gives you great potential power, and it can be lifesaving. Despite their suicidal states, the vast majority of persons reach out for help rather than following through with suicide, or they manage to get lifesaving help in the aftermath of a suicide attempt.

Above all, one point merits emphasis: the vast majority of persons who commit suicide—90% to 95%—have a diagnosable mental illness.[390] In the long run, the best way to prevent suicide is to obtain treatment for the illnesses that conspire to put you into a vulnerable state—not least, depression, anxiety, and substance abuse. Jamison's[390] advice exemplifies agency:

> Patients and their family members can benefit by actively seeking out books, lectures, and support groups that provide information about suicide prevention, depressive and psychotic illnesses, and alcoholism and drug abuse. They should question their clinicians about their diagnosis, treatment, and prognosis and, if concerned about a lack of collaborative effort of progress in their clinical condition, seek a second opinion. (p. 258)

As the complexity of depression and suicidal states attests, intervention and prevention entail working on many fronts, all of which entail variations of catch-22. This brings us to the next and final part of this book: coping.

Part V

COPING WITH CATCH-22

• C h a p t e r   1 1 •

HEALTH

In coping with depression, you may need to work on many fronts, contending with problems in sleeping, eating, activity, positive emotions, thinking, and relationships. Above all, you'll need to cultivate hope. I discuss all these fronts. However, you cannot work on all fronts at once; you will need to prioritize. If you're severely depressed, I think the first priority should be your *physical health*. As discussed in Chapter 10 ("Related Disorders"), when you become depressed, you should consider having a thorough physical evaluation not only to investigate general medical conditions that might contribute to depression but also to treat any such condition that may be undermining your health in any way. To recover from depression, you will need all the strength you can get.

Three cornerstones of physical health are adequate sleep, good nutrition, and physical fitness. Depression may interfere with all three. As discussed in Chapter 9 ("Brain and Body"), depression involves persistent changes not only in the nervous system but also in the rest of the body. Excess stress hormones can interfere with sleep, appetite, and energy. In addition, working on any front requires motivation, and motivation requires a capacity to be moved by rewards—to be interested, enthusiastic, and excited. Thus I view impaired capacity for positive emotional experience as a fundamental health problem. As we've seen, depression can interfere with the brain circuitry that supports your capacity to be moved by pleasure and rewards, and you may need to get this circuitry working again.

In this chapter I launch the discussion of coping by considering four domains of health: sleeping, eating, activity, and positive emotion. Of course, direct physiological intervention with medication often will play a crucial role in restoring your health. Yet, in my view, it's crucial for you to be an active agent in this process, in effect, assisting the medication not only by taking actions that bolster your physical health but also by working actively on your thinking and relationships. Consider Andrew Solomon's[114] counsel:

> We would all like Prozac to do it for us, but in my experience, Prozac doesn't do it unless we help it along. Listen to the people who love you. Believe that they are worth living for even when you don't believe it. Seek out the memories depression takes away and project them into the future. Be brave; be strong; take your pills. Exercise because it's good for you even if every step weighs a thousand pounds. Eat when food itself disgusts you. Reason with yourself when you have lost your reason. These fortune-cookie admonitions sound pat, but the surest way out of depression is to dislike it and not to let yourself grow accustomed to it. Block out the terrible thoughts that invade your mind. (p. 29)

SLEEPING

If you're depressed, you're likely to feel exhausted. I often think a few nights of solid sleep might be the single most therapeutic intervention for depression. Catch-22: you need sleep to recover from depression, and you need to recover from depression so you can sleep.

I think sleep problems are among the most daunting challenges of depression, and I cover several topics here: characteristics of sleep, the conflict between the drive to stay awake and the drive to sleep, the range of sleep disturbance associated with depression and related psychiatric disorders, the potential role of insomnia in precipitating depressive episodes, the importance of sleep hygiene, and treatment interventions for insomnia. Fortunately, given the prevalence of sleep problems, there are excellent guides for the afflicted. My favorite books are *The Promise of Sleep*[398] by William Dement, a pioneer in sleep research, and *No More Sleepless Nights*[399] by Peter Hauri, former director of the Mayo Clinic Sleep Disorders Center.

CHARACTERISTICS OF SLEEP

Our daily need for sleep is perhaps the most conspicuous sign that circadian rhythms organize our bodily functioning. These daily cycles affect a wide range of physiological processes, including body temperature, hormone secretion, cardiovascular activity, and gastrointestinal functioning; the fantastically complex brain organization that regulates them is being increasingly understood.[400] These rhythms are entrained by light, that is, synchronized to the daily light/dark cycle; such cues are called *zeitgebers* (from the German, time givers).

Although there are wide individual differences, most persons need to sleep about a third of the day (7–8 hours). As we all know from episodes of dreaming, sleep isn't homogeneous. The changing patterns of brain waves during sleep (measured by electroencephalography) reveal that we cycle through different levels throughout the night, each marked by a distinct pattern of brain electrical activity:[398] stages 1 and 2 are light sleep from which we are relatively easily aroused; stages 3 and 4 are relatively deep sleep, with stage 4—slow-wave sleep—being the deepest. After we fall asleep, we progress fairly quickly from stage 1 to stage 4; then we remain in stage 4 for a longer period. After about an hour, we enter into rapid eye movement (REM) sleep, during which we dream. After a relatively short first bout of REM sleep, we drift back into deep sleep (stages 3 and 4). We cycle through the stages from non-REM back to REM sleep about every 90 minutes, typically five times a night; yet over the course of the night, the periods of REM sleep become progressively longer and more frequent.

A TUG-OF-WAR

We have a drive to sleep, just as we have drives for food and sex.[398] The longer we're awake, the greater the drive to sleep. Dement[398] proposed that *clock-dependent alerting*, one of many circadian rhythms, opposes the drive to sleep. Largely kept in line by light-darkness cycles, clock-dependent alerting is high in the morning and wanes in the night, although there's a dip in alertness in the early afternoon as well, conducive to napping after lunch. Engaging in absorbing, exciting, demanding, or anxiety-provoking activities also opposes sleep by fostering arousal and alertness.

Over the course of the day, the drive to stay awake and the drive to sleep compete with each other more and more strongly. After a night's sleep, during the hours you are awake, you are building up a stockpile of *sleep debt*, which must be paid off by sleeping. You accumulate about 1 hour of sleep debt for every 2 hours you are awake. However, if you have difficulty sleeping, you may accumulate a large sleep debt. With a high load of sleep debt, you're stuck with a high sleep drive opposed by alerting, and the result is a compromise: you function in a state of fatigue. Fatigue and sleepiness are indications of the extent of sleep debt, and a good measure of sleepiness is the time it takes to fall asleep if you lie down, close your eyes, and allow yourself to sleep. If your sleep debt is extreme, you fall asleep in a few minutes; if it's low, you cannot fall asleep.

Sleep disturbance is part and parcel of ill health, and the added fatigue associated with sleep disturbance erodes several aspects of your mental functioning: alertness, reaction time, concentration, memory, and problem solving. Thus fatigue not only interferes with performance; it can be downright dangerous. We pay a great deal of attention to driving drunk but too little attention to driving tired. Falling asleep at the wheel is a common cause of traffic accidents and fatalities. Fatigue and monotony can conspire to put you to sleep in moments. We can only wonder how many accidents are connected with sleep disturbance related to depression and anxiety.

SLEEP DISTURBANCE

Sleep disturbance is one of the cardinal symptoms of depression, and it typically takes the form of insomnia—sleeping too little. To depressed persons, the various forms of insomnia are all too familiar: longer time to fall asleep (initial insomnia), awakening in the middle of the night with difficulty falling back asleep (middle insomnia), awakening early in the morning with inability to return to sleep (terminal insomnia), restlessness, and nonrestorative sleep.[401]

Extensive research on brain electrical activity shows a range of changes in sleep patterns associated with depression: decreased amount of slow wave (deep) sleep, more rapid onset and longer duration of REM (dreaming) in the first sleep period, and greater proportion of REM sleep throughout the night.[402] Psychologist Rosalind Cartwright[403] also observed that the dreams of depressed persons are more unpleasant; she views dreaming as an effort at problem solving and speculates that stress is overloading the dreaming system.

Although insomnia is typical, a sizeable minority of depressed persons—estimates vary widely from 15% to 33%—show a profile of reverse vegetative symptoms:[404] instead of symptoms of insomnia, lowered appetite, and weight loss, they show hypersomnia (sleeping too much) along with increased appetite and weight gain. Hypersomnia may be an effort to compensate for inadequately restful sleep. Many depressed persons also use sleep deliberately as an escape from stress.

Not only depression but also a wide range of other psychiatric disorders are associated with sleep disturbance. Although none of the symptoms or brain changes I've enumerated are unique to depression, these alterations are more widespread and pronounced in depression than in other psychiatric disorders.[402] Of course, as described in Chapter 10 ("Related Disorders"), many depressed persons also have other psychiatric disorders, and these other disorders can compound the problems with sleep.

As we have seen throughout this book, depression is a high-stress state often accompanied by anxiety. Anxious arousal interferes with sleep,[405] as it should: sleep is incompatible with the fight-or-flight response.[406] Trauma-related anxiety problems, which may be intertwined with depression, are especially disruptive of sleep, with symptoms including nightmares, awakening in a state of panic, fear of sleep, and abnormal movements (e.g., sudden jerking) during sleep.[407] In addition to anxiety, substance abuse is often associated with depression, and substance abuse also contributes to sleep disturbance.[402] Alcohol, for example, might be employed to combat anxiety or to induce sleep, yet alcohol interferes with the continuity of sleep.

A RED FLAG

Sleep disturbance is not just a symptom of depression; it's also a precipitating factor.[401] Plainly, insomnia can contribute to stress pileup in a number of ways. Moreover, insomnia can be a marker of vulnerability to depression,[408] and it's a harbinger of relapse, progressively worsening over the weeks preceding a depressive episode.[409] For persons vulnerable to depression, insomnia nearly every night for a period of 2 weeks can be taken as a warning sign of an impending episode and an indication that preventive steps should be taken.

With a vulnerability to depression, you should be especially alert to insomnia during times of social stress. Although light remains our primary zeitgeber, our biological rhythms are also entrained by social relationships. For example, marital partners tend to synchronize their mealtimes, bedtimes, and rest-activity cycles. As I described in discussing manic episodes (see Chapter 10, "Related Disorders"), disruptions in relationships—a breakup or a death—often disrupt routines and thus circadian rhythms as well.

Schedule-disrupting events can play an important role in triggering depressive episodes.[410] Given the role of insomnia in triggering depression, we can envision a cascading series of stressors: a breakup in a relationship disrupts routines, disturbs circadian rhythms, leads to insomnia, and ultimately triggers a depressive episode. Conversely, persons who are able to maintain their routines in the aftermath of losses are less likely to experience depression.

SLEEP HYGIENE

Catch-22 is perhaps nowhere more frustrating than in the area of sleep. You cannot force yourself or will yourself to sleep; the harder you try, the more you fail. Yet there are many things you can do to facilitate your ability to sleep; these strategies all go under the rubric of sleep hygiene.

Dement[398] provided a comprehensive strategy for managing sleep, and I summarize a few of his key points here. As I've already emphasized, sticking to a routine sleep schedule is crucial. Sleeping during the daytime—as many depressed persons are prone to doing—also interferes with nighttime sleep, contributing to many of the disturbances in sleep architecture associated with depression.[411] Winding down by engaging in relaxing activities prior to bedtime is also essential. Soothing bedtime rituals such as a hot bath, quiet music, or reading may help facilitate relaxation. Your bed and bedroom also should be conducive to relaxation; it should be a comforting place, quiet and properly heated or cooled. Developing *skill* in relaxation may be one of the most important aspects of coping with sleep problems. Relaxation techniques include deep breathing, progressive muscle relaxation, and guided imagery.[412] Like any skill, becoming proficient at relaxation requires extensive practice—and 3 A.M. is no time to start practicing! The more skilled you become, the better you are able to implement these skills in a pinch, both to help you settle down to fall asleep initially as well as to help you return to sleep if you wake up in a state of anxiety in the middle of the night.

Engaging in activating or stressful activities (e.g., discussing problems or arguing) before bedtime is counterproductive. Routine exercise can enhance sleep, but exercise is activating, so it should not be done within a few hours of bedtime. It's best not to eat a full meal within a few hours of going to sleep. It's obvious that you should avoid caffeine or other stimulants in the evening, but you may not be aware that it can take *several hours* for the caffeine to clear your system. Although alcohol is a relaxant, excess alcohol can cause rebound insomnia as it wears off in the middle of the night.

Thus you can do many things to improve the amount and quality of your sleep. However, Dement noted that 70% of Americans do not sleep alone. If your roommate or bedmate has habits that conflict with yours, or if the relationship is fraught with conflict and tension, the challenges of sleep hygiene are greatly magnified. This area may call for complex negotiations, and the benefits of a good bedmate cannot be underestimated.

TREATMENT

The best treatment for depression-related insomnia is optimal treatment for depression,[413] ranging from psychotherapy to antidepressant medication and including all the coping strategies discussed in this book. Yet as the extensive work on sleep hygiene attests, sleep problems often need to be tackled directly. Of course, as is true for depression more generally (see Chapter 10, "Related Disorders"), it's important to be sure that general medical conditions or prescribed medications aren't contributing to your insomnia.[399,413]

One of the most common problems associated with chronic insomnia is a conditioned anxiety response. Going to bed makes you anxious, because you anticipate the frustration of being unable to sleep. Peter Hauri[399] summarized a strategy to undo this conditioned anxiety:

1. Go to bed only when you are sleepy.
2. Use the bed only for sleeping; do not read, watch TV, or eat in bed.
3. If you're unable to sleep, get up and move to another room. Stay up until you are really sleepy, then return to bed. If sleep still does not come easily, get out of bed again. The goal is to associate the bed not with frustration and sleeplessness, but with falling asleep easily and quickly.
4. Repeat step 3 as often as necessary throughout the night.
5. Set the alarm and get up at the same time every morning, regardless of how much or how little you slept during the night. This helps the body to acquire a constant sleep-wake rhythm.
6. Do not nap during the day. (p. 88)

Hauri cautioned that you'll initially get little sleep when you employ this strategy. Yet as your sleep debt increases, you'll find it easier to fall asleep, and your sleep pattern will gradually become more normal.

A wide variety of medications—antianxiety, sedative, and hypnotics—are commonly prescribed to treat insomnia. Yet as psychiatrist Thomas Neylan[413] counseled, "Depressed patients who are receiving adequate treatment for depression ideally should rely on nonpharmacologic interventions for their sleep disturbance" (p. 59). Sleeping medications are best used on a short-term basis. Over the long term, your nervous system can become habituated, such that the medication is no longer helping but discontinuing it provokes insomnia.[399] Nonetheless, as Dement[398] detailed, there are very wide differences among sleeping medicines and many recent improvements; misguided prejudices against them often interfere with persons getting all the help they need. To reiterate, sleep deprivation is harmful in many ways, not least because it can play a significant role in the unfolding of a depressive episode or interfere with recovery. Thus the best thing you can do is work closely with a psychiatrist to be sure that you're taking the optimal medication if you need it and that you're not overusing it.

EATING

Typically, depression is associated with a decrease in appetite and weight loss, although the atypical pattern includes overeating and weight gain. Fundamentally, as described in Chapter 9 ("Brain and Body"), disturbance in appetite and eating is symptomatic of chronic stress. In addition, lack of enjoyment in eating is also part and parcel of the generalized inability to experience pleasure. Considering that good nutrition and proper weight are essential to health, and that physical health is crucial to resilience to stress, we must attend to catch-22: you should eat well, even if you have no incentive to do so. Of course, as it is with sleep, all effective treatment interventions, from psychotherapy to medication, will help restore your appetite. Meanwhile, you'll need to cope with catch-22.

When you have no appetite, there's no alternative to going against the grain, making a concerted effort to eat three meals a day. You might benefit from planning daily meals, following the plan, and keeping track of what you eat. One of the best ways to regulate your behavior is to monitor it by keeping a written record. Some depressed persons find that eating with others helps. Some make a point of selecting especially tasty foods. Some find that eating a little bit sparks their appetite to eat more. Many just plain force themselves to eat despite the lack of pleasure, knowing they need to do so.

Although lack of appetite goes with extreme stress and severe depression, more moderate depression is often associated with overeating. Food is a substance like alcohol or stimulants that can be employed to boost mood. Like alcohol or stimulants, the boost will be temporary, and it can backfire: eating can increase your energy immediately but then lower your energy an hour later. Most problematic, chronic overeating to control mood can lead to being overweight and thereby contribute to fatigue as well as undermining your health in many other ways.

Psychologist and mood researcher Robert Thayer[414] described the relationship between mood and food in his book *Calm Energy*. Thayer found that we are most vulnerable to overeating—what he calls emotional eating—when we're in a state of *tense tiredness:* anxious and depressed. High-energy foods—high in sugar and fat—are both mood elevating and calming, just as alcohol can be. Temporarily. Thayer is convinced that our high-stress lifestyle plays a major role in epidemic overweight. Eating is an easy and quick way to regulate your mood. He noted that, as the stress of the day wears on and tense tiredness increases, the likelihood of bingeing and overeating increases. Late afternoon and evening are therefore high-risk times for overeating.

Keep in mind that sleep disturbance will contribute to these states of tense tiredness, thereby increasing your inclination to overeat. The challenge is to get yourself into states of calm energy, the opposite of tense tiredness. As Thayer argued convincingly, one of the best ways to get into a state of calm energy is exercising, which brings us to the next topic.

ACTIVITY AND EXERCISE

Like sleeping well and eating properly, activity is basic to physical health. Catch-22: if you're depressed, you don't have the energy or motivation to do much of anything. It's a vicious circle: inactivity contributes to feelings of lethargy and unproductiveness. As I discuss shortly, we know that exercise is a good antidepressant, but you're not likely to have the energy to engage in vigorous exercise if you're severely depressed. You'll need to work up to it. Some profoundly depressed persons have difficulty even sitting up in bed, much less getting out of bed. Getting bathed and dressed can feel like climbing a mountain.

Take small steps. A cornerstone of cognitive-behavioral therapy for depression is developing an hour-by-hour schedule of activities and sticking to it as best you can.[236] Involvement in activities counters feelings of lethargy and also serves as a distraction from distressing preoccupations. Following the schedule provides an experience of success and promotes feelings of mastery. Activity is basic to agency: you gradually develop the sense that you can do something about your depression. I'm not talking about *enjoying* activity here, just being active. In the early phase of recovery, the goal is to get yourself going and to stay as active as you can throughout the day. Of course, developing a schedule puts you at risk for not carrying through with all of it—an expected occurrence when you're depressed. As with all else in life, some failures are inevitable; all you can do is persist.

When your energy begins increasing, you can begin physical exercise. Small steps. The beauty of exercise like brisk walking or jogging is that it readily lends itself to very gradual increases. For example, you can begin by walking slowly and for short distances and gradually build up to walking more briskly and for longer distances. You might proceed to more vigorous exercise like jogging, swimming, or bicycle riding. Ultimately, as your energy builds, you can adhere to a regular exercise schedule, a foundation of recovery and wellness. The potential benefits of exercise are legion: improved physical health, stress resilience, enhanced mood, and decreased anxiety.

Thayer's research[414] indicates that exercise is among the best strategies for getting yourself out of a bad mood, but there's relatively little experimental research on the effectiveness of exercise as an intervention for major depression, and the physiological mechanisms by which exercise might alleviate depression are unclear.[415] Yet one recent study yielded provocative findings.

Researchers at Duke University Medical Center[416] compared the effectiveness of exercise and antidepressant medication for older persons with major depression. Participants in the exercise group engaged in 30 minutes of cycling, brisk walking, or jogging at an aerobic level three times weekly. Those in medication group received the selective serotonin reuptake inhibitor Zoloft. A third group both exercised and received medication. Patients treated with medication responded more rapidly; yet after 4 months the majority of patients were no longer clinically depressed, and the extent of improvement was comparable in all three groups. A follow-up evaluation 6 months later revealed that the improvements were generally sustained for all three groups. Moreover, functioning at the follow-up point was related to the extent to which the individuals had *continued regular aerobic exercise*: each 50-minute increment in exercise per week was associated with a 50% decrease in the likelihood of being clinically depressed at the 10-month point. The authors of this study concluded provocatively that "exercise is a feasible therapy for patients suffering from MDD [major depressive disorder] and may be at least as effective as standard pharmacotherapy" (p. 636). More specifically, they noted,

> The present findings suggest that a modest exercise program (e.g., three times per week with 30 minutes at 70% of maximum heart rate reserve each time) is an effective, robust treatment for patients with major depression who are positively inclined to participate in it and that clinical benefits are particularly likely to endure among patients who adopt exercise as a regular, ongoing life activity. (p. 637)

Yet the authors also introduced a number of qualifications. Participants were recruited for a study of the effects of exercise on depression, and some were disappointed to be assigned to a group in which medication was prescribed. During the follow-up period, many of the patients who had been prescribed medication stopped taking it, and many who had not been exercising started to do so. Thus I would not interpret this study to mean that you can substitute exercise for medication. Rather, I consider exercise to be a cornerstone of a healthy lifestyle that counters depression.

POSITIVE EMOTIONS

Perhaps the most annoying advice for depression: "If you'd just go out and have more fun, you wouldn't be so depressed!" A truism. Catch-22: you can't easily experience pleasure or enjoyment. Just as people advise, you've probably tried to do things that will be enjoyable, but it hasn't worked. Activities that you've enjoyed in the past no longer provide any pleasure.

I find it helpful to think of this problem very concretely: the pleasure circuitry in the brain isn't working properly; metaphorically, you're low on cerebral joy juice,[6] and you need to jump-start the circuits. To some degree, despite your diminished energy, you can force yourself to be more active. But I don't believe that you can force yourself to feel pleasure; all you can do is make an effort to engage in activities that will provide an *opportunity* for enjoyment.

In this section, I start by reviewing the benefits of positive emotions and then discuss strategies for enhancing them. I conclude by drawing your attention to the variety of positive emotions.

FUNCTIONS OF POSITIVE EMOTION

I have referred to the functions of positive emotions throughout this book and merely include a reminder here. I'm partial to the concept of a *seeking system* that yields pleasure as an incentive to keep us engaged in activities that satisfy basic needs ranging from hunger, thirst, and sex to social contact and secure attachment.[7] Our memories of specific events are saturated with emotions, because we need to remember what to approach and avoid in the future. Anticipating reward is pleasurable; looking forward to enjoyable activities brightens our mood. The bane of depression is that you don't look forward to anything.

Keeping in mind the dual problems of too much negative emotion along with too little positive emotion, it's worth noting that enjoyable emotions also serve to dampen stress—what's been called an *undoing* function.[417] When you're in a state of stress, amusement can decrease your physiological arousal—the basis of gallows humor, perhaps.

Flying in the face of catch-22, a few strategies for cultivating positive emotion are worth considering: scheduling pleasant events, finding positive meanings in stressful circumstances, and paying attention to positive emotions.

SCHEDULING PLEASANT EVENTS

Over the course of decades, psychologist Peter Lewinsohn[418] has developed a behavioral treatment that includes a systematic strategy for countering depression by enhancing your involvement in pleasurable and satisfying activities. He developed the Pleasant Events Schedule to guide a comprehensive self-assessment. This schedule includes 320 activities, many of which you might find enjoyable (if you weren't depressed). The list is long, because there's a tremendous variety in the activities that people find enjoyable, and there are also enormous individual differences in what people enjoy. Lewinsohn found three general types of activity to be particularly helpful in combating depression: enjoyable interactions with others, such as being with friends; activities that enhance a sense of competence and achievement, such as completing a project; and inherently pleasurable activities that directly counter depression, such as laughing.

For each activity, you first indicate how often you have engaged in the activity recently, and then you indicate how characteristically enjoyable the activity has been for you. Next you select from the 320 activities those 100 that are most enjoyable for you. Then, to learn how your mood relates to your activities, for 1 month you keep track of your pleasant activities and your mood. You're likely to find that engaging in more pleasant activities will be associated with more positive mood. The final step is planning a *gradual* increase in enjoyable and satisfying activities to further enhance your mood. Lewinsohn and colleagues' book, *Control Your Depression*, clearly lays out the specifics.[419]

Lewinsohn recognized catch-22: feeling depressed, you engage in few pleasant activities and you are unable to enjoy them when you do; engaging in few activities means you're experiencing little reward, which is depressing. Yet he emphasized the possibility of turning this vicious circle around by systematic effort. I think you'll do best by respecting catch-22 and keeping your expectations modest. If you believe that you should find delight in the activities, you're likely to feel frustrated and disappointed. Then the whole strategy will backfire.

At first, being depressed, you may find little enjoyment in any of the activities you attempt. You're accomplishing a lot merely by getting yourself engaged in something that will take your mind off your suffering for a bit. Pleasure will increase in frequency and duration over time. Another bit of caution: some persons who've been depressed hit on something they enjoy. Then, understandably, they do it in an addictive way. They overdose on the activity, it becomes stressful, and the pleasure wears out. Go slowly with pleasure; it's best not to try to force it.

FINDING POSITIVE MEANING

Making an effort to find positive meaning in daily events can enhance your mood when you're coping with stress.[420] Psychologists Susan Folkman and Judith Moskowitz investigated this phenomenon in their study of persons caring for loved ones with AIDS.[421] They noted that positive emotions serve as psychological and physiological buffers, potentially short-circuiting the spiral of negative rumination that can plunge a person who is coping with stress into depression. Surprisingly, persons coping with stress may be *more* likely than others to experience positive emotions during the stressful period: they actively draw on positive emotions as a way of attempting to offset the distress.

Folkman and Moskowitz identified three kinds of coping that were associated with positive emotions. First, caregivers employed *positive reappraisals*, that is, ways of seeing a stressful situation in a positive light (i.e., the glass half full instead of half empty). In the caregiving situation, such reappraisals involved caregivers' awareness of their loving qualities and how their efforts preserved the dignity of their ill partners. Second, caregivers engaged in *problem-focused coping*, that is, efforts to gather information, make decisions, make plans, resolve conflicts, and acquire resources. Such coping required setting realistic goals and focusing on tasks that could be accomplished (e.g., performing caregiving tasks rather than curing their partner's disease). Such problem-focused coping combated feelings of helplessness and hopelessness by promoting a sense of mastery. Of course, effective coping is extremely important to the extent that it alleviates the problems that contribute to stress and depression. Third, caregivers *infused ordinary events with positive meaning*. Interestingly, virtually every one of the participants was able describe some meaningful event that made them feel good and helped them get through the day. Examples included preparing a special meal, getting together with friends, seeing a beautiful flower, or receiving a compliment.

Thus, the meaning of events plays a major role in positive coping, just as it does in becoming depressed. Folkman and Moskowitz emphasized that participants in their research were *not* clinically depressed, and they believed that the positive emotions caregivers were able to summon in these stressful circumstances may have served to prevent clinical depression. I believe that efforts to summon positive emotions may facilitate recovery from depression and help prevent relapse and recurrence. Some depressed patients, for example, benefit from listing a few things for which they are grateful each day.

ATTENTIVENESS TO POSITIVE EMOTIONS

As you're aspiring to restore your capacity to experience positive emotions, you're likely to find it slow going. When you do begin to experience pleasure, it's likely to be subtle. You are more likely to feel a spark of interest, involvement, or absorption in something rather than outright excitement or playful joy. I think it's important to pay attention to such subtle feelings that might signal the return of pleasure—a harbinger of recovery.

In his marvelous book *Emotions Revealed*,[422] psychologist Paul Ekman advocated *attentiveness* to emotions. Nowhere is such attentiveness more important than in cultivating positive emotions when you're depressed. You might try to be more aware of moments of interest or slight glimmers of pleasure. They won't last—you're depressed. But I think it's useful to turn up the dial on subtle glimmers of positive emotion: notice them, linger over them, and amplify them. I worked with a man who was hospitalized with profound depression after a pileup of losses. In one of his therapy sessions, he talked about how he had gotten involved in a board game with some other patients; in telling the story, he was animated, and there was a sparkle in his eye. He wasn't aware of the significance of this event as a sign of his improvement; only when I drew his attention to it did he recognize its importance. Then he was duly encouraged.

In sum, it's important not just to engage in pleasant activities but also to learn to *pay attention to your positive feelings* as they arise so as to cultivate and enhance them. You might think of each moment of pleasure as a dose of antidepressant. Savor these moments. In addition, you can benefit from attending to the sheer variety of positive emotions you might experience—pleasure, interest, enthusiasm, excitement, joy, love, pride, compassion, and contentment, to name a few. I discussed these emotions at greater length in the book *Coping With Trauma*[95] and will hit a few highlights here.

VARIETIES OF POSITIVE EMOTION

We can start with *pleasures* associated with the satisfaction of bodily needs and appetites, such as thirst, hunger, and sex. It's no surprise that evolution has wired us to experience pleasure in these life-sustaining activities. We also can distinguish between anticipatory pleasure and consummatory pleasure, for example, the contrast between pleasurable anticipation of a good meal and the enjoyment of eating it. Of course, anticipatory and consummatory pleasures often intermingle; the enjoyment of the first swallow of a tasty meal raises the anticipatory pleasure of the next bite. Regretfully, depression undermines the satisfaction of consumption as well as the excitement in anticipation. Neither food nor sex may be appealing or enjoyable.

In addition, we can distinguish between sexual pleasure and sensual pleasure.[163] Sensual pleasure, beginning in infancy, comes from being touched, held, stroked, and soothed. Sensual pleasure may spark sexual excitement, but it stands on its own. Sensual pleasure also may be extended to aesthetic pleasure, as evident in the powerfully pleasurable responses we may have to nature, art, and music.

Although we often think of positive emotions in conjunction with such highly arousing states as excitement and joy, we should also pay attention to the other end of the pleasure continuum. Many terms capture various shades of *contentment*: tranquility, peace, relaxation, calm, stillness, and quiet—the opposite end of the negative emotion spectrum. Contentment often follows pleasurable arousal, for example, as in the calm feeling after orgasm or the pleasurable feeling of being tired after vigorous activity. The safe haven of secure attachment also fosters a feeling of profound contentment, the comfortable feeling that everything's all right.[7]

What is depressed by depression? Simply put, interest and excitement, the emotional fuel of the seeking system. To be depressed is to be disengaged from the world. Engagement entails interest at the mild level and excitement at the more intense level. I've mentioned the importance of paying attention to glimmers of positive emotion as a harbinger of recovery from depression. You might think that merely being interested in something is insignificant. On the contrary, finding yourself interested in a conversation, a news item, or an appealing sight is an indication that the seeking system is becoming active—a sign of the of the lifting of depressed mood. Enthusiasm and excitement will follow.

Going for the gold, psychologist Mihaly Csikszentmihalyi proposed the term *flow* to capture human experience at its best.[553] Activities exemplifying flow entail a high level of interest and excitement; they're completely absorbing. Examples are mountain climbing, sailing, skiing, and racing. The formula is simple: you must balance challenge with skill. Thus to be in flow is to be on a tightrope: if the challenge is too low, you'll be bored; if your skill is too low, you'll be anxious—or in big trouble! Thus flow doesn't require a high level of skill, just the right level of challenge.

You don't need to be moving at high speed to be in flow; the level of challenge is crucial. More quiet activities conducive to flow include writing, lively conversation, or any sort of effective problem solving. Reading or meditating may involve flow, as do routine activities of daily living when they are engaging. Perhaps surprisingly, Csikszentmihalyi found that you're more likely to be in flow at work than in leisure, especially if you have a challenging occupation. Unsurprisingly, watching television usually counts as a low-flow activity.

Of course, whatever form it takes, you'll have a hard time getting into flow when you're depressed. These activities require not only interest and excitement but also good concentration. You might best seek flow in the quieter activities and work your way into increasingly active pursuits. However, the potential antidepressant benefits are especially clear with flow. Csikszentmihalyi noted that the deep and effortless absorption in flow activities blocks worries and frustrations.

WELLNESS

I assume you would have put this book down right away if I had told you flatly that, to recover from depression, you must sleep well, eat well, be active, and enjoy yourself. Catch-22: not easy. All the coping strategies in this chapter, along with all the strategies in the chapters to follow, are more easily employed when you're no longer depressed.

Pointing this out isn't as ludicrous as you might think, because you can employ these strategies preventively to maximize your chances of staying well once you've recovered from depression. Then you can sleep, eat, exercise, and enjoy yourself. However, you shouldn't take these capacities for granted; you'll do best to pay special attention to all these aspects of health. If you find yourself slipping—most notably, having trouble sleeping for several days running—you can make a concerted effort to regain your balance before you slide deep into depression, at which point you'll revisit catch-22.

Chapter 12

FLEXIBLE THINKING

Emotion and reason are entangled—most often, helpfully so. We're moved and guided by feeling and thought, all at once. We rely heavily on intuition, an amalgam of feeling and thought. Often, without awareness, we rely on information provided by our gut feelings,[423] especially in relating to each other. Contemporary philosopher Martha Nussbaum[263] poignantly described her experience of *emotional knowing* when she learned of her mother's death: "This news felt like a nail suddenly driven into my stomach" (p. 19). She elaborated:

> My mother has died. It strikes me, it appears to me, that a person of enormous value, who was central in my life, is there no longer. It seemed to me as if a nail from the world had entered my insides; it also felt as if life had suddenly a large rip or tear in it, a gaping hole. I saw, as well, her wonderful face—both as tremendously loved and as forever cut off from me. (p. 39)

Emotion and reason are entangled in your immediate appraisals of situations that usher forth full-blown emotions. In a split second, in response to an oncoming car, you can appraise a situation as dangerous and feel fear. You respond by hitting the brakes and feeling afraid, far more quickly than you can think the situation through. Fortunately, you not only appraise; you continually re-appraise. You avert the crash and feel relief. Then you might think about the carelessness of the other driver and start feeling angry. Very often, in response to an emotion-provoking situation, you have a whole cascade of appraisals, emotions, and feelings. Think about all the thoughts and feelings that might unfold if you learned that you'd been let down or betrayed by your best friend or spouse.

Feelings and thoughts are thoroughly entangled in depression. It's a chicken-and-egg problem: depression and negative thinking go together, and it's hard to know which comes first. Does depressed mood evoke negative thoughts? Yes. Do negative thoughts evoke depressed mood? Yes. The whole process begins with a more or less conscious emotional appraisal of a situation, then depressed mood and negative thinking become part of the cascade. Events per se are not depressing; the *meaning* of events depresses us.

Psychiatrist Aaron Beck[102] made a monumental contribution to disentangling feeling and thinking as they unfold in depression. Beck[102] and his colleagues[236] developed a broad understanding of depression and a correspondingly comprehensive treatment approach. Most importantly, Beck pinpointed certain thought processes that fuel depressed mood, and he developed a treatment approach—cognitive therapy—to reverse this process.

The development of cognitive therapy stimulated a wealth of research on thought processes in depression. The knowledge gained is immensely useful to depressed persons: knowing how your thinking worsens your depression, you can exert some influence over your mood by working to modify your thinking. Of course, it's not easy; you're depressed. Catch-22.

In this chapter I describe how negative thinking, ruminating, and memory disturbance contribute to depression, then I summarize the cognitive therapy techniques that have been developed to enable you to become more aware of these problems so as to interrupt them. Yet recovery from an episode of depression doesn't necessarily eliminate your cognitive vulnerability to additional episodes. Thus you'll benefit from knowing about cognitive approaches to relapse prevention. I conclude with a comment about how cognitive therapy can be a means to improve your relationship with yourself.

NEGATIVE THINKING

In practicing psychotherapy, Beck noticed that depressed patients' experiences of emotional distress often were preceded by fleeting negative thoughts of which the patients were only dimly aware. A common example: "I can't do anything right!" Beck observed that such thoughts were on the periphery of the stream of consciousness, and they often came to mind quickly, in a reflexlike manner, flitting through the mind with little notice. These thoughts carried depressing themes: deprivation, disease, and defeat. Beck called them *automatic negative thoughts*.[236,424] In developing cognitive therapy, Beck began drawing his patients' attention to these thoughts, bringing them to the center of consciousness. Enhanced awareness of the connection between their thoughts and feelings put his patients in a position to reconsider their thinking and thereby exert some influence over their feelings. In the course of investigating these depressing thought patterns, Beck identified a *negative cognitive shift*.

NEGATIVE COGNITIVE SHIFT

Beck was struck by a pervasive change in thinking that comes about in conjunction with depression: whereas nondepressed persons tend to have a positive, optimistic bias in their thinking,[425] depressed persons tend to filter out the positive and exaggerate the negative. Receiving compliments on a successful performance, a depressed person might think, "They don't know what they're talking about! Anyway, it was just luck, and I'll never manage to pull it off again."

More specifically, Beck identified a *cognitive triad* of negative thoughts about the self, the world, and the future.[236,426] Stressful events amplify your negative view of your *self*. Self-criticism takes over; you feel inadequate, defective, and deprived. Depression also colors your view of the *world*, especially your relationships. Being depressed, you're likely to perceive others as being critical of you,[427] making exorbitant demands. Finally, being depressed, you're liable to see the *future* as bringing only unrelenting hardship, frustration, and deprivation. As I discuss shortly, your perception of the future is especially important in relation to feeling hopeless.

Reading about negative thinking in depression, you might feel like protesting: "Things *really are* bad!" Beck would be the last to deny the reality of stress, but he homed in on the *unrealistic aspects* of thinking about stressful circumstances that add fuel to the depressive fire. For example, he observed a wide range of *cognitive distortions* that can make a truly bad situation seem even worse.[236,426] Common examples are *overgeneralizing* (e.g., having been turned down for a date, concluding that you'll be alone for the rest of your life); *all-or-none thinking* (e.g., either you must succeed at everything you do or you're a total failure); *mind reading* (e.g., believing without evidence that someone is critical of your performance); and *emotional reasoning* (a failure of mentalizing—for example, confusing the *feeling* that you're inadequate with actually *being* inadequate). All such distortions amplify depressive feelings; bringing these distortions to light and reappraising the situation can tone down depression. In short, given that you naturally feel discouraged about serious, real problems, you can learn how the way you think can either turn the dial up or down on your depressive feelings.

HOPELESSNESS

We associate feelings of helplessness with anxiety and feelings of hopelessness with depression. We've seen throughout this book that anxiety typically accompanies depression; you can feel helpless *and* hopeless—certain that your helplessness cannot change.

It's crucial to distinguish your *feeling* of hopelessness from your circumstances actually *being* hopeless. A number of cognitive therapists have investigated how the feeling of hopelessness stems from your characteristic *explanatory style*, a way of explaining the causes of stressful events in which you're involved.[428,429] You're most likely to feel hopeless when you explain your plight as being due to factors that are *stable*—"Things will never change!"—and *global*—"My whole life is ruined!"[272,430] You're more likely to feel hopeful if you view your situation as temporary—"This will pass!"— and specific—"This project may be doomed, but I can do others." Explaining negative events on the basis of *internal* as opposed to external factors also contributes to hopelessness. The internal focus construes negative events as stemming from fundamental flaws in the self, such as being unalterably deficient, worthless, or unlovable. An external focus doesn't lead to such enduring self-blame but rather construes events as being due to outside factors beyond your control.

To reiterate, the meaning you attribute to stressful events, the way you explain their occurrence, and your view of their consequences, will determine whether you come to feel hopeless—trapped, defeated, and perpetually helpless. Hopelessness is depressing. Moreover, if your characteristic explanatory style is conducive to hopelessness (attributing negative events to factors that are stable, global, and internal), you're more vulnerable to recurrent depression. By addressing these problematic thought patterns, cognitive therapy promotes hope.

CHILDHOOD MALTREATMENT

Why would you develop an explanatory style conducive to depression? There are many developmental pathways to negative thinking, but I want to highlight one that keeps us mindful of harsh realities as we also consider exaggerations and distortions in thinking.

As we've seen earlier in this book (Chapter 6, "Childhood Adversity"), childhood trauma is a significant risk factor for depression. Correspondingly, childhood maltreatment—family discord, abuse, and neglect—is conducive to developing negative cognitive styles that persist into adulthood.[431] The connection is direct in psychological abuse,[211] when the child who is humiliated and cruelly castigated develops a negative self-image:[144] "I'm bad, worthless, good for nothing." Keep in mind that hopelessness entails an expectation of unending helplessness. Repeated trauma can lead to *learned helplessness*.[41] This learning may be a natural evolution of the child's experience: painful events did happen continually, the child was blamed for them, and the child was helpless to prevent them. Thus maltreatment is conducive to all the ways of thinking that promote hopelessness, and it is not surprising that—now grown up—the individual tends to interpret ongoing stressors in much the same way. Becoming aware of the roots of this explanatory style in childhood and recognizing that you are no longer helpless in the present can be crucial in coping with depression.

RUMINATING VERSUS PROBLEM SOLVING

Many depressed persons ruminate, turning over depressing thoughts in their mind, becoming more mired in depression in the process. My colleague, psychologist John Hart, explains ruminating as follows: if you ask yourself questions that cannot be answered, or the answer is always the same no matter how much you think about the question, you're ruminating. If you're prone to ruminating, consider this saying: when you're in a hole, the first thing to do is stop digging!

RUMINATION

Psychologist Susan Nolen-Hoeksema[147] and her colleagues have studied depressive rumination thoroughly, and their findings have clear-cut practical implications. Not everyone is disposed toward ruminating when depressed; some are more inclined to engage in distracting activity. Yet a number of persons show a pattern of *ruminative responses to depressed mood*, namely, focusing attention on the symptoms of depression as well as their causes and consequences. As I've been discussing, it's natural to attend to these matters; yet merely cycling through the same thoughts over and over, spinning your wheels in a rut, does more harm than good.

Examples of ruminating are thinking about how tired you feel, worrying about whether you'll be able to sleep, thinking about the impact of your depression on your relationships, and wondering what's wrong with you.[432] Of course, such thoughts are natural and to some degree essential in coping. Yet the *inability to disengage* from ruminating causes trouble. Ruminating typically intermingles depressive thinking with anxious worrying; not surprisingly, persons with a combination of anxiety and depressive symptoms may be especially prone to ruminating, and ruminating makes both depression and anxiety worse.[433] Put crassly, ruminating can be viewed as "recycling cognitive trash" (p. 243).[275]

Nolen-Hoeksema and her colleagues observed several problems associated with ruminating:

- Ruminating amplifies depressive symptoms and is associated with more severe and prolonged depression as well as with increased risk for recurrence of depressive episodes.[147,433]
- Ruminating is motivated by ruminators' experience of gaining insight into their problems; ironically, while generating a feeling of self-understanding, ruminating increases pessimism, leaving the person "sadder but wiser" (p. 346).[432]
- Ruminating interferes with the person's willingness to engage in distracting activities that would improve mood, even when ruminators realize they'd feel better if they did something to free up their mind.[432]
- Ruminating interferes with effective problem solving, as exemplified by ruminators' generating fewer effective solutions to interpersonal problem situations and being less willing to implement solutions.[434,435]
- Ruminating is conducive to seeking social support following a loss and, when ruminators receive support, they benefit from it. Yet ruminators are more likely to feel that others are not supportive; indeed, they perceive their relationships as becoming increasingly less supportive, more characterized by friction and criticism. Perhaps they believe that others are becoming worn down with their ruminations. A vicious circle may ensue: ruminating about social rejection fans the flames of distress.[436]

To summarize, in ruminating, you may feel you're gaining insight and have the illusion of getting somewhere. I've presented these research findings in attempt to dispel that illusion; rumination interferes with coping and effective problem solving. The best strategy: distract yourself from ruminating by engaging your attention with something outside yourself, such that your mood lifts and your concentration improves; in short, take a break.[434] This strategy requires effort, due to the changes in patterns of brain activity associated with depression (see Chapter 9, "Brain and Body"), but getting unstuck from ruminating will put you in a better position to engage in effective problem solving. You may well need the help of others in this process, both to distract you from ruminating and to help you think more objectively about problem solving. Keep in mind, however, that ruminating in these interactions also may wear others out; in the hole, stop digging.

PROBLEM SOLVING

Throughout this book I have emphasized how depression stems from stress, much of which is related to interpersonal conflicts. I have also emphasized how recovering from depression and remaining well entails minimizing stress as well as coping with stress more effectively (see Chapter 7, "Stressful Events"). Here's a straightforward—and effective—approach to treating depression: helping patients identify and solve distressing problems.[437] Problem-solving therapy promotes agency, and the first step is mentalizing: learning to label distressing emotions and to use them as signals to identify the existence of a problem.

I've noted that depressive thinking tends to be global: "No one cares about me!" The problem-solving approach gets down to specifics, broken down into seven steps:[438] identifying and defining feasible problems described in objective terms; setting achievable goals in behavioral terms; brainstorming to generate alternative solutions; evaluating each solution in terms of pros and cons; selecting solutions that best satisfy goals; implementing the solution by engaging in relevant tasks; and evaluating the outcomes and revising problem-solving strategies as necessary.

You are encouraged to start with relatively simple problems (e.g., procrastinating on a particular household chore) and work up to more complex problems (e.g., feeling ignored by your spouse). Succeeding at simpler problems fosters confidence, and the therapy fosters a *problem-solving attitude* that counters helplessness and hopelessness. Solving problems is crucial in developing self-efficacy (see Chapter 3, "Agency and Elbow Room"); in the process, you learn, "I can *do something* about this!" This problem-solving spirit is inherent in cognitive therapy as discussed in this chapter and in interpersonal psychotherapy as discussed in Chapter 13 ("Supportive Relationships").

REMEMBERING

We've just seen that depression promotes negative thinking about recent, ongoing, and future events. Moreover, when you're depressed, negative memories also come to mind more readily. For example, you might be inclined to mull over past losses, failures, and interpersonal problems.[427] In addition, when you're depressed, you find it harder to remember events associated with positive emotions—just as it's harder to experience positive emotions in general.

Depressive memories of stressful events often have an intrusive, unwanted quality, not unlike the intrusiveness of memories in posttraumatic stress disorder.[439] Furthermore, like persons with posttraumatic stress disorder, depressed persons try to avoid remembering and thinking about stressful events—expending considerable effort to do so. Sadly, intrusive memories may serve to reinforce negative thinking; for example, memories of embarrassments or failures may fuel feelings of inadequacy. In addition, intrusive memories interfere with concentration and problem solving, further undermining self-confidence.

The tendency to remember painful life events will be all too familiar to many depressed persons. Psychologist Mark Williams[440] identified a more subtle problem: *overgeneral memory*. Depressed persons are prone to remembering events in a global, abstract way, for example, "I was never invited to parties in high school." They have difficulty remembering specific events in detail, for example, "The time I had a falling out with my best friend and was told to go home when I arrived at her birthday party."

Research has identified some problems associated with overgeneral memory:

- Vivid memories, which entail being able to imagine yourself in the scene, are associated with strong feelings.[441] Thus remembering events in an overgeneral way serves the defensive function of toning down painful feelings. Persons with a history of trauma also are prone to remembering in an overgeneral way.[442] Yet this memory style doesn't protect you from depression; on the contrary, it's associated with greater vulnerability to depressive episodes.[443] Moreover, difficulty recalling detailed pleasant memories also blocks access to positive feelings.

- Overgeneral memory goes hand in hand with ruminating; both involve mulling over abstract ideas.[444] Like ruminating, being stuck at the level of overgeneral remembering blocks you from practical problem solving.[445] To bring the past to bear on the future, you need to remember specifics—what worked and what didn't in particular situations.[446]

- The tendency to remember in an overgeneral way is characteristic of persons who are prone to depression—not just when they're in the midst of a depressive episode.[447] Yet you're not irrevocably stuck in this overgeneral mode of thinking. When depressed persons are distracted from ruminating about abstract ideas about themselves for several minutes, they become more capable of recalling specific and vivid memories.[444] Focusing on concrete outer reality frees up the mind; it's an entrée into problem solving.

COGNITIVE THERAPY

Beck and his colleagues[236] developed a comprehensive approach to treating depression, *cognitive-behavioral therapy*, that includes not just working with negative thinking but also fostering behavior change conducive to improving mood. I've discussed activity and pleasure in Chapter 11 ("Health"), and I focus on the cognitive part here. However, I want to emphasize that cognitive-behavioral therapy fosters agency by encouraging you to take action, changing your behavior and patterns of thinking. By employing methods of cognitive-behavioral therapy, you learn that you can do something to change your mood, and cognitive-behavioral therapy provides some tools to do so.

The central premise of cognitive therapy dates back two millennia. Epictetus,[448] a Roman Stoic philosopher, proclaimed: "It is not things that disturb people but their judgments about things" (p. 213). The Stoics believed that whereas we cannot control external events, we can decide how to think about them and thereby control our emotional reactions. It's not the course of events but rather our beliefs and values that get us into emotional trouble. By changing our beliefs and values, we can achieve greater emotional equanimity. Roman emperor Marcus Aurelius[449] counseled, "I can control my thoughts as necessary; then how can I be troubled? What is outside my mind means nothing to it. Absorb that lesson and your feet stand firm" (p. 85).

There's great wisdom and consolation in Stoicism, but I think the Stoics went too far in believing that we can fully control our mental states. Consider Epictetus's[450] strong claim: "Remember, for example, when you embrace your child, your husband, your wife, you are embracing a mortal. Thus, if one of them should die, you could bear it with tranquility" (p. 7). Short of extremes such as preventing ourselves from becoming emotionally attached, we can benefit from reconsidering values and beliefs that engender unnecessary emotional pain. You're bound to be miserable if you want everyone to be pleased with you all the time and believe that you're inadequate if they're not. Yet your control over your emotions will be limited. I believe you're better off striving to *influence* your judgments and emotions rather than believing that you can *control* them. While you cannot fully control external events, you certainly spend a lifetime trying to influence them—especially when you're not depressed.

Quite often, we're in the position of exerting influence over our emotions after the fact. The Stoics focused on our judgments; contemporary psychologists home in on the cognitive *appraisals* that influence our emotional responses.[451] Yet our thoughts and emotions are utterly entangled, and our immediate appraisals are so fast as to seem reflexlike, as Nussbaum's reaction to the news of her mother's death illustrates: the news felt like a nail driven into her stomach. We don't have much leverage over such immediate appraisals, but we can create some elbow room in our *reappraisals*, thus influencing the *course* of our emotional responses. Here's where cognitive therapy comes in.

Cognitive therapy has been researched and refined over the course of four decades, and I can only provide the gist of it here. Fortunately, given its deserved popularity among clinicians and patients, a great deal has been written for lay persons; *Feeling Good*, by psychiatrist David Burns, is a classic.[452]

The techniques of cognitive therapy can be broken down into four basic steps:[426]

1. Cognitive therapy begins with *identifying the automatic negative thoughts* associated with distressing emotions. Fleeting thoughts don't lend themselves to emotional reappraisals; bringing these thoughts into full awareness helps underscore the relation between thoughts and feelings and sets the stage for new considerations. Having learned the technique of identifying automatic negative thoughts during therapy sessions, patients are instructed to keep a daily record of negative thoughts to facilitate awareness and change.

2. Having brought the automatic thoughts into awareness, the next step is to evaluate their accuracy. Thus the essence of cognitive therapy is identifying and *questioning* automatic thoughts, rather than letting these unquestioned thoughts dominate your mood. Patients are taught to think like scientists, to consider the evidence that supports the thoughts—or the lack of evidence.

3. Having become aware of automatic thoughts and learned to question them, patients learn to *develop more rational alternatives*. Like scientists, patients are encouraged to consider alternative explanations. Failing an exam, you might automatically think, "I'm stupid." On reflection, you might realize there's much evidence to the contrary and consider an alternative explanation: "I wasn't prepared." Thus you go from global negative thinking to more refined negative thinking that points toward problem solving (e.g., planning adequate time for study). The goal is not to eliminate negative thinking but rather to engage in *useful* critical thinking. Awareness of various cognitive distortions, such as all-or-none thinking and catastrophizing, can facilitate such reappraisals. The daily thought records structure this process: you identify the situation that evoked the distressing emotion; you identify the automatic thoughts associated with the emotion; you identify the specific emotions you felt; you examine the reasonableness of the automatic thoughts, the evidence for them, and possible alternative explanations; then you indicate how strongly you believe the automatic thoughts after having reevaluated them and notice the corresponding changes in your emotions.

4. After identifying a range of automatic thoughts associated with various situations and emotions, the patient and therapist pinpoint *core negative beliefs* and recurrent themes associated with depression. Often the exploration of automatic thoughts leads from the tip of the iceberg ("I really messed up that interview!") into the more unconscious depths ("I'll never amount to anything, just as my father kept telling me!"). As we've seen repeatedly, core themes are likely to revolve around dependency (feeling unwanted and unloved) and self-criticism (feeling like a failure).[159] Modifying these core beliefs in the context of the therapeutic relationship is a main agenda in cognitive therapy.

You should not equate cognitive therapy with the power of positive thinking; Beck and colleagues[236] were adamant about this point:

> An obvious problem with "positive thinking" is that the positive thoughts are not necessarily valid or accurate. A person may deceive himself for a while with unrealistically positive thoughts, but he will eventually become disillusioned…. Positive thoughts lead to positive feelings only when the person is convinced they are true. Cognitive therapy can be called the power of *realistic* thinking. (p. 299)

Plainly, persons who become depressed in the aftermath of extremely stressful events will have plenty of realistic negative thoughts. Negative consequences may abound, and we all have personal limitations and shortcomings that may play a role in the stress we experience. Cognitive therapy comes into play when unreasonable thinking makes a bad situation seem worse than it is, fanning the flames of depression. Fully recognizing that depression stems from very real life problems, cognitive therapy—just like all other forms of therapy—involves working actively on problem solving. Of course, problem solving will go more smoothly when you're thinking reasonably and when you're not mired in ruminating, spinning your wheels in the world of global depressing ideas.

COGNITIVE VULNERABILITY

There's a wealth of evidence that negative thinking goes with the depressed state; whereas after individuals have recovered from depression, their negative thinking may no longer be evident—or at least less prominent as it was during the depression. Yet, in cognitively vulnerable persons, the negative thinking is latent, in the background, and easily *activated* by stressful events or sad mood.[275] Accordingly, improvement in depression, such as occurs with successful treatment of any sort, may *deactivate* negative thinking rather than eliminating it.[453] In effect, negative thinking goes underground, only to resurface when things go badly.

It's crucial to distinguish depressive *feelings*—being bummed out or having the blues—from depressive *illness*—major depression, for example. Cognitive vulnerability—your tendency to get down on yourself when something goes wrong—can transport you from depressive feelings to depressive illness. Notably, the diagnosis of a major depressive episode requires a 2-week duration of symptoms;[8] this period might reflect the role of cognitive vulnerability: a tendency to ruminate over time can create a spiral from depressive feelings to depressive illness.[275]

Here's what researchers have learned about cognitive vulnerability:

- Cognitive vulnerability to depression can be established by late childhood.[272]
- A predisposition to negative thinking has been shown to put both adolescents[454] and young adults[431] at higher risk for episodes of depression.
- A pattern of negative thinking during an episode of major depression impedes recovery from that episode.[455,456]
- A history of episodes of depression is associated with ongoing cognitive vulnerability and a propensity to ruminate.[457]
- Cognitive vulnerability puts individuals with a history of depression at greater risk for recurrence of depression,[252] especially when negative thinking is coupled with a propensity to ruminate.[431]
- Cognitive vulnerability to depression isn't an all-or-none phenomenon; it's a matter of degree.[458] Life stress evokes negative thinking and rumination in cognitively vulnerable persons and, the more cognitively vulnerable you are, the less stress it takes to trigger depression.[272]

These findings are sobering: a disposition toward negative thinking and rumination can increase the risk for a depressive episode, prolong the episode, and leave you vulnerable to further episodes. Fortunately, you can do something about your cognitive vulnerability. As we've seen, Beck and others have developed and refined cognitive therapy to facilitate recovery from depression, and recent research has gone a step farther, decreasing cognitive vulnerability for the sake of relapse prevention.

RELAPSE PREVENTION

Extensive evidence shows that cognitive therapy facilitates recovery from episodes of major depression.[459] Yet one of the most troubling aspects of depression is the likelihood of relapse and recurrence, especially for persons with a history of multiple previous episodes.[66] As we've just seen, recovery from depression may still leave in its wake a significant level of cognitive vulnerability: in response to stressful events or feelings of sadness, negative thinking can return and fuel a spiral back into depression. Might cognitive therapy have any protective effect?

INTERRUPTING SPIRALS

Evidence from several studies suggests that cognitive therapy provides some protection against relapse.[460] How so? One experimental study of re-covered patients illustrates.[461] One group of patients had recovered with antidepressant medication, the other with cognitive therapy. The research-ers experimentally induced a sad mood by asking all participants to listen to sad music and to recall a time in their lives when they felt sad. The par-ticipants also filled out a questionnaire assessing negative thinking before and after the mood-induction procedure. The two groups of patients did not differ from one another in negative thoughts prior to the mood induc-tion. The difference between groups emerged only in response to the mood induction: the patients who had recovered with medication showed a greater increase in negative thinking than those who had recovered with cognitive therapy. Apparently, the patients who had learned cognitive ther-apy techniques were able to feel sad without engaging in negative thinking. Moreover, a follow-up study showed that participants who had engaged in negative thinking in response to their sad mood during the experiment were more likely to relapse into depression over the course of the next 30 months. The experiment had revealed their cognitive vulnerability.

These findings regarding the potentially protective effects of cognitive therapy are instructive in suggesting that you can learn to interrupt the spi-ral from a sad mood into a full-blown depression. Yet a comprehensive re-view of current research on treatment of depression suggests several caveats.[17] First, cognitive therapy during the acute phase of illness may have some protective advantages compared with medication only when medica-tion is discontinued after the acute phase; continuing medication also pro-tects against relapse. Second, it's not clear that, compared with other forms of psychotherapy, cognitive therapy has any *uniquely* protective effects. Third, neither cognitive therapy nor any other form of treatment abso-lutely prevents relapse; rather, treatment can prolong the length of recovery and decrease the *risk* of relapse. Regardless of the type of treatment, con-tinuing care is often the best protection against relapse.

MINDFULNESS-BASED COGNITIVE THERAPY FOR DEPRESSION

Recognizing the potentially protective effects of cognitive therapy, clinicians have developed specific techniques to bolster resilience. Psychologist John Teasdale and his colleagues[460,462] borrowed from stress-reduction research to develop a novel approach to relapse prevention in depression, *mindfulness-based cognitive therapy*. Building on knowledge gained about the psychological processes involved in relapse, this intervention is appealing in respecting catch-22: the intervention is employed *after* patients have recovered from depression, at which point their improved mental functioning puts them in the best position to learn the cognitive techniques. Then they develop cognitive skills that can further reduce their cognitive vulnerability to stress, with the intention of preventing recurrences of depression.

Teasdale and colleagues augmented cognitive therapy with mindfulness meditation, an ancient practice that cultivates awareness of the present. Such awareness can be focused on your state of mind, such as your thoughts or feelings, or on something outside yourself, such as an object like a flower or an activity like walking or washing the dishes. The essence of mindfulness is "keeping one's consciousness alive to the present reality" (p. 11).[463] Mindfulness practice is a promising strategy for treating depression, because it's been employed successfully in stress-reduction programs.[464,465] Mindfulness is an intuitively appealing approach to cognitive vulnerability, because mindfulness enhances mental flexibility and openness—an antidote to being stuck in the mental groove of depressive rumination.

Mindfulness-based cognitive therapy takes a subtly different tack: it doesn't aim to change the content of thoughts; moreover, it's antithetical to fighting depressive thoughts, for example, by struggling to find clever arguments against them. Instead, mindfulness entails cultivating a different *relationship* to your thoughts, feelings, and bodily sensations.[460] Specifically, you're encouraged "to 'allow' difficult thoughts and feelings simply to be there, to bring to them a kindly awareness, to adopt toward them a more 'welcome' than a 'need to solve' stance" (p. 55). The welcoming and allowing attitude toward depressive thoughts and feelings discourages avoidance of painful experience; it "encourages 'opening' to the difficult and adopting an attitude of gentleness to all experience" (p. 58).

Participants develop the core skill of observing their thoughts and feelings, letting them go rather than grabbing onto them and ruminating. Mindfulness practice is conducive to this process because in meditation you become aware of the unceasing flux in your thinking. Ordinarily, when you're not severely depressed and you don't get locked into rumination, depressive thoughts, feelings, and sensations pass through, floating by in the endless stream of consciousness. Mindfulness actively cultivates the experience of *mental states changing*, the antidote to feeling stuck. Consistent with cultivating attentiveness to the details of experience, mindfulness also decreases the propensity to overgeneral thinking.[445] In addition, mindfulness enhances attentiveness to pleasant mental states that, sadly, might go unnoticed otherwise. Of course, it's not easy to become mindful; thought patterns are deeply ingrained habits. As stress researcher Jon Kabat-Zinn[466] remarked about mindfulness meditation, "Try it for a few years and see what happens" (p. 104).

Clinicians have developed mindfulness-based cognitive therapy into an 8-week group intervention. The treatment involves education about the role of thinking in depression coupled with training in mindfulness meditation.[460] Like any skill, practice is crucial; participants meditate on a daily basis throughout the therapy. The treatment respects the fact that you can develop your skill most easily when you're not in the throes of depression; having developed it, you can put it to use when the going gets tough. Thus you can turn cognitive vulnerability into cognitive resilience. The research results are encouraging: for patients who had experienced three or more previous episodes of depression, mindfulness-based cognitive therapy substantially reduced the risk of relapse and recurrence over a 5-year period.[467] Although this approach is promising, keep in mind that we lack sufficient research to declare any one approach to relapse prevention superior to any other, and at least periodic ongoing care with treatments of proven effectiveness will provide the best protection.[17] Cognitive therapy and mindfulness-based cognitive therapy in particular are instructive in illustrating ways in which you can exert influence over your vulnerability to relapse. However, like any other facet of wellness, you must keep working at it. What happens when you lose weight by exercising then quit exercising?

MENTALIZING

Cognitive therapy promotes mentalizing with respect to yourself: you become more aware of your thoughts and feelings. Cognitive therapy also promotes mentalizing in relation to others: instead of making automatic negative assumptions about what others are thinking, you adopt a more open-minded, inquisitive, and experimental approach, considering alternatives and testing them out. Taking action, you might ask a friend who seemed distant what was on her mind rather than assuming the worst. You might learn that she was worried and preoccupied about her mother's health, not annoyed with you.

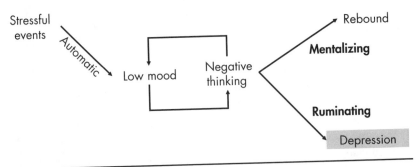

FIGURE 12-1. Cognitive resilience through mentalizing.

Mindfulness-based cognitive therapy promotes mentalizing by drawing your attention to depression as a *mental state*.[460] States change. You're encouraged to recognize that thoughts are not facts but rather mental events. Thus you can learn to identify, for example, "the-mental-state-in-which-I-view-myself-as-utterly worthless" (p. 31).[462] When you catch yourself ruminating, you might think, "I'm recycling cognitive trash" and refrain from taking your thoughts too seriously. You can learn to think of depressive feelings not as a sign of inadequacy but rather a normal mental state to be dealt with. That way you rebound to feeling well rather than spiraling into an episode of depressive illness (see Figure 12–1).

RELATING TO YOURSELF REVISITED

I discussed the importance of your relationship with yourself in Chapter 8 ("Internal Stress"). You might think of cognitive therapy and mindfulness practice not just as a means to change your patterns of thinking but also as a way to improve your relationship with yourself. Thinking is a way of relating to yourself. You can discourage yourself with pessimistic thoughts. You can oppress yourself, continually berating yourself and putting yourself down. You can torment yourself with cruel self-criticism. You'd be depressed if you were in a close relationship with someone who discouraged, oppressed, berated, and tormented you. No relationship is closer or more pervasive in its influence than your relationship with yourself. In short, you can create a depressing relationship with yourself, perhaps based on the model of depressing relationships you've had with others.

Of course, in principle, you can also encourage and support yourself, giving yourself a sense of freedom rather than oppressing yourself. I find the language used in mindfulness-based cognitive therapy suggestive of a secure attachment relationship. A welcoming, allowing, and gentle attitude toward feelings is just what we would hope an emotionally attuned parent would offer to a distressed child. Zen master Thich Nhat Hahn[468] made this link explicit:

> You calm your feeling just by being with it, like the mother tenderly holding her crying baby. Feeling his mother's tenderness, the baby will calm down and stop crying. The mother is your mindfulness, born from the depth of your consciousness, and it will tend the feeling of pain. A mother holding her baby is one with her baby. If the mother is thinking of other things, the baby will not calm down. The mother has to put aside other things and just hold her baby. So don't avoid your feeling. Don't say, "You are not important. You are only a feeling." Come and be one with it. (p. 54)

To tie all this together: we know that secure attachment promotes mentalizing,[157] and a secure attachment relationship with yourself is essential to a mindful attitude toward your thoughts and feelings. We want to move from a vicious circle of cognitive vulnerability and depression to a benign circle: cognitive therapy can improve your relationship with yourself, and improving your relationship with yourself will promote more cognitive resilience.

Chapter 13

SUPPORTIVE RELATIONSHIPS

Supportive relationships—connections with others that provide emotional comfort, practical help, and companionship—unquestionably promote physical and mental health.[124,469] The range of potentially supportive relationships is considerable, including friends, family members, therapists, and a host of informal social contacts;[470] yet there's no substitute for the support of a close, confiding, intimate relationship.[93,471]

Among other benefits, supportive relationships—especially attachment relationships—are an antidepressant. Conversely, conflict in attachment relationships and social isolation are depressing. Catch-22 takes two forms here: first, stressful relationships play a paramount role in generating depression; second, depression often exacerbates existing relationship stress by creating additional conflicts.

I begin this chapter by describing problematic interpersonal behavior associated with depression and its impact on relationships. Then I focus on the impact of depression on attachment relationships, using marital relationships as a model. Next, I discuss how relationship problems associated with depression create a vulnerability to relapses. Then I review interpersonal and psychodynamic psychotherapy, two forms of therapy for depression that address relationship problems. I conclude with dilemmas that caregivers face in striving to be supportive to depressed persons, noting the role of marital and family therapy in this context.

INTERPERSONAL BEHAVIOR

To reiterate catch-22: recovering from depression requires supportive relationships, and depression can undermine these potentially supportive relationships. Keeping these pitfalls in mind can help you avoid them and thus prevent you from alienating persons whose support you need.

When you're not depressed, you take for granted your ability to interact with others in a lively way. When you're depressed, you appreciate how much energy and effort social interactions require. Moreover, as I have reiterated throughout this book, depression diminishes your capacity for pleasure and enjoyment. Ordinarily, interacting with others is a major source of pleasure; when you're depressed, you don't have the same incentive to interact. Even when depressed persons do make the effort to interact with others, they're likely to find the interactions relatively unrewarding—less intimate and less enjoyable.[472] Finally, mentalizing interactively is one of the most complex things we do, and it's hard to keep the other person's mind in mind when you're depressed.

NONVERBAL AND CONVERSATIONAL BEHAVIOR

Psychologists have meticulously examined the interpersonal behavior of depressed persons interacting with others, ranging from strangers to marital partners.[473,474] None of these findings are likely to surprise you. Depression is evident in your facial expressions: you're less animated, not moving your facial muscles, and you're more likely to be furrowing your brow, squinting or closing your eyes, and turning down your mouth. Depression is also evident in your tone of voice, which is lower in pitch and volume, as well as less varied in pitch—monotonous. Overall, your voice has a sad, tense quality. Depression is evident in your speech: you speak less and more slowly; you also hesitate more and pause for longer periods. You're less interactive: you tend to keep your head down, nod less, and show less eye contact. You also smile less often and don't gesture much.

Depression also has a significant impact on the content of your conversations—what you talk about. Your conversations tend to be nonreciprocal; you tend to be self-absorbed and don't take an interest in what's going on with the other person. You're likely to talk about your emotional distress. You tend to be highly disclosing, often inappropriately so, talking about your troubles when others aren't eager to listen. You focus on the negative, particularly talking about your own flaws and failures. Ironically, you might seek out criticism, a process called *negative feedback seeking*.[475] Although such criticism is painful, it provides self-validation; the need to maintain a coherent sense of self can override the desire for positive feedback that would conflict with your negative beliefs.[476] Accordingly, you might spend more time with people who are critical, actively elicit criticism from them, or at the very least selectively attend to whatever criticism comes your way.

Given the nature of depressive behavior, it's not surprising that—like other emotions—depression can be contagious.[170] In interactions, the non-depressed person's behavior comes to match that of the depressed person. As I described in Chapter 6 ("Childhood Adversity"), this matching process occurs early, as evidenced by infants interacting with their depressed mother. For nondepressed persons, interacting with depressed persons is difficult because it's not rewarding; it violates social expectations.[477] When we interact with each other, we expect reciprocity and responsiveness, give-and-take. The ordinarily animated, lively, and responsive give-and-take makes interacting with other persons rewarding. Interacting with de-pressed persons is less rewarding owing to their diminished vitality and re-sponsiveness; moreover, their painful disclosures and lack of interest in others can feel burdensome and be upsetting.

REASSURANCE SEEKING

We've just seen how the lack of responsiveness, animation, and give-and-take creates difficulties in interactions; this difficulty can be compounded by pervasive negativity. Yet an additional interpersonal dynamic associated with depression can be the last straw: repeatedly seeking reassurance and rejecting it.[475,478] Seeking reassurance is natural and healthy; we all do it. Yet when you're depressed, the reassurance may not assuage your negative views, partly because of your proneness to ruminating, which continues to fuel your self-doubt and need for reassurance. Perpetual reassurance seek-ing wears out those who aspire to help; they feel burdened, frustrated, and helpless when you ask them incessantly if they love you, if they're going to stick with you, if you're doing things adequately, if they still think you're a good person, and so on.

We've seen that depressed interpersonal behavior creates strain in rela-tionships, yet it's the combination of depression and repeated reassurance seeking that is most problematic for other persons.[479] At worst, you're caught in a vicious circle:[478] others offer reassurance, but their efforts fail, and then their reassurance becomes increasingly disingenuous, intermin-gled with irritation. As a result you feel dismissed and rejected—accurately so—which only escalates the depression and anxiety and hence your need for reassurance.

COPING

As just described, being depressed potentially creates a multitude of problems in relationships. You may be perceiving others as critical, rejecting, and withdrawing from you. If so, you would be mistaken to chalk up your perceptions entirely to cognitive distortions.[473] Nonetheless, there may be *some* distortion in your perception; research shows that depressed persons are more self-critical of their interpersonal behavior than others are.[477]

In addition, I have looked at only the negative side of the coin so far; depression also elicits caring and compassion. True, others may be frustrated with your depressed behavior, but they may be even more frustrated when you don't reach out for their help. Most people have a strong desire to help their friends and loved ones; frustrating their desire to do so is no favor to them. Others who care about you may feel rejected when you shy away from seeking their support. They may feel more helpless and guilty. The fact that many persons are inclined to be caring and helpful justifies your effort in trying to cope with these interpersonal challenges.

Catch-22: because you're depressed, it's not easy to reach out for support, and you'll need to go against the grain in doing so. Here are some suggestions:

- First, to cope with the challenges, you must be aware of your own behavior and its impact on others—you must mentalize, keeping their mind in mind. You can exert extra effort, for example, to be more animated, responsive, and inquisitive about them. Most important, you can be aware of your tendency to seek negative feedback and especially your desire for reassurance. Of course, there's nothing wrong with seeking reassurance; we all need it. The problem comes with ruminating and continually seeking reassurance from the same person for the same matters. By doing this repeatedly, you are, in effect, rejecting the other person's efforts.
- It's helpful to acknowledge and discuss relationship problems surrounding your depression, for example, with friends.[473] Depressed persons can respond positively to frank feedback about their behavior,[480] and you might ask others you trust to provide it so as to bolster your awareness.
- You might also benefit from widening your network of social support, that is, spreading your needs around more rather than allowing fewer relationships to become increasingly burdened. Many people feel they must do something actively to help; then, failing to respect catch-22, they give unhelpful advice. You can also lighten their burden and guilt feelings by conveying that they don't need to *do* anything; just listening

and being there helps. You also can decrease others' sense of being burdened or helpless by conveying that you're coping actively and that you also have other sources of support.[481]

- When you're depressed, you may find it especially difficult to be with people who are particularly cheerful or upbeat; interacting with such people will require a high level of energy, and they may find it hard to relate to your depression. It's easiest to be with people who have a relatively *high tolerance for depression;* they're less likely to try to just cheer you up. Self-help groups composed of persons who have struggled with depression can be valuable for this reason.

- Finally, when you're depressed, it's best to focus on low-key activities that don't require a lot of energy. You might feel even more isolated if you go to a lively party where everyone seems to be having a riotously good time. Instead, you might do better by going to a movie, a concert, or a play, where you won't be expected to interact or converse much.

CONFLICTS IN ATTACHMENT RELATIONSHIPS

The interpersonal problems I've discussed pertain to a wide range of relationships, including relatively casual social contacts. Yet these problems are all intensified in close relationships, particularly attachment relationships, and they are especially evident when you're living together—married, for example. One reason for the intensity of the difficulty in close relationships is that depressed persons progressively withdraw from a range of other relationships, becoming increasingly dependent on fewer relationships. Those remaining—sometimes only the spouse or partner—become ever more burdened.[478]

Here we face the perennial chicken-and-egg conundrum: relationship problems and depression are intertwined, often in a vicious circle, and it's hard to know which came first. As we've seen, many persons who develop depression have experienced problems in attachment relationships since childhood, and these problems can persist into later relationships. In addition, many persons who have a history of relationship problems and depression tend to select partners who are also troubled. For example, women who are vulnerable to depression are likely to marry earlier and more hastily,[475] and they are likely to marry men who struggle with substance abuse and relationship problems.[473] Thus the stress of a troubled relationship can evoke depression, and the behavior associated with depression can exacerbate an already strained relationship.

As discussed in Chapter 8 ("Internal Stress"), problems with anger and resentment contribute significantly to the unfolding of depression. Again, vicious circles:[480] depressed persons alternate between stifling their anger and expressing it in irritable outbursts. Guilt feelings for expressing anger, along with fear that their anger will drive their partner further away, lead to further stifling of anger. Resentment builds as the depressed person not only stifles anger but also submits to the partner's criticism and demands in order to avoid even more criticism. Escalating depressive behavior also sometimes temporarily suppresses the partner's criticism; partners feel guilty for contributing to the depression, so they stifle their frustration and anger to avoid making the depressed person feel even worse.[482]

Over time, both partners continue to build up resentment. Angry interchanges alternate with depressive retreat and isolation. Moreover, it is not uncommon for both partners to be depressed,[483] such that vicious circles intermingle with vicious circles. A pattern of mutual alienation can ensue; gradually, the emotional distance and mutual resentment increases.

Catch-22: the single most important buffer against depression is an intimate, confiding relationship, yet the single most potent perpetuator of depression is a stable bad relationship—one in which conflict and a sense of alienation prevails. Commonly, depressed persons in a troubled marriage face a terrible dilemma: should I stay in the marriage or end it? Such decisions are fraught with conflict, including the choice between intolerable stress and major loss—each of which is potentially depressing. Ironically, this dilemma is especially troubling in connection with abusive or battering relationships: frightening and depressing as they may be, breaking the emotional bonds can be particularly difficult.[95,144]

There are no general prescriptions for the dilemma of whether to stay or leave; individual situations call for individual resolution. Sometimes it may be easiest to recover from depression by ending a chronically bad relationship, despite the loss this entails.[473] However, there is an alternative, which I discuss at the end of this chapter: marital therapy is particularly helpful when a troubled relationship is playing a significant role in perpetuating the depression.[17] This alternative, of course, requires willing collaboration of both partners.

INTERPERSONAL VULNERABILITY

Just as conflict in relationships can trigger depression and perpetuate it, ongoing conflict after recovery from an episode of depression can contribute to relapse and recurrence. In Chapter 12 ("Flexible Thinking"), I described how ongoing cognitive vulnerability increases risk for relapse; here I focus on the interpersonal counterpart.

As I described earlier, depression tends to be a recurrent illness, and a history of multiple episodes places a person at especially high risk for further episodes.[484] Like cognitive vulnerability, interpersonal vulnerability also contributes to this risk. We have seen how troubled relationships contribute to depression and, notwithstanding recovery from the acutely depressed state, ongoing relationship difficulties can contribute to relapse.[239,485] I described in the previous chapter how stresses can evoke depressive *feelings* that, in turn, can trigger rumination and thus lead back into depressive *illness*. The same process happens in relationships: experiencing and expressing depressive feelings can evoke relationship conflicts that trigger the escalation back into depressive illness.

To reiterate, two intertwined problems create a risk for relapse: isolation and conflict. A sense of alienation in a relationship is a major stressor: one study found that, for both men and women, being married and unable to confide in the spouse was associated with a 25-fold increase in the risk of depression.[242] Similarly with marital conflict, criticism of the depressed spouse dramatically increases the likelihood of relapse after recovery.[486] Criticizing symptomatic behavior (e.g., staying in bed) is not especially problematic, but criticizing the *person* is. For example, during a psychiatric interview, the spouse might remark that the depressed patient *always* has been selfish, spoiled, moody, or impossible to get through to. Such criticism of the depressed spouse's personality indicates a risk for relapse. Indeed, in one study, relapse was strongly predicted by the depressed person's answer to one question: "How critical is your spouse of you?"[487]

These findings don't show that criticism per se triggers relapses but rather suggest that such criticism is indicative of a characteristically troubled relationship. Thus addressing such relationship problems is a crucial facet of remaining well. Catch-22: a history of depression and relationship conflict calls for interpersonal problem solving, actively addressing and resolving conflicts. Yet depression interferes with problem-solving skills, and difficulty with problem solving in relationships increases the risk of depression.[488] Accordingly, if you're in this plight, you need help.

INTERPERSONAL PSYCHOTHERAPY

Gerald Klerman, Myrna Weissman, and their colleagues[489,490] developed interpersonal psychotherapy specifically to address the kinds of relationship problems discussed in this chapter, problems that precipitate and perpetuate depression and contribute to vulnerability to relapse. Interpersonal psychotherapy is a well researched, effective treatment for depression.

Interpersonal psychotherapy is designed to "change the way the patient thinks, feels, and acts in problematic interpersonal relationships" (p. 15).[489] Like cognitive therapy, interpersonal psychotherapy promotes agency. The therapist provides help with interpersonal problem solving, helping the patient consider alternative courses of action with the expectation that the patient will take an active role in the process: "To make real life changes, and to help alleviate the symptoms of depression, the patient will have to *do* things in his or her life between therapy sessions" (p. 53).[490]

Emphasizing active problem solving is consistent with the fact that interpersonal psychotherapy is designed as a time-limited treatment, typically consisting of 12–16 weekly sessions. Interpersonal psychotherapy is also highly focused, concentrating on one or two of four interpersonal problem areas: grief, role disputes, role transitions, and difficulty maintaining relationships.

GRIEF

As Freud,[267] Bowlby,[198] and many others recognized, the death of a loved one is a common trigger for depression. Interpersonal psychotherapy identifies two problematic grief reactions. *Delayed grieving* may not be recognized as such. For example, a woman whose husband died many years earlier might become depressed when she must leave the family home; she might not be aware that belated grief is contributing to her despondency. *Distorted grieving* may involve a lack of awareness that distress is related to the loss, for example, when a widower focuses all his attention on stress-related physical symptoms instead of his emotional reactions to the loss. Another form of distorted grieving is interminable grief, as evident in ongoing preoccupation with the loss to the exclusion of other interests (e.g., spending hours gazing at photographs of the deceased or remaining in their former room among their belongings). Interpersonal psychotherapy helps the grieving patient to recognize the significance of the loss and to explore and express the full range of emotions associated with the loss—including suppressed ambivalence, resentment, and guilt feelings. This process ultimately enables the grieving person to develop new supportive relationships and interests.

ROLE DISPUTES

Role disputes involve nonreciprocal expectations in a key relationship, most commonly in marital relationships. For example, a woman might become depressed when she expects her husband to be more emotionally involved with her and their children as well as to be more helpful with household responsibilities, whereas her husband expects her to be relatively self-sufficient owing to his demanding work life, because he is providing financial support for the family. Such role disputes can be depressing for a variety of reasons: they can damage self-esteem, evoke a sense of being helpless and trapped, and contribute to resentment and emotional distance. Interpersonal psychotherapy helps patients identify the dispute, make choices about potential courses of action, and communicate their needs and wishes in a clear and assertive way. Changes involve negotiating, resolving conflicts, and readjusting expectations. Alternatively, the patient might identify irreconcilable differences, terminate the relationship, and cultivate other sources of support.

ROLE TRANSITIONS

Many role transitions come about as part of the normal life cycle: leaving home, marrying, having children, children leaving home, and retirement. Others include job promotion, marital separation, divorce, adverse economic changes, loss of status, moving, and changes due to illness in oneself or a family member. Such stressful life changes can precipitate depression because they entail losses and dissatisfaction with the new role or evoke a sense of helplessness in relation to coping and a feeling of failure in relation to being able to manage the new role. Interpersonal psychotherapy helps patients express emotions related to the changes, give up the old role, acquire new skills, and develop new attachments and sources of social support.

DIFFICULTY MAINTAINING RELATIONSHIPS

Difficulty developing and maintaining relationships can contribute to depression by virtue of promoting social isolation and chronic feelings of loneliness. Interpersonal psychotherapy helps patients overcome isolation by examining the associated interpersonal problems, for example, problems stemming from troubled childhood relationships with family members or peers. Often, the patient's problems in relating to the therapist can be addressed as exemplifying difficulties in other relationships; experimenting with new ways of relating in the psychotherapy—for example, expressing concerns and frustrations assertively—can be generalized to other relationships. The therapist also encourages the patient to develop new relationships while providing assistance in identifying and solving problems that emerge in the course of these efforts.

Like cognitive therapy, the effectiveness of interpersonal psychotherapy has been supported by extensive controlled research.[190,490] Although typically a 3- to 4-month intervention, for persons with recurrent depression, maintenance sessions may be added. For example, weekly sessions for 6 months or monthly sessions for 3 years have been shown to be effective in preventing relapse. In addition, patients who experience persistent problems that require more extensive treatment may be referred for longer-term treatment, for example, psychodynamic psychotherapy.

PSYCHODYNAMIC PSYCHOTHERAPY

Psychodynamic psychotherapy focuses on internal conflicts, some of which are unconscious.[491] Yet internal and interpersonal conflicts are thoroughly intertwined: internal conflicts stem largely from interpersonal relationships—most prominently, attachment relationships in childhood—and internal conflicts also contribute to interpersonal conflicts. As we saw in Chapter 5 ("Attachment"), for example, being continually criticized by a parent in childhood can lead to relentless self-criticism and perfectionistic strivings. In turn, perfectionism can lead you to believe that others are equally demanding and critical, such that you resent them. At the same time, you also might be demanding and critical of others, incurring their resentment, thereby generating active relationship conflicts. These conflicts are depressing, adding to internal and interpersonal stress pileup. Psychodynamic psychotherapy aims to unravel such conflicts and thereby alleviate stress and depression.

By addressing conflicts, psychodynamic psychotherapy aims not only to promote recovery from depression but also to diminish vulnerability to relapse and recurrence. Psychodynamic psychotherapy can be particularly helpful when persistent personality problems perpetuate depression and limit your capacity to benefit from other forms of treatment, such as cognitive therapy or medication. If you're highly perfectionistic—for example, self-critical and critical of your therapist—you might need a substantial period of time to develop a relationship that can ameliorate problems that interfere with treatment.[159]

Not all individuals are suited to psychodynamic psychotherapy.[491] This approach is best if you are reflective, motivated to explore and understand the psychological origins of your depression, and able to develop a trusting relationship with a therapist that you can use as a secure base for such exploration. You will also need a relatively stable life situation that makes extended psychotherapy possible. Like cognitive therapy and interpersonal psychotherapy, psychodynamic psychotherapy promotes agency:[492] by making your unconscious conflicts conscious, you can be more self-reflective; rather than responding in habitual ways, you can become more flexible, able to make conscious choices. Two unconscious processes of concern for psychodynamic psychotherapy are transference and resistance.

TRANSFERENCE AND RESISTANCE

Although cognitive therapy and interpersonal psychotherapy often include some exploration of childhood origins of depression, these developmental contributions are a central focus of psychodynamic psychotherapy. Conflicts stemming from earlier experience become evident in the patient–therapist relationship in the form of *transference:* you attribute to your psychotherapist characteristics from persons in your past, prototypically, your parents. Thus you reenact earlier relationship patterns in the psychotherapy. For example, you might perceive the psychotherapist unrealistically as being critical, demanding, withholding, cold, or indifferent. Correspondingly, you might be cautious and reticent or perhaps hostile and challenging. Examining such responses in the treatment process enables you to mentalize, that is, to see that your perceptions are based on past experience more than current reality. Mentalizing, you come to perceive the psychotherapist more accurately and to relate more collaboratively.

Of course, the point of psychodynamic psychotherapy is not to develop a good relationship with your psychotherapist. Rather, you can learn from conflicts and problems identified in that relationship to develop increasingly stable and secure attachments in other relationships. In this way, psychodynamic psychotherapy becomes a laboratory for change.[491] You cannot influence what you cannot see. By exploring connections among your childhood relationships, your relationship with your psychotherapist, and your current attachment relationships, you bring unconscious patterns into awareness.[493] Consciousness affords choice: identifying problematic relationship patterns puts you in a position to change them.

Psychodynamic psychotherapy also examines unconscious *resistances,* that is, obstacles to change based on ambivalence and fear. Transference and resistance often go hand in hand, for example, when you're blocked from exploring and expressing painful feelings for fear of your therapist's harsh judgments.

CORE THEMES

Psychiatrist Fredric Busch and colleagues articulated five core themes commonly addressed in psychodynamic psychotherapy for depression: narcissistic vulnerability, conflicted anger, severe superego, idealization and devaluation, and defenses against painful emotions.[494] All these themes are intertwined:

- *Narcissistic vulnerability* entails exquisite sensitivity to injuries to self-esteem. Such injuries might stem from losses, rejections, or failures. Psychodynamic psychotherapy addresses the origins of your vulnerability along with its manifestations in the patient–therapist relationship and other relationships. The therapy also brings to light the counterproductive ways in which you attempt to defend against injury or to compensate, for example, by striving for perfection or by putting others in a dominant position, seeking their approval, and then resenting their control.
- *Conflicted anger* is a common response to narcissistic injury. Such anger might be abetted by envy, for example, when you perceive others as being more competent, powerful, and independent. The conflict stems from the dangers you associate with expressing anger. You might fear, for example, that expressing anger—or even *feeling* it—will disrupt already tenuous sources of support and nurturance. You might suppress your anger or even block awareness of it. You might also turn your anger inward in the form of self-criticism. Attacking yourself is depressing and puts you in a vicious circle: you aggravate your low self-esteem and thereby fuel your narcissistic vulnerability.
- In psychoanalytic theory, the ego is the self or the "I." The *superego* is, in effect, over the ego; it's your conscience, and it embodies your ideals and values. What Blatt[159] characterized as self-critical depression also could be called "superego depression." A punitive superego, often internalized from childhood relationships, is the epitome of anger turned inward; the associated self-oppression is profoundly depressing. Hallmarks of a harsh superego are feelings of guilt and shame, which also fuel low self-esteem.
- *Idealization and devaluation* are ways of compensating for narcissistic vulnerability and low self-esteem. You can attempt to raise your self-esteem by establishing relationships in which you idealize the other person; then you can bask in reflected glory. Yet idealizing others is bound to lead to disappointment when they fail to live up to your unrealistic expectations. Moreover, idealization can generate envy and thus escalate your feelings of inadequacy and inferiority. Consequently, idealization flip-flops: when you're disappointed, or your envy becomes unbearable, you can triumph by devaluing the person whom you idealized. Yet this psychological maneuver leaves you feeling resentful and depressed—and alone.

- *Defenses* against painful feelings leave you tied in emotional knots, creating continual stress and strain. Fear, anger, shame, and guilt may be defended against. Defenses, like the emotions defended against, operate unconsciously: you're not fully aware of the internal knots you're tying. As noted throughout this book, conflicted anger plays an important role in depression. You can block anger from awareness by repression and denial; you can project your anger onto others, believing instead that they're angry at you; or you can express your anger indirectly through passive aggression, for example, by procrastinating, stonewalling, and withholding what others desire. Psychodynamic psychotherapy provides a safe climate for you to explore and express painful feelings; doing so can be liberating, and it can set the stage for change.

Psychodynamic psychotherapy can be conducted as a relatively short-term treatment, for example, in twice-weekly meetings over the course of 3–6 months. Yet, as I noted earlier, psychodynamic psychotherapy is widely employed as a longer-term treatment for more enduring personality problems. It's not uncommon for psychodynamic psychotherapy to extend from several months to a couple of years—or even longer if need be.

Psychodynamic psychotherapy is widely practiced, but compared with cognitive therapy and interpersonal psychotherapy, its effectiveness has been less extensively researched.[17] Logistically, it's most challenging to research long-term treatment; hence most of the controlled research that has been done has focused on brief psychodynamic treatment. Although there is not nearly as much research as we would like, a small number of well-conducted studies suggest that psychodynamic psychotherapy can be comparable in effectiveness with better-researched interventions such as cognitive and interpersonal therapy.[495]

THE CAREGIVER'S TIGHTROPE

Seeking support when you're depressed can become a minefield if your relationships have become fraught with conflict and you're exquisitely vulnerable to feeling wounded. In addition to working on your own conflicts, appreciating the perspective of persons from whom you seek support may allow you to avoid setting off some of the mines. You'll need to mentalize, keeping their mind in mind. Admittedly, this isn't easy when you're depressed.

Being in a close relationship with a depressed person is a strain. One study found a significant positive correlation between the level of depression in the patient and the level of depression in the spouse.[483] Another

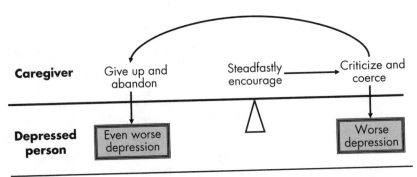

FIGURE 13–1. The caregiver's tightrope.

Source. Reprinted from Allen J: "Depression," in *Coping With Trauma: Hope Through Understanding.* Washington, DC, American Psychiatric Publishing, 2005, p. 170. Used with permission. Copyright 2005 American Psychiatric Publishing.

study found that 40% of persons living with depressed patients were showing a level of symptoms indicating a need for professional help.[496] Thus caregivers often are under considerable emotional strain as they face the challenge of supporting their depressed loved ones. They walk a tightrope (see Figure 13–1).

THE TIGHTROPE

There's a delicate balance that people need to maintain to be of help to a depressed person. I think of the caregiver as being on a tightrope in the sense that it's easy to fall off in one direction or the other.[95]

Staying on the tightrope entails providing steadfast encouragement. Providing support doesn't necessarily require *doing* anything, much less *fixing* anything. Rather, it requires an accepting attitude and a willingness to *be there* so that the depressed person at least doesn't feel so totally alone.

When caregivers' support fails to be effective, there are two ways they can go wrong. I think the natural inclination is to push harder and to become critical ("If you'd just get up off your..."). After criticism also fails—indeed, makes things worse—the caregiver may be inclined to give up and withdraw. This leaves the depressed person being alternately criticized and feeling abandoned, both of which fuel depression. As discussed earlier in this chapter, just as the depressed person is likely to alternate between conflict and withdrawal, so too is the caregiver. Each may attempt to engage, then become frustrated, then withdraw.

Quite often, caregivers feel they must *do* something to pull you out of your depression, and they may have a strong urge to do so, because your depression is depressing, distressing, or frustrating to them. If you're suicidal, those who care deeply about you will feel downright frightened. In any case, when you don't recover quickly despite their efforts, caregivers may feel frustrated, guilty, helpless, and inadequate. Ironically, the more they care about you, the more frustrated and anxious caregivers will become.

It's a lot to ask of you when you are depressed, but you may need to coach your caregivers, letting them know what's more and less helpful. This coaching won't be easy for you to do, and it may not be easy for the caregiver to receive. To feel criticized for not helping in just the right way also can be discouraging and frustrating. Yet caregivers need reinforcement; they need to hear that they're being helpful and to know *what* they're doing that helps. Here's Andrew Solomon's[114] advice:

> What can you do when you see someone else trapped in his mind? You cannot draw a depressed person out of his misery with love (though you can sometimes distract a depressed person). You can, sometimes, manage to join someone in the place where he resides. It is not pleasant to sit still in the darkness of another person's mind, though it is almost worse to watch the decay of the mind from outside. You can fret from a distance, or you can come close and closer and closest. Sometimes the way to be close is to be silent, or even distant. It is not up to you, from the outside, to decide; it is up to you to discern…. So many people have asked me what to do for depressed friends and relatives, and my answer is actually simple: blunt their isolation. Do it with cups of tea or with long talks or by sitting in a room nearby and staying silent or in whatever way suits the circumstances, but do that. And do it willingly. (pp. 436–437)

MARITAL AND FAMILY THERAPY

Sometimes, recovering from depression can undo problematic interactions, but not always. The relationship may need to be renegotiated. Both persons may need to change their pattern of interaction. Otherwise the spiral into depression is easily restarted. Oftentimes, staying in a bad relationship can be more conducive to remaining depressed than facing the loss associated with breaking off the relationship. Alternatively, marital therapy can help repair relationship problems when both spouses are willing to work together for the sake of change.

Marital therapy is a logical extension of interpersonal psychotherapy for depression, and a conjoint version of interpersonal psychotherapy has been developed to focus on marital disputes.[490] The therapy focuses on a limited number of key problems and fosters renegotiation of the marital contract. Partners examine interactions that create conflict and learn to express their feelings assertively as well as to negotiate constructively. An initial study indicated that marital therapy was as effective as individual interpersonal psychotherapy for resolving the depressed spouse's illness; not surprisingly, compared with individual psychotherapy, marital therapy also led to more improvement in marital functioning.

Although marital therapy is not as refined as individual psychotherapy for depression, a number of approaches in addition to the interpersonal psychotherapy version have been developed.[482,497] Naturally, marital therapy is particularly likely to be helpful when marital problems are strongly related to the patient's depression—either as causes, consequences, or both—and when both partners agree that relationship problems play this central role. Both partners must be willing to make changes. Agreement to participate in marital therapy itself can have an antidepressant effect by promoting hope in a fresh start. Going beyond resolving marital disputes, engaging in positive interactions can buffer depression. For example, partners can be supportive by spending enjoyable time together, listening to each other in a positive manner, confiding in each other, supporting each other's self-esteem, and providing practical help and assistance.[482]

Of course, family conflicts that play a role in depression are not limited to marital disputes; problems with children also can be significant contributors. Depression can stem from parent–child problems, and it can exacerbate these problems. As described in Chapter 6 ("Childhood Adversity"), research suggests that maternal depression creates a risk for infant depression; similarly, parental depression is associated with adolescents' behavior problems. At any stage of child development, depressed persons who are having difficulty with parenting might benefit from specific help, for example, as provided by parent training and family therapy tailored specifically to these problems.[497]

As I hope this chapter has made plain, depression frequently is more than an individual problem; it's often a symptom of persistent relationship problems. In a family, depression in one or more members can be symptomatic of a whole network of relationship problems. Accordingly, overcoming depression may require the active involvement of others in the treatment process—sometimes, the whole family. A crucial part of educating yourself about depression is identifying just where the stressors lie as well as where you have the greatest leverage for change. The more allies you have in the process of change, the better. The fact that there are so many potential avenues for intervention—and so many treatment approaches—is a mixed blessing. Much potential help is available, but figuring out just what kind of help to seek is not so easy. This problem brings us to the next chapter, "Integrating Treatment."

Chapter 14

INTEGRATING TREATMENT

As the previous three chapters indicate, to recover from depression you will need to work on many fronts: sleeping well, eating properly, staying active, cultivating pleasurable experience, thinking flexibly, and maintaining supportive relationships. As I've described, clinicians have developed specific therapies to help you on each of these areas: behavior therapy, cognitive therapy, interpersonal psychotherapy, psychodynamic psychotherapy, and marital therapy. As I discuss in this chapter, medication also can be of considerable help on all these fronts.

In principle, when you are struggling with severe or protracted depression, you have a wide range of possible treatments from which to choose. In practice, you'll be constrained by a number of factors: availability of treatments in your region, financial limitations, and—not least—the number of things you can do at any one time. This chapter addresses considerations that enter into making choices among treatments as you strive to recover and stay well.

I start with medication and then summarize research comparing the effectiveness of medication and psychotherapy. I present conclusions of research on the advantages of combining medication with psychotherapy as well as research contrasting different types of psychotherapy. I also discuss the role of hospitalization in the treatment of depression. I conclude with some thoughts about integrating various forms of treatment with lifestyle changes.

MEDICATION

Medication has played a central role in the treatment of depression for several decades, and its role will become increasingly refined as the research on neurobiology of depression progresses. It is tempting to regard medication as treating the biological aspects of depression and psychotherapies as treating the psychological aspects, but this is misleading: mind and body are entirely integrated. Any intervention that improves your mood—medication or psychotherapy—will affect both your mind and body for the better.[498] Thus, by improving your mood, medication can improve your physical health, your thinking, and your relationships. Ditto for psychotherapy. Yet to say that medication and psychotherapy overlap in their effects on depression is not to say that they are equivalent; you need to appreciate their differences as well.

This chapter is intended to help you think about the role of medication in treating depression, not to provide guidance as to whether you should take medication, much less what particular medication you should take. You must make decisions about medication in collaboration with your family physician or psychiatrist; informing yourself about the options puts you in the best position to collaborate. Plenty of consumer-oriented publications provide more detailed information on medication.[69,499,500] Fortunately, this field is rapidly evolving, so new publications are pouring out continually. Unfortunately, information about depression available on the Internet is plentiful but generally poor in quality, dominated by for-profit sites promoting nonprofessional interventions.[501] Here I wish merely to make the point that there are many potential avenues of help and to alert you to some challenges you might face in making the best use of medication.

ANTIDEPRESSANTS

Broadly, antidepressant medications influence brain systems involved in modulating the stress response[350] by enhancing the function of the monoamine neurotransmitters norepinephrine, serotonin, and dopamine (see Chapter 9, "Brain and Body"). Antidepressant medications differ from one another in their mechanism of action. Although all these medications are generally equivalent in their effectiveness,[498] there are substantial individual differences in response; you might benefit much more from one medication than another. The differences among medications in mechanisms of biological action account for differences in individual response and the specific nature of their effects. These differences in mechanisms also influence the nature and extent of side effects, and much of the impetus for developing new medications is based on minimizing side effects as well as enhancing overall antidepressant effectiveness. There are about a dozen commonly used antidepressant medications, some additional experimental antidepressant medications and devices, and other medications employed adjunctively. I give a few examples of differences in mechanisms of action here to illustrate the range of antidepressant action.[350]

The earliest antidepressant medications, monoamine oxidase inhibitors (MAOIs) and tricyclic antidepressants (TCAs), were developed in the 1950s. The MAOIs, such as Nardil and Parnate, inhibit the action of the enzyme that degrades the monoamines (norepinephrine, serotonin, and dopamine), thus MAOIs increase the levels of these neurotransmitters in the synapses between neurons. Because the MAOIs have significant side effects and entail strict dietary restrictions, they are usually employed only after other antidepressants have been found to be ineffective. Like the MAOIs, the TCAs, such as Elavil and Tofranil, increase the availability of neurotransmitters in the synapses, but they have a different mechanism of action: they are reuptake inhibitors that block the action of transporters that otherwise would transfer the neurotransmitters from the synaptic cleft back into the secreting neurons.

The most commonly prescribed antidepressants are selective serotonin reuptake inhibitors (SSRIs), such as Prozac, Zoloft, Paxil, Celexa, and Lexapro. As their classification implies, SSRIs selectively block the reuptake of serotonin. Some antidepressants, such as Wellbutrin, block reuptake of norepinephrine and dopamine; others, such as Effexor and Cymbalta, block reuptake of serotonin and norepinephrine. Other newer antidepressants function more directly by blocking and/or stimulating various neuronal receptors for the various neurotransmitters.

The mechanisms of action I have just described account for only the immediate effects of the medications. For example, the SSRIs increase the synaptic levels of serotonin within hours of administration of the first dose, but the therapeutic response does not begin for 1–2 weeks, and the full response may take many weeks. The therapeutic benefit depends on a fantastically complex cascade of molecular effects that neurobiologists are just beginning to fathom.[311,350] The increased availability of serotonin, for example, initiates changes in the expression of genes in the neurons that, in turn, increase and/or decrease the number of receptors available to respond to neurotransmitters. Thus, over the long term, the neurons adapt to the changes in stimulation associated with the presence of the medication, fundamentally changing their pattern of responsiveness. Accordingly, although antidepressants target serotonin and/or norepinephrine initially, the molecular cascade and the therapeutic effects depend on broad changes in patterns of brain activity associated with these adaptive changes in the neurons. As discussed in Chapter 9 ("Brain and Body"), neuroimaging research is now clarifying how depression alters patterns of brain activity and how medications and psychotherapy can help normalize patterns of brain functioning.

LIMITATIONS AND COMPLICATIONS

Extensive research has demonstrated the effectiveness of a wide range of antidepressants, but as many patients know all too well, their effectiveness can be limited. As I've already mentioned, unlike other medications (e.g., stimulants and antianxiety medications), antidepressants initiate a complex cascade of effects that must unfold over time before therapeutic effects can occur.[350,498,502] You might begin to notice some benefit in 1–2 weeks; usually, 2–3 weeks is required for discernable clinical improvement. Yet it may take longer: 4–8 weeks may be required for an adequate trial and, especially if you have been depressed for a long time, the full benefit might not be realized for 12 weeks or even several months.

Although the therapeutic benefits may take considerable time to emerge, side effects become evident more rapidly. To reiterate, the nature of the side effects depends on the type of medication; these potential side effects are variable from one individual to another and are often temporary. Examples of side effects with the newer antidepressants include nausea, sedation, nervousness, insomnia, and sexual dysfunction. Some side effects are relatively short lived, whereas others may be persistent. Side effects can be managed to some degree by adjusting dosages; when side effects are intolerable, switching medication or trying alternative forms of treatment, such as psychotherapy, may be indicated.

Widespread media attention reflects heightened concern about the possibility that antidepressants might paradoxically increase suicidality (i.e., suicidal thinking and behavior), especially in children and adolescents with major depression; this concern is being addressed in systematic research.[503] One possible explanation for this paradoxical effect is the typical pattern of response to antidepressant medication, which includes relatively rapid improvement in energy levels compared with somewhat delayed improvement in symptoms of low self-esteem, feelings of worthlessness, guilt, and suicidality.[504] During this early time window of increased energy with ongoing depression, the individual might be more inclined to take action on suicidal thoughts. Yet we must keep this potential problem in perspective; the vast majority of persons who commit suicide are not taking antidepressants when they probably should be.[504] Furthermore, the proportion of young patients who experience increased risk of suicidality is relatively small: the U.S. Food and Drug Administration (FDA) estimated the risk of increased suicidality to be 4% with antidepressant medications compared with 2% with placebos.[505] Moreover, no deaths related to suicidality occurred in any of the 24 research studies the FDA reviewed. Nonetheless, a small increase in risk for such a serious effect merits concern, especially because most antidepressants have not been shown to be of benefit in children and adolescents with depression.[506]

In sum, the increased risk of transient suicidal states must be weighed against the benefits of demonstrably effective antidepressants such as Prozac for children and adolescents; effective medication decreases the risk of suicidal thinking and behavior over the course of treatment.[503] The take-home message: rather than depriving children and adolescents of antidepressant treatment when it's needed, we should employ only medications with demonstrated effectiveness, and we should monitor the response carefully, especially in the early stages of treatment. In addition, prescribing physicians should be alerted to any indications of bipolar disorder, including a family history, because the increase in agitation some young patients experience might be associated with an antidepressant-triggered switch into a manic or mixed episode (see Chapter 10, "Related Disorders"). Finally, in weighing risks versus benefits, the options of individual psychotherapy and family therapy also merit consideration.

Although the potential benefits of antidepressant medication are well demonstrated in research, many patients have only a limited response. In medication research, a significant response is defined as a 50% reduction in symptoms (for example, as measured by depression rating scales). Although such a response is of considerable benefit, patients who start out at a severe level of depression may nonetheless continue to experience troubling symptoms despite having shown a response to medication. The persistence of such symptoms is a significant problem for many reasons: you don't feel well, your relationships and ability to work may remain compromised, and ongoing symptoms also render you more vulnerable to relapse into more severe depression. Commonly, patients settle for limited benefit or stop taking medication when they feel somewhat better; yet, for all the reasons just stated, it's best to persist in treatment until you recover fully.

As I've made plain throughout this book, however, full recovery is often far from easy. Essential as it may be, there are two significant limitations to medication. First, only two-thirds of patients show a response to antidepressant medication (compared with one-third who respond to a placebo).[498] Second, only 30%–50% show full remission; the remainder only experience a partial response.[502] Plainly, considering both quality of life and vulnerability to relapse, full remission should be the goal of treatment. Yet

when we consider the limited number of patients who experience full remission in conjunction with those who relapse after full remission, only a
minority of patients achieve recovery with a single acute intervention.[502]
Take heart: if you are in need of complicated treatment, you are in the majority. If you're beginning treatment, you might keep in mind the likelihood
of needing to try more than one intervention.[507]

All is not lost. There are many strategies for enhancing the likelihood
of recovery, although all take time and may try your patience.[189,502] The
first strategy is optimization: although 4–8 weeks is considered an adequate
trial of an antidepressant, if you've been depressed for a long time, a longer
period (e.g., 10–12 weeks) as well as higher dosages may be warranted. Another strategy is augmentation, that is, adding a nonantidepressant medication such as lithium, thyroid supplements, stimulants that enhance
dopamine, and antianxiety agents. In addition, switching medications is an
option (e.g., switching from an SSRI to dual reuptake inhibitor). Finally,
combinations of antidepressants can be employed (e.g., an SSRI and Wellbutrin). Moreover, new medications are continually being developed, so
you should stay informed and not give up hope of finding more effective
treatment in the future. As I discuss later, adding psychotherapy to medication—or vice versa—is often a good strategy.

As I discussed in Chapter 10 ("Related Disorders"), many patients experiencing severe depression also struggle with other psychiatric disorders,
and such combinations of disorders also call for complex medication strategies. For example, in depressed patients with bipolar disorder, treatment
with antidepressant medication alone can trigger a manic episode;[508] accordingly, treatment requires a mood stabilizer (e.g., lithium or Depakote),
anticonvulsant (e.g., Lamictal), or an atypical antipsychotic medication
(e.g., Seroquel). In addition, psychotic depression is often treated with a
combination of antidepressant and antipsychotic medications.[502] Electroconvulsive therapy (ECT) is also highly effective.[509]

Given that the nature of your symptoms as well as the presence of psychiatric disorders besides depression will affect the choice of medication, it
is essential that you receive a careful diagnostic evaluation as a first step. In
addition, the choice of medication also will be affected by the presence of
general medical conditions and any other medications you are taking. Such
considerations enter into the decision to seek medication treatment with a
primary care physician versus a psychiatrist.[507] Indications that you should
see a psychiatrist include diagnostic complexity; severe, recurrent, or
chronic symptoms; suicidal states; history of bipolar disorder; poor response to initial trials of treatment; or the need for complex combinations
of medications or ECT.

Although we have the benefit of extensive research on individual medications, there is relatively little research on the complications: matching medications to different symptom profiles, combining medications, and switching medications, not to mention how best to sequence this process. Employing research to date, general clinical guidelines have been proposed,[510] and more specific treatment algorithms and care pathways also have been developed; these specific strategies are carefully designed step-by-step procedures adjusted to the individual patient's response along the way. These treatment algorithms have been developed to standardize optimal practice, and they have been shown to be more effective than standard treatment.[511,512]

As you might have inferred from this brief review, although the number of antidepressant compounds is burgeoning and will continue to do so, research on how they might be used most effectively in light of their limitations lags far behind. Finding the best medication or combination often will take a considerable period of time with a fair amount of experimentation. Patients and psychiatrists alike wish that a simple test would indicate the best choice. The quest for such a test has been going on for many years. We now have reason to be encouraged that functional neuroimaging research will be of help. At the time of this writing, neuroimaging researchers have begun observing different patterns of brain activity associated with major depression; identifying different neurobiological subtypes of depression might guide choice of medication as well as psychotherapy.[331] We're not there yet, but we're going there.

CONTINUATION AND MAINTENANCE

Acute-phase treatment includes the period from the low point of the illness to the point at which full remission (freedom from significant symptoms) has been achieved. After a stable period of remission—variously defined as 2–6 months—we can speak of recovery. We know there's a high risk of relapse after the initial response as well as after remission, thus patients are urged to follow acute-phase treatment with continuation treatment—typically 6–9 months—during which treatment gains are consolidated.[350]

Unfortunately, antidepressant medication is not curative and, even after recovery, you run the risk of recurrence—a new episode of illness. Thus, for many patients, the continuation phase is followed by maintenance medication; typically, the medication employed to achieve remission is maintained at the same dosage through the continuation and maintenance phases. Maintenance medication would be especially important to consider if you are at high risk of recurrence; pertinent factors include a family history of depression, early age of onset, multiple previous episodes, ongoing stressors, and residual symptoms of depression.[30,350,507] Unfortunately, there's relatively little research on the optimal duration of maintenance treatment. Yet one careful study of patients with a history of recurrent depression who had been maintained on antidepressant medication for 3 years found a high level of recurrence over the following 2 years when medication was discontinued.[513] Thus some persons with a history of chronic and recurrent depression may need to remain on medication for a decade or longer.[507] If you decrease or discontinue medication, you'll need to work closely with your physician and monitor your condition carefully, especially during the first several months.

Understandably, you might be averse to remaining on medication for a long time. Consider Andrew Solomon's[114] response to people who ask him why he's still on medication when he seems to be fine:

> I invariably reply that I seem fine because I am fine, and that I am fine in part because of medication. "So how long do you expect to go on taking this stuff?" people ask. When I say that I will be on medication indefinitely, people who have dealt calmly and sympathetically with the news of suicide attempts, catatonia, missed years of work, significant loss of body weight, and so on stare at me with alarm. "But it's really bad to be on medicine that way," they say. "Surely now you are strong enough to be able to phase out some of these drugs!" If you say to them that this is like phasing the carburetor out of your car or the buttresses out of Notre Dame, they laugh. "So maybe you'll stay on a really low maintenance dose?" they ask. You explain that the level of medication you take was chosen because it normalizes the systems that can go haywire, and that a low does of medication would be like removing half of your carburetor. (pp. 79–80)

Yet it is not uncommon for patients on maintenance medication to experience some return of symptoms short of a major depressive episode, a process called roughening.[502] Often these periods of roughening can resolve without changing the treatment, but these potential harbingers of recurrence may call for stepping up your efforts at wellness, reevaluating medication, or obtaining additional psychotherapeutic help. Unfortunately, maintenance treatment with antidepressants does not always prevent recurrence; up to a third of patients might experience new episodes despite ongoing treatment.[514] Plainly, there might be many reasons for recurrence, not least, encountering additional severe stressors. Yet clinicians have raised the possibility that medications might lose their effectiveness over time, a prospect technically called acquired tolerance. Paralleling strategies for coping with lack of full response during acute-phase treatment, options employed to deal with acquired tolerance include augmenting the antidepressant with other medications or switching to a different medication. Adding psychotherapy to medication treatment also merits consideration, especially when you are contending with new stressors.

AGENCY

Throughout this book, I have emphasized the importance of agency in recovering from depression. You might think that medication treatment involves little agency; you merely take a pill. As all the foregoing attests, most patients who employ medication to recover from depression and remain well exercise a great deal of agency, and exercising this agency when you are in the throes of severe depression will be especially challenging.

Consider all the things you might need to do. First, you will need to find a physician. You'll have to give a clear account of your symptoms, their history, and your current life situation. You may need to participate in diagnostic tests to rule out general medical conditions that could play a role in your symptoms. Then you will need to educate yourself about medication options and collaborate with your physician in deciding what to do. If you take medication, you'll need to carefully monitor side effects and improvement in your symptoms. If you fail to respond fully, you may need to try different dosages, medications, and combinations while continuing to monitor side effects and symptoms. If this whole process becomes unduly complex, you might need to find a specialist (i.e., a psychiatrist if you've been working with an internist or family practitioner). You might also need to consider psychotherapy, if you are not already involved in it, and you will need to continue taking the medication for a period after remission as well as possibly employing maintenance medication. All the while, you'll have to keep track of your mood so as to optimize your treatment.

Thus taking medication is likely to be anything but simple. You'll do best if you learn all you can about medications, and you'll need to deliberate about costs versus benefits. Above all, if you're among the majority for whom taking one medication does not suffice to produce recovery, you'll need patience, persistence, and endurance—often in the face of ongoing illness. There's no substitute for a good working relationship with your psychiatrist as you go through this process.

OTHER SOMATIC INTERVENTIONS

Antidepressant medication is almost always the first-line somatic (physical) treatment for depression, but medication is not always fully effective. When you have received limited benefit from medication, there are other alternatives, the most demonstrably effective being ECT. Just as new medications are being developed continually, researchers are developing other kinds of somatic treatments. I mention two of these here: transcranial magnetic stimulation and vagus nerve stimulation.

ELECTROCONVULSIVE THERAPY

Many of us who've been around for awhile indelibly associate ECT with *One Flew Over the Cuckoo's Nest*. ECT might seem like punishment, torture, or a brutal form of treatment at best. To the contrary, in contemporary practice, ECT is safe when carefully prescribed, and it's widely regarded as the most effective treatment for major depression as well as producing the most rapid benefit.[189,509,515] ECT has the benefit of a half-century of practice and research, and the past decade has seen major advances in refinement of administration. If you or a family member are considering ECT, it makes sense to educate yourself, and good information is available.[516]

ECT entails an electrically induced generalized seizure following the administration of a general anesthetic and a muscle relaxant. Depending on the patient's condition, ECT may be administered on either an inpatient or outpatient basis. The typical course of treatments is three per week for a period of 2–4 weeks, although fewer or more treatments may be employed depending on the individual's response. A wide range of dosages and electrode placements have been studied. Perhaps most important is the distinction between bilateral ECT, which generally has the greater antidepressant effect, and unilateral right-hemisphere ECT, which is less disruptive to memory. Relatively high doses of unilateral ECT also have been used to maximize the antidepressant effect while minimizing the memory impairment.[517]

Despite its safety and effectiveness, ECT is rarely employed as a first-line intervention for depression, although there are exceptions: when a patient is extremely ill or suicidal and a rapid response is urgently needed; when alternative treatments involve higher risk; and when the patient has responded best to ECT in the past or has a strong preference for ECT. Most often, ECT is employed after extensive trials of medication have failed. Unfortunately, failure to benefit from antidepressant medication is also an indication of less likelihood of benefiting from ECT. Yet many patients who have not responded to medication respond positively to ECT. Like medication, ECT is not curative; remission can be followed by relapse or recurrence. Accordingly, continuation and maintenance treatment are often employed, most often with antidepressant medication. Some patients also benefit from continuation and maintenance ECT.

Careful medical and psychiatric evaluation must precede administration of ECT, as is true for antidepressant medication. When medical contraindications (e.g., certain forms of cardiovascular disease) have been ruled out, ECT is a safe treatment with minimal lasting side effects.[509] Commonly, however, patients will experience a period of confusion lasting up to 1 hour after the seizure, and a sizeable minority of patients experience memory problems, which take two forms. Retrograde amnesia entails forgetting of information preceding the treatment, primarily during the months before ECT. Apart from the time immediately preceding each seizure, this retrograde amnesia abates over the weeks or months following the treatment. Some patients experience anterograde amnesia, difficulty retaining new information after the course of ECT. This form of amnesia also abates in the weeks following ECT.

Occasionally, however, patients report more extensive and persistent memory problems associated with ECT, and potential adverse effects on mental functioning continue to be investigated. Of course, any potential adverse effects must be weighed against potential treatment benefits, and the adverse effects of continuing depression are all too obvious. Moreover, because depression is associated with problems in concentration and memory, ECT also can improve general memory functioning, just as any other successful treatment can do.

REPETITIVE TRANSCRANIAL MAGNETIC STIMULATION

Repetitive transcranial magnetic stimulation (rTMS) employs a handheld electromagnet to induce an electrical current in the brain without causing seizures.[502,515] Depending on the frequency of the current, rTMS either increases or decreases neuronal excitability in the brain region stimulated. rTMS is a relatively new intervention that has shown promise in treating patients who have not responded fully to multiple trials of antidepressants and ECT,[518] and it has been employed to augment medication. Clinicians and researchers are exploring a wide range of rTMS procedures with widely varying results; at this point, it remains an experimental treatment.

VAGUS NERVE STIMULATION

Vagus nerve stimulation (VNS) requires that a battery-operated stimulator be surgically implanted in the chest, with leads attached to the vagus nerve. The vagus nerve has widespread connections to the autonomic nervous system as well as to the subcortex and cerebral cortex. VNS was initially employed as an anticonvulsant but was discovered also to have mood elevating effects. Hence it is currently being investigated as an intervention for severe and chronic depression that has been unresponsive to other treatments, with some preliminary evidence of success for a sizeable minority of patients.[515]

MEDICATION AND PSYCHOTHERAPY

When you are considering treatment options for depression, you face a broad choice: medication or psychotherapy or both? We know from extensive research that medication, psychotherapy, and combinations of the two are effective; are all viable options. Unfortunately, we have not advanced very far on the question of concern to each individual: which is best for me? As psychologists Anthony Roth and Peter Fonagy[17] aptly put it, the most important question is not, what works? but rather *what works for whom?*

MEDICATION VERSUS PSYCHOTHERAPY

If we had only one form of psychotherapy and one antidepressant medication, researchers doubtlessly would have discovered by now if one were generally more effective than the other. However, we have a number of different therapies as well as many medications and innumerable combinations; research has been conducted on a tiny fraction of possible combinations. Current research indicates that medication and psychotherapy are often equivalent in their effectiveness, but we need to take differences into account.

The National Institute of Mental Health (NIMH) Treatment of Depression Collaborative Research Program was the most ambitious experimental comparison of the effectiveness of medication and psychotherapy. Outpatients in three research sites were randomly assigned to one of four treatment groups: medication (the TCA Tofranil), placebo, interpersonal psychotherapy, and cognitive therapy. The medication and placebos were administered in the context of weekly 20–30 minute supportive therapy sessions conducted by experienced psychiatrists. The interpersonal and cognitive therapy was provided in weekly 50-minute sessions. In all groups, the length of treatment was around 16 weeks.

The complex results of this landmark study defy simple summary.[519–521] Most broadly, medication was most effective and placebo least effective; the two psychotherapies were intermediate in effectiveness and not greatly different from one another. Medication led to more rapid improvement than the other treatments. Yet the severity of the patients' condition proved to be an important factor in the effectiveness of the treatments. For the less severely depressed patients, all four treatments were equally helpful—including the placebo condition, which included weekly supportive contact with a psychiatrist. For the more seriously ill patients (those who were severely depressed and whose daily functioning was impaired), medication was superior to psychotherapies and placebo.

Disconcertingly, however, an 18-month follow-up study showed that only 24% of the patients had both recovered and remained well, and there were no differences among treatments in their long-term effectiveness.[522] Only a minority of patients continued in further treatment after the initial 16-week period, and the researchers[522] concluded "that 16 weeks of these particular treatments is insufficient treatment to achieve full recovery and lasting remission for most outpatients with [major depressive disorder]" (p. 786).

Yet this story is incomplete; later investigations of findings from this study went beyond symptom improvement to examine life adjustment.[523,524] Patients who had participated in some form of psychotherapy reported better functioning in relationships, better ability to control their self-critical thinking, a greater sense of agency, and better understanding of the relation of their thinking and relationships to their depression. Moreover, the quality of the patient–therapist relationship contributed to enhanced adaptive capacities; patients may have benefited from internalizing the therapist's acceptance, thereby becoming more self-accepting.

If the NIMH study were your only guide, you might conclude that, if you're severely depressed, medication would be preferable to psychotherapy for symptoms of depression for two reasons: it's more effective, and its effects are more rapid. This conclusion would be consistent with recent trends in outpatient care: with the advent of SSRIs, the proportion of patients using medication increased dramatically (from 37% to 74%) in the decade between 1987 and 1997, whereas the proportion engaging in psychotherapy decreased somewhat (from 71% to 60%).[525] Yet ongoing research does not yield straightforward conclusions about which is best. Several carefully controlled studies revealed equal effectiveness of medication and psychotherapy for patients with mild to moderate depression,[526] and some reviewers have concluded that psychotherapy is equivalent in effectiveness to medication even for severe depression.[527]

Thus, to the potential frustration of consumers, research conducted to date leaves clinicians in no position to make absolute declarations as to whether or when you should choose medication versus psychotherapy. Yet most clinicians, myself included, favor using antidepressant medication to treat moderate to severe depression. Research is limited to comparing large groups of participants; in clinical practice, a wide range of individual factors must be considered, and increasingly sophisticated guidelines that take more individual factors into account are being developed.[528] Meanwhile, your clinician's judgment and your individual preferences will prevail. There's some reassurance in this; you can exercise choice. Furthermore, if you cannot take medication for some reason (e.g., a medical condition that precludes it), psychotherapy is a viable alternative. In addition, barring severe depression, you might begin with whichever one you prefer, and if you find it to be insufficient, you might switch to the other or combine the two.[17]

COMBINING MEDICATION AND PSYCHOTHERAPY

Although questions abound, one thing is clear: antidepressant medications and various therapies designed to treat depression are effective. If either is effective, you'd be inclined to think that combining the two would be even better. Surprisingly, it's not been easy for researchers to demonstrate that the combination is better than either one alone.[17,528] Yet one major study yielded convincing evidence of the benefit of combining treatment for adults with a history of severe and chronic depression (i.e., major depression and 2-year duration of depressive symptoms at some level).[529] This 12-week study compared the antidepressant Serzone (which is no longer in regular use) with the Cognitive Behavioral Analysis System of Psychotherapy, a form of cognitive therapy developed specifically to treat chronic depression.[530] This cognitive treatment is specifically designed to promote agency and interpersonal problem solving; patients learn how changing their thinking and behavior relieves their feelings of depression. The comparison revealed that antidepressant medication and cognitive therapy were equally effective and that their combination was even more effective: among those who completed treatment, 55% responded positively to medication, 52% to cognitive therapy, and 85% to both. Notably, patients responded more rapidly to medication than cognitive therapy. Nearly twice the proportion achieved full remission of symptoms with the combination (42%) compared with medication alone (22%) or cognitive therapy alone (24%). Although the fact that a minority of patients achieved full remission might be discouraging, keep in mind that this treatment was for a relatively short-term for patients who had been depressed for years.

Research on medication treatment for children lags behind that for adults; thus a major study comparing cognitive-behavioral therapy and the SSRI Prozac in the treatment of adolescents with major depression is noteworthy.[503] The results were clear-cut: medication was more effective than placebo, and combining cognitive-behavioral therapy with medication was even more effective. Notably, the cognitive-behavioral therapy was multifaceted, including education and family sessions as well as behavioral strategies for improving mood and interpersonal relationships along with ways of improving thought patterns.

Practice guidelines suggest combining medication and psychotherapy for adults with severe and recurrent depression.[510] If you're combining treatments, there are advantages to having both provided by one psychiatrist who can provide integrated care;[531] yet it is increasingly common for psychotherapy to be provided by a nonphysician therapist, and in that case, collaboration between the two treatment providers is essential.

Although experimental research does not invariably show an advantage for combining treatments, there are several cogent reasons to do so.[17,532] First, combined treatment can increase the magnitude of response, for example, with chronic depression. Second, combined treatment can increase the probability of response. Given that you might respond to one or the other, you might start them together so as to maximize the potential benefit. Third, combining treatments may enhance the breadth of response. For example, medication might yield the most rapid effects on symptoms of severe depression, whereas psychotherapy might be additionally helpful with problems in relationships and capacity to cope with stress. Psychotherapy might also help stabilize your response to medication to the extent that psychotherapy can help you resolve conflicts, manage stress, and learn coping strategies that will decrease the likelihood of relapse or prolong the duration of recovery.

One series of studies illustrates the potential role of psychotherapy in enhancing the effectiveness of treatment with antidepressant medication. The research compared two groups of patients who had shown a response to antidepressants; one group continued in standard treatment, and another group was provided with 10 sessions of cognitive-behavioral therapy focused on symptoms that had not responded fully to medication treatment.[533–535] The therapy was designed to modify symptoms such as anxiety and irritability that might contribute to the development of a new episode as well as to reduce long-term stress and foster lifestyle modifications that would enhance well-being. Over the course of a 6-year follow-up period, patients who had engaged in cognitive-behavioral therapy showed fewer residual symptoms and less likelihood of relapse and recurrence.

COMPARING PSYCHOTHERAPIES

Researchers have been comparing various types of psychotherapy for decades, and studies typically show a wide variety of approaches to be roughly equivalent in effectiveness.[536,537] Thus, it's not surprising that the same holds true of psychotherapies for depression.[17] Some therapies such as cognitive therapy and interpersonal psychotherapy rest on a far more solid research foundation than others. Yet to the extent that they have been properly researched, the various therapies structured specifically to treat depression that I have discussed in this book have been shown to be generally comparable in effectiveness. Moreover, many approaches to therapy can be administered effectively in group psychotherapy as well as individual psychotherapy.

BRAND NAMES

Extensive research showing comparable effectiveness casts doubt on how seriously we should take brand names of therapies, such as behavior therapy, cognitive therapy, interpersonal psychotherapy, and psychodynamic psychotherapy. Rather than taking these brand names at face value, psychotherapy researchers have begun examining what therapists and patients are actually doing in the psychotherapy, regardless of the brand name. In addition, researchers are investigating which components of the multifaceted brand-name therapies account for their effectiveness:

- Illustrating a brand-name effect, one study found that cognitive therapy included vigorous encouragement and reassurance coupled with employing intellect and rationality to control distressing emotions. In contrast, psychodynamic psychotherapy involved bringing disturbing feelings into awareness and expressing them, relating current problems to previous life experiences, and focusing on the patient–therapist relationship as a vehicle for change.[538]
- Similarly, another study showed that interpersonal psychotherapists focused more on relationship problems, asked for more elaboration, and were seen as more sensitive to the patient's feelings, whereas cognitive therapists exerted more control over the interaction and gave more explicit advice. Yet the features of the therapeutic process that determined the outcome did not relate to the difference in cognitive versus interpersonal emphasis but rather to the patient's experience of the therapy: in both interpersonal and cognitive therapy, patients benefited more if they experienced a sense of trust, effectiveness, and comfort coupled with a positive view of the therapist and a sense of closeness. Thus, regardless of the brand name, the patient's positive attachment made the difference.[539]
- In another study, leading experts representing cognitive-behavioral therapy and interpersonal psychotherapy were asked to indicate what characterizes the ideal psychotherapy process. Ironically, in practice,

both forms of therapy adhered more closely to the experts' ideal prototype of cognitive therapy, and greater adherence to the cognitive therapy ideal was associated with a better outcome in both forms of therapy.[540]

- It's not always clear in complex treatments what elements account for the benefit. A study of cognitive-behavioral therapy showed that the behavioral component alone was as effective as the standard procedure that combines behavioral and cognitive interventions.[541] The behavioral intervention was quite elaborate, including a systematic effort to facilitate engagement in activities that engender a sense of enjoyment or mastery along with enhancing social skills. Interestingly, the behavioral intervention was just as effective in altering negative thinking as the interventions that focused specifically on cognitive distortions. When your mood improves, your thinking becomes more reasonable.

We can infer from such studies that what the therapy is called is merely a rough guide to what the therapist and patient will actually do and little guide as to how effective it will be. In practice, many therapists are eclectic, drawing on interventions from a wide range of brands. For example, as Beck and colleagues developed it,[236] cognitive-behavioral therapy focuses on behavior, thinking, and relationships. The version of cognitive therapy developed specifically for chronic depression[530] is even more eclectic; it emphasizes interpersonal relationships, considers trauma history, and addresses the patient–therapist relationship. There's a potential tradeoff here: a more eclectic therapist can flexibly adapt the approach to your specific problems, but it's also helpful for the therapy to maintain a relatively consistent focus rather than jumping from pillar to post. A specific focus with corresponding practical accomplishments promotes a sense of agency, and a clear agenda is especially crucial in time-limited therapies.

COMMON FACTORS

One interpretation of the finding that different psychotherapies have similar effectiveness is that they all share some common factors. The therapist's empathy and positive regard for the patient play a significant role in all therapies,[542] including highly focused, problem-oriented therapies such as cognitive therapy.[543] Similarly, the therapeutic alliance, a solid working relationship between patient and therapist,[544] plays a major role in the outcome of psychotherapy. In the study comparing medication and cognitive therapy for chronic depression, for example, a good therapeutic alliance established early in the treatment predicted greater improvement in symptoms of depression, regardless of the type of treatment received.[529]

I have also suggested that a range of different therapies promotes agency, actively changing patterns of behavior, thinking, and relationships as well as working to resolve internal emotional conflicts. Moreover, agency is central to the therapeutic alliance, which we've construed as the patient's active collaboration with the therapist in working toward constructive change.[545]

In thinking about what form of psychotherapy is best, we might make an analogy with medication. Research compares groups, averaging across individuals. Although one group may do as well as the other, wide differences may still exist among individuals within each group. You are an individual. You will need to find a good match not just with a type of therapy (based on brand name) but also with an individual therapist. The interpersonal chemistry will play a significant role in your developing an effective working relationship.

MAINTENANCE PSYCHOTHERAPY

While placing stock in the value of medication in treating depression, I have also emphasized a specific benefit of psychotherapy: you can learn something—perhaps a number of things—that not only will help you recover but also can better enable you to remain well. But I do not want to overstate the case for psychotherapy; as I've also noted, many patients experience recurrence after benefiting from time-limited treatment, whether it be medication or psychotherapy. Here's a sobering assessment from Roth and Fonagy[17] based on a meticulous review of extensive research on the treatment of depression:

> The pattern of results for a structured therapy (and for pharmacotherapy) is quite consistent; a simple rule of thumb would be that, in around 50% of cases, symptoms will have remitted posttherapy, but that over 1 year of follow-up, around half of those who recovered will relapse. On this basis, only about one-fourth of patients treated using a *brief* therapy remain well. (p. 133; emphasis mine)

Thus we must consider not only trying different forms of treatment and combining them to enhance remission but also employing maintenance treatment to minimize the risk of recurrence and relapse. Maintenance medication provides substantial, although not absolute, protection against relapse or recurrence. Might maintenance psychotherapy do the same?

Unfortunately, research on long-term maintenance psychotherapy is even sparser than research on medication. One noteworthy study found that maintenance treatment provided over the course of 3 years to patients with a history of multiple episodes of depression substantially decreased the likelihood of recurrence.[546] Antidepressant medication (the TCA Tofranil) was most effective, but monthly interpersonal psychotherapy sessions without medication were more effective in preventing recurrence than was placebo. The research left open the question as to whether more frequent psychotherapy sessions might have provided more protection against relapse.

As I have noted in discussing research combining medication and psychotherapy, a number of studies have employed cognitive-behavioral therapy as a continuation treatment, often as a booster intervention when medication has not led to full remission of symptoms. Such studies generally show that the addition of cognitive-behavioral therapy reduces the risk of relapse.[17] However, we have little information on long-term maintenance treatment and no research that provides guidance as to whether any particular brand of psychotherapy might be more effective than any other as a maintenance treatment. Generalizing from research on medication, we might think that whatever therapy facilitated recovery might also be helpful as a continuation and maintenance treatment. Yet new kinds of problems might also call for a switch in psychotherapy approach.

HOSPITALIZATION

Patients and clinicians alike should heed author William Styron's experience with hospitalization.[2] After a several-month spiral into deepening depression, Styron developed the conviction that he would take his own life, and he sought psychiatric help. He entered twice-weekly psychotherapy and took antidepressant medication. Yet, as he wrote, "Neither medications nor psychotherapy were able to arrest my plunge toward the depths" (pp. 54–55). He deteriorated:

> The mornings…were becoming bad now as I wandered about lethargic, following my synthetic sleep [with sleeping medications], but afternoons were still the worst, beginning at about three o'clock, when I'd feel the horror, like some poisonous fog bank, roll in upon my mind, forcing me into bed. There I would lie for as long as six hours, stuporous and virtually paralyzed, gazing at the ceiling and waiting for that moment of evening when, mysteriously, the crucifixion would ease up just enough to allow me to force down some food and then, like an automaton, seek an hour or two of sleep again. *Why wasn't I in the hospital?* (pp. 58–59; emphasis mine)

Styron had disclosed his suicidal thinking at the outset of treatment and broached the option of hospitalization—he had had a friend whom hospital treatment had helped. Sadly, his psychiatrist discouraged it, saying it would be stigmatizing. Only after Styron had begun to make concrete preparations for suicide was he hospitalized; in his view, "I'm convinced I should have been in the hospital weeks before" (p. 68). He characterized the hospital as "an orderly and benign detention where one's only duty is to try to get well" and wrote that "the real healers were seclusion and time" (p. 69).

I have emphasized the importance of agency—initiating action—in recovering from depression. As Styron did, you can get to the point where your agency is at rock bottom; he was stuporous and virtually paralyzed. You can get to the point where you can't pull yourself out of it; you need a great deal of help to get going. Hospitalization can provide such help. Hospitalization also provides safety in the midst of suicidal states; Styron[2] wryly commented on the safety "of being removed to a world in which the urge to pick up a knife and plunge it into one's own breast disappears in the newfound knowledge, quickly apparent even to the depressive's fuzzy brain, that the knife with which he is attempting to cut his dreadful Swiss steak is bendable plastic" (p. 69).

In today's managed care climate, hospital treatment is typically brief, a matter of a few days to help the patient through an acute crisis. Styron was hospitalized for nearly 7 weeks, a length of treatment now available at a relatively small number of specialized inpatient programs such as The Menninger Clinic. As Styron described, such hospitalizations provide safety and sanctuary. By engaging patients in a structured routine, they promote activity and counter lethargy. Most important, in my view, they counter the profound sense of alienation and isolation that persons in the throes of severe depression experience. You recognize that you are not alone; others can comprehend what you are going through and provide solace. The sanctuary of the hospital also enables you to take stock of your stressful situation and to get a fresh start. Also, given the complexity of working with medications, hospitalization can allow for adequate trials with careful monitoring. Specialized inpatient programs also can capitalize on the extended period of hospitalization to provide patients with thorough education about depression and treatment options so as to promote self-care over the long haul.

As Styron's experience attests, profound depression can make it impossible to benefit from psychotherapy. Often, medication treatment might lead to sufficient improvement that psychotherapy can be undertaken, although not in Styron's case. Sometimes, hospitalization is required to make psychotherapy possible.

Geoff was virtually bedridden with depression, even in the hospital. He was so depressed he could hardly bathe, shave, dress properly, or eat. He could not talk much either, and he was quite irritable when he did. Fortunately, the weather was decent, and I suggested to Geoff that we hold our sessions outside. For some weeks, we sat in the sun, chatting a bit. I figured that, even if the psychotherapy didn't do him much good, the sun might. Sun therapy—with companionship. Gradually, with the help of hospitalization and medication, his depression improved to the point that we eased into a highly productive psychotherapy process. He responded well to all his treatment, and he was able to use all he had learned to continue his recovery process very effectively on an outpatient basis.

RECOVERY AND WELLNESS

You're approaching your depression in the right way: you're taking agency by learning about your illness and treatment options. If—like most patients—you have not recovered fully from a reasonable course of treatment, or you are continuing to struggle with relapses and recurrences along with ongoing symptoms, you will need to approach depression intelligently, keeping abreast of treatment developments and using your knowledge to obtain the best care. You face two challenges: recovering fully and remaining well.

RECOVERING

You will do best to aim for freedom from depression rather than settling for partial relief. Freedom from symptoms of depression puts you in a position to function best in your relationships and your daily responsibilities. Freedom from depression also will enhance your physical health and overall quality of life. Finally, full recovery is the best protection against relapse. As all the research shows, however, full recovery is harder to achieve.[30] A small minority of depressed persons receive adequate treatment, and many discontinue treatment prematurely. Notoriously, many patients quit taking medication after they feel somewhat better, then they relapse. Depressed and discouraged, they go without further treatment.

As with many things in life, in aspiring to recover from depression, the key will be persistence, which is asking a lot of you when you're depressed. Considering the potential complications in finding the best medication, it's little wonder that so few people are adequately treated. You also have the further complication of deciding between psychotherapy and medication or combining them. If you decide to seek psychotherapy, you have many brands to choose from, not to mention the viable options of individual, group, or marital therapy. I don't take the brand names too seriously; the crucial factor is that you feel you have a good working relationship with your therapist and that you believe the therapy is addressing your individual concerns. I've intended the chapters in this last part to highlight the range of problems associated with depression so as to help you identify where your therapeutic focus should be.

Your therapist will rely on you to identify the specific problems and to steer the course of the therapy, although finding the best focus for therapy is a joint effort that often requires some period of exploration. I worked with an extremely depressed man who, after giving a brief synopsis of his plight, demanded, "Therapize me!" Would that I could. That's not how it works. Assuming you've found a good match with a therapist, psychotherapy is like anything else: what you get out of it will depend on what you put into it. The key to using therapy is simple and not easy: being open and honest.

Reiterating, I think you'll do best if you proceed intelligently, armed with knowledge and prepared to experiment. Whatever treatment you choose, you'll need to give it an adequate trial, although medication will often have more rapid effects than psychotherapy. For either form of treatment, an adequate trial will be several weeks, and you'll need to consult with your clinician about what constitutes "adequate." You'll need to strike a balance. On the one hand, you'll be struggling with ongoing symptoms while you give the treatment adequate time to take effect. On the other hand, you won't want to struggle with symptoms too long if the treatment is not helping and there's a good likelihood that another treatment will be more effective. You'll need to wrestle with the trade-off between persisting and switching. You're best advised not to settle for partial response, whether you're taking medication, working with a psychotherapist, or both. For example, if you are averse to taking medication and you begin psychotherapy instead, you might reconsider if the therapy is not fully effective—either switching to medication or adding medication. Agency will rule the day: you'll do best by actively experimenting. The ultimate question is finding out what works for you. Trying different options is the norm.

Regardless of the treatment you employ, treatment is not enough. Recovering involves more than taking medication or going to psychotherapy sessions. I cannot overstate the importance of working on your health: being as active as you can, attending to your diet, obtaining regular sleep, and maintaining a steady routine. Strengthening and making use of social support also is crucial. In addition, the surest way to undermine your chances of recovering from depression is to abuse alcohol and drugs. Thus of paramount importance is refraining from substance abuse and seeking whatever help you might need to do so. As Figure 14–1 depicts, how you live your life is the main factor in your battle with depression; engaging in treatment is merely one facet of how you live your life, and ideally, treatment can be helpful in living your life with more freedom from depression.

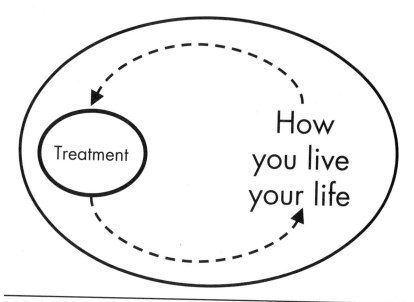

FIGURE 14–1. What matters most.

REMAINING WELL

You'll work hard to recover as fully as you can from depression. Yet your work isn't finished when you've recovered. I have been focusing on depression as the primary problem, but depression is typically a response to other problems, the resolution of which is critical to durable recovery and remaining well. In some ways, recovering from depression is only the first step—it can give you back the energy and the mental wherewithal to cope with the problems that brought on or perpetuated your depression. Thus recovery can help return you to a more effective problem-solving mode. Tackling and resolving problems can decrease the stress that renders you vulnerable to depression.

Furthermore, rebounding from depression does not mean that you are finished with treatment. Even when your symptoms have abated, you will be wise to continue in treatment. Especially if you have had recurrent episodes or chronic depression, you'll need to consider maintenance treatment, which may include some combination of medication and psychotherapy over a long period of time. The likelihood of recurrence for major depressive episodes can be discouraging, but you are an individual, not a statistic. Keep in mind that the vast majority of depressed persons do not obtain adequate treatment. Agency is central here: you can influence your risk of recurrence, even if you cannot fully control it.

Here's how I interpret the benefits and limitations of treatment revealed by research: a brief dosage of treatment—16 weeks, for example—is unlikely to have lasting effects unless you use it to make enduring changes—in your health, patterns of thinking, and relationships. You also may need ongoing help, at least periodically, to reinforce these changes or to reinstate them when you've slipped. Here's Andrew Solomon's[114] succinct advice for relapse prevention: "Act fast; have a good doctor prepared to hear from you; know your own patterns really clearly; regulate sleep and eating no matter how odious the task may be; lift stresses at once; exercise; mobilize love" (p. 86).

I've emphasized catch-22 in so many parts of this book that you may be as tired of reading it as I am of writing it. When you're relatively well, you're not dogged by catch-22, and you can more easily do all you need to do to stay well—be active, have your fill of positive experience, eat well, sleep well, maintain a routine, and do whatever else you must to take care of your physical health. You'll be able to think reasonably, flexibly, and creatively, and you'll be in the best position to develop and maintain secure attachment relationships.

I think a history of depression requires that you care for yourself in an ongoing way, with help from others as you need it. There are worse fates! Having tackled the daunting challenges of recovery, you're in a good position to take care of yourself. When and if you need it, you can seek treatment sooner rather than later, so that you don't become mired in catch-22. In short, there's hope, which brings us to the last chapter.

Chapter 15

HOPE

I can't think of anything more important than maintaining hope when you're striving to recover from depression. Catch-22: at its worst, depression promotes hopelessness. I believe that thinking clearly about hope can be of some help. This chapter gives some definition to hope and describes how depression can undermine it. Yet my main aim is to stimulate your thinking about what might give you hope.

I have proposed repeatedly that catch-22 makes recovery from depression difficult but not impossible. Here's author William Styron's[2] perspective: "Men and women who have recovered from the disease—and they are countless—bear witness to what is probably its only saving grace: it is conquerable" (p. 84).

UNDERSTANDING HOPE

As my mentor, psychologist Paul Pruyser,[547] advocated, we can best start defining hope by distinguishing it from optimism and wishful thinking. Hope, wishful thinking, and optimism are all forward-looking: they involve desiring and anticipating positive events and outcomes. Compared with having hope, wishing is easy: you can wish for anything, effortlessly. It's not so easy to be optimistic, especially when you're depressed; then, you're likely to be pessimistic. I think depression and optimism are downright incompatible, but hope and depression are not. I don't want to minimize the importance of optimism; its widespread benefits for physical and emotional well-being are well demonstrated.[548] However, optimism is too light-hearted a concept to be brought to bear on severe depression.

Unlike wishing and optimism, Pruyser[547] construed hope as pertaining to serious concerns, a response to felt tragedy:

> "To hope...one must have a tragic sense of life, an undistorted view of reality, a degree of modesty vis-à-vis the power and workings of nature or the cosmos, some feeling of commonality, if not communion, with other people, and some capacity to abstain from impulsive, unrealistic wishing." (p. 465)

The profoundly depressed patients I work with need hope in just this sense. They have been terribly mistreated, their marriages are threatened or have been dissolved, their careers are in jeopardy, they feel completely alienated, or they've battled depression for months, years, or decades. Some patients face all these at once—and more. In this context, a buoyant, optimistic stance makes no psychological sense. Yet hope is essential.

Because hope pertains to tragic circumstances, hope is always haunted by fear and doubt. Without fear and doubt, you would have no need for hope. Hope can be unstable: you alternate between hope and doubt, hope and hopelessness. You strive, you feel defeated, you give up, then you pull yourself together, rekindle hope, and strive some more. To the extent that you can maintain it, hope sustains striving, and persistence is the key to recovery.

REALISM

You can wish for anything, realistic or unrealistic. Hope is far more challenging: hope requires facing reality. Oncologist-hematologist Jerome Groopman[549] addressed this facet of hope squarely:

> Many of us confuse hope with optimism, a prevailing attitude that "things turn out for the best." But hope differs from optimism. Hope does not arise from being told to "think positively," or from hearing an overly rosy forecast. Hope, unlike optimism, is rooted in unalloyed reality. Although there is no uniform definition of hope, I found one that seemed to capture what my patients had taught me. Hope is the elevating feeling we experience when we see—in the mind's eye—a path to a better future. Hope acknowledges the significant obstacles and deep pitfalls along that path. True hope has no room for delusion. (p. xiv)

Like other serious medical illnesses, depression must be faced with a realistic attitude. We must acknowledge catch-22 in all its manifestations. We must face the findings of careful research showing the level of impairment in functioning associated with depression, the likelihood of experiencing ongoing symptoms of depression despite benefiting from treatment, and the potential for relapse and recurrence. We must face the limited effectiveness of various treatments along with the need to try different treatments and combinations as well as the need to persist in treatment—despite all its limitations. The whole point of this book has been to urge you to take the seriousness of depression seriously so you can cope as intelligently and effectively as possible.

You need hope, because you're likely to spend considerable time struggling with some level of depressive symptoms, episodically, as you strive to get well and stay well. You need to find a way of living with the sheer seriousness of depression as you work with it and against it. Author Andrew Solomon[114] captured the spirit of maintaining hope in the midst of depression in this eloquent advice:

> The most important thing to remember during a depression is this: you do not get the time back. It is not tacked on at the end of your life to make up for the disaster years. Whatever time is eaten by a depression is gone forever. The minutes that are ticking by as you experience the illness are minutes you will not know again. No matter how bad you feel, you have to do everything you can to keep living, even if all you can do for the moment is to breathe. Wait it out and occupy the time of waiting as fully as you possibly can. That's my big piece of advice to depressed people. Hold on to time; don't wish your life away. Even the minutes when you feel you are going to explode are minutes of your life, and you will never get those minutes again. (p. 430)

AGENCY AND PATHWAYS

Hope requires a marriage of emotion and reason. Karl Menninger[550] neatly construed hope as providing a motive force (emotion) for a potentially successful plan of action (reason). Psychologist Rick Snyder and colleagues[554] captured the same idea in pinpointing two components of hope: *agency* (the motive force) and *pathways* (the plan of action). I've emphasized the importance of agency throughout this book. Although agency is essential for hope, it's not sufficient. You also need a pathway: a sense of direction, a way forward, something specific to do or to hope for.

I always include discussions of hope in the educational groups I lead on depression and trauma; I've learned that hope will not be pinned down. In one group, after I'd made the case for the importance of pathways—a sense of direction—a patient protested that she sometimes relied on *blind faith*. Who was I to argue? Subsequently, I came across this passage in philosopher John Dewey's[97] writing; he'd have agreed with her:

Man continues to live because he is a living creature not because reason convinces him of the certainty or probability of future satisfactions and achievements. He is instinct with activities that carry him on. Individuals here and there cave in, and most individuals sag, withdraw and seek refuge at this and that point. But man as man still has the *dumb pluck* of the animal. He has endurance, hope, curiosity, eagerness, love of action. These traits belong to him by structure, not by taking thought. (pp. 199–200; emphasis mine).

Dumb pluck. I love that. I gave this quote to one of my most depressed patients the day after I discovered it; he'd lost just about everything and had no sense of direction. He appreciated the idea of dumb pluck too. Sometimes you just put one foot in front of the other. Granted, some people become so hopeless as to consider suicide, attempt it, or do it. Yet many people keep going *despite* hopelessness. Sometimes I ask patients, "What keeps you going?" They answer: "Survival instinct, I guess." A shred of agency, no pathway. Dumb pluck. Sometimes, we must bank on dumb pluck until a pathway can be found.

IMAGINATION

A compromise: full-fledged hope requires a sense of direction—pathways. Blind faith is fledgling, essential as it may be. Put more strongly, hope requires *imagination*. Things could be different. As contemporary philosopher Colin McGinn[551] construed it,

> Imagination is what presents the mind with alternative courses of action—the envisaging of possible futures. There is some merit in the idea, favored by the Romantics, that imagination is the *primary* locus of human freedom: it is what makes our overt actions free by offering us alternatives, and it is in itself an instance of free action, as we use it spontaneously to create all manner of marvelous mental products (literature, music, science, philosophy, etc.). Certainly, imagination is the most weightless and unconstrained of human faculties, the most fleet and feathery. (p. 195)

The fleet and feathery imaginativeness required for hope stands in stark contrast to the sluggishness and heaviness of depression. Yet as you recover from depression, your imaginative capacity returns, and you can begin envisioning what you can do to influence the future for the better—the practical steps toward concrete improvements. Sometimes the path isn't so clear. A depressed man I worked with had felt utterly trapped, and midway in the treatment, I asked him to create a visual image of his present situation. He said he'd walked out of the trap, but all he could see was fog. As he continued in treatment, his depression lifted further, and the fog began to clear.

In group discussions I ask patients what basis they have for hope. In one of these discussions, a young woman in the throes of depression replied imaginatively, "I can be surprised." She could imagine the unimaginable. Hearing her, Pruyser[547] would have smiled. Here's what he wrote:

> The person who hopes is future oriented in a special sense, namely, by seeing reality as a process of unfolding, and therefore essentially open-ended. This is precisely what may make waiting peaceful, and such a state of calmness stands in sharp contrast to the restlessness and impatience that typically accompany strong wishing. If reality is seen as open-ended, it is also likely to be seen as resourceful, and possibly as novelty producing. (p. 467)

HOW DEPRESSION UNDERMINES HOPE

Depression can undermine both pillars of hope, agency and pathways. Agents initiate action. Initiating action requires energy, oomph. Depression is enervating, sapping energy and motivation. You can be so depressed that you can hardly move. You're in a state of inertia, passive rather than active.

Depression also undermines your ability to find pathways. Envisioning pathways requires imagination and creativity. To have hope, you need to engage in problem solving, considering alternative courses of action and anticipating their outcomes. Yet we have seen from both neurobiological and psychological perspectives that depression undermines flexible thinking. When you're depressed, you tend to focus on the negative, perhaps ruminating, going around in circles.

Groopman's[549] work with cancer patients led him to believe that hope and hopelessness are grounded in the body. As it metastasizes, cancer can affect many vital organ systems, undermining the vital functions of respiration, circulation, and digestion. Groopman surmised that the brain registers the body's compromised state in the feeling of hopelessness. Depression, too, consists of a generalized state of physical ill health. If Groopman is right, the physiological state of depression might also contribute to the experience of hopelessness. As Groopman avers, there's hope in this: restoring your physical health also restores hope.

Many severely depressed patients feel hopeless, some for a considerable period of time. Alone, they cannot pull themselves out of this hopeless, depressed state. They need help. Physical help, for example, through medication, can begin restoring hope by giving you more energy and improving your mental functioning. Supportive relationships also restore hope. You may not be able to get going on your own, but the encouragement of others can inspire you to do so. You may not be able to imagine alternatives—or even to remember that you once felt better—but others can help you do so.

Sometimes you may need to rely on *borrowed hope*—the hope that others can hold out for you. I sometimes lend patients hope, on good grounds: I know it's possible to rebound from suicidal despair and hopelessness to feeling grateful to be alive; I've seen patients do it. I, too, rely on blind faith at the beginning of treatment. I may not be able to envision any pathways for my patients, but I know I can be surprised. Indeed, I count on it: pathways emerge as agency is restored.

BASES FOR HOPE

I have written this book to provide some basis for hope, grounded in the reality of the seriousness of depression. It's not some unfathomable failing on your part that accounts for the difficulty you're having with the illness; difficulty recovering and remaining well is intrinsic to the illness. As discussed in Chapter 2 ("Between a Rock and a Hard Place"), depression is an extraordinarily disabling disease, ranked fourth worldwide.[51] One of the main reasons depression remains so disabling is the failure to obtain adequate treatment. In part, this failure can be attributed to limitations in healthcare delivery. In part, the failure can be attributed to the illness: by depleting energy and undermining hope, depression interferes with seeking treatment.

KNOWLEDGE

Respecting catch-22, I've emphasized how hard it can be to recover from depression. Yet I've also described the wealth of things you can do to facilitate your recovery as well as a multitude of treatment interventions that can help you do all these things. Knowledge is power, and we have a wealth of knowledge. We are not in the dark. Of course, we always want to know more—and we will. Monumental effort, intelligence, and creativity are all going into understanding the development of depression from the womb to senescence as well as into creating and researching treatments. Brain research, ranging from molecular biology to neuroimaging, holds great promise. However, neurobiologists also recognize what Freud observed a century ago: early experience in attachment relationships plays a major role in vulnerability to illness and resilience, shaping the course of physiological and emotional development. Fortunately, as we're now glimpsing, we have a two-way street: biological treatments influence the mind as well as the brain, and psychological therapies influence the brain as well as the mind.

To the extent that our society will support further research and effective treatment, we will continue to learn at a rapid pace. It's realistic to hope for more effective treatments, and it's essential to stay informed as you care for yourself. Don't give up. Imagine the unimaginable.

BENEVOLENCE FROM WITHOUT

Of all the perspectives on hope, the one I've found most compelling over the years is Pruyser's[547] conclusion that "hoping is based on a belief that there is *some benevolent disposition toward oneself somewhere in the universe, conveyed by a caring person*" (p. 467; italics in the original). Pruyser captured the crux of hope in a marvelously open-ended way. Many depressed persons maintain hope through their spiritual connection with God or some other greater power. Many persons in the throes of depression also find their faith in God shaken. The loss of faith can engender guilt feelings and compound depression, in which case sensitive religious and spiritual counseling can be of inestimable value. Some persons, religious or not, benefit from a spiritual connection with nature. In discussing hope, one patient responded to Pruyser's definition by stating that she found benevolence in the sun and the rain: both are nourishing. She, as part of nature, was nurtured by nature.

Hope has deep religious significance; it's one of the theological virtues (with faith and charity). It is rightly regarded as a virtue: it's difficult, it's rare, and it's precious. Intriguingly, psychoanalyst Erik Erikson[552] regarded hope as the *virtue associated with basic trust*, the first stage of development. Erikson's view dovetails with Pruyser's; both authors predicated hope on the model of secure attachment. Pruyser[547] construed hope as developing out of the infant's ability to depend on the mother: "Eventually, the infant comes to *hope*, that is, gains the ability to accept peacefully some inevitable waiting, in the firm belief that the mother herself has a need to give her child what she can and is benevolently disposed toward him" (p. 467).

We have seen throughout this book that troubled attachment relationships play a major role in vulnerability to depression and that secure attachment relationships are a cornerstone of recovery. Attachment and hope are intertwined from an early age. In his struggle with hope, Styron[2] was blessed by the presence of his loving wife, Rose. Yet, mired in depression, he couldn't connect with her. He returned to his Connecticut home in October but remarked that the "fading evening light...had none of its familiar autumnal loveliness, but ensnared me in a suffocating gloom." He continued, "Physically, I was not alone. As always Rose was present and listened with unflagging patience to my complaints. But I felt an immense and aching solitude" (pp. 45–46). (He subsequently traced the origins of his depression to earlier sorrow; his mother died when he was 13.) Yet his attachment to Rose was not unendingly elusive: "Not for an instant could I let out of my sight the endlessly patient soul who had become nanny, mommy, comforter, priestess, and, most important, confidante—a counselor of rocklike centrality to my existence" (p. 57). No doubt, as Styron[2] made plain, attachment can be lifesaving:

> It has been shown over and over again that if the encouragement is dogged enough—and the support equally committed and passionate—the endangered one can nearly always be saved.... It may require on the part of friends, lovers, family, admirers, an almost religious devotion to persuade the sufferers of life's worth, which is so often in conflict with a sense of their own worthlessness, but such devotion has prevented countless suicides. (p. 76)

BENEVOLENCE FROM WITHIN

Styron is surely right: you'll need to rely on others' conviction of your worth when you feel utterly worthless. Yet cultivating your sense of worth is crucial to hope. Pruyser's view of hope as depending on a benevolent disposition toward yourself from somewhere in the universe might include your own benevolent disposition toward yourself.

As I construed it in Chapter 8 ("Internal Stress"), your relationship with yourself could be a powerful source of hope. Bonding with yourself gives you strength and vitality. Imagine having *a secure attachment relationship with yourself*: being emotionally attuned to yourself, keeping your mind in mind, with a benevolent and compassionate spirit.

> Marilyn had been cruelly abused by her mother, hated for being born and, most excruciatingly, castigated and beaten for being raped by neighbors when she was in her early teens. Throughout her adult life, despite many achievements and successes—not least raising children she loved—Marilyn felt utterly worthless. In childhood, her loving grandmother was her saving grace. Marilyn beamed as she talked about her grandmother, although her loving feelings were intermingled with deep sadness as she recalled the death of the one person with whom she had been close. As she talked about her grandmother, it became evident that Marilyn shared many of her grandmother's best attributes, including her kindness and compassion. I remarked that she had her grandmother's spirit. Marilyn then recalled that she'd occasionally felt a deep spiritual connection with her grandmother. Over the course of several weeks of hospital treatment, she had established a stronger sense of self-worth than she'd ever recalled having, and there were many contributors to this. But I believe that, in her identification with her grandmother and her sense of connection with her grandmother's spirit inside, Marilyn had found a benevolent disposition toward herself from within herself.

INDIVIDUAL CREATIVITY

Hope is an individual matter; I offer some general concepts but no prescriptions. I've discussed hope merely to encourage you to think about it and wrestle with it. Of all the topics we consider in educational groups on depression, hope is the most intriguing. I encourage participants in the group to describe their current basis for hope, if they have any—and not all do. I'm struck by the unpredictability and idiosyncrasy—sometimes the sheer quirkiness and creativity—in individuals' responses to this question. Table 15–1 lists some answers to the simple but difficult question, What gives you hope? These examples illustrate how hope is a way of relating to the world. It's an active process. Finding hope in the sight of a monarch butterfly, a sliver of sunlight, or a tiny yellow rose requires an imaginative connection with the world; it's a way of seeing. Noticing the grocery clerk's smile and taking it as a sign of hope is an active process. Hoping is something you *do*.

What basis do you have for hope? If you can, think of specific experiences that contribute to hope. Keep in mind that hope is infused with fear and doubt; it doesn't stay still. Your basis for hope is likely to shift from one time to another. You might be afraid to hope, fearing that, if you allow yourself to have hope, you'll wind up disappointed and disillusioned. Hoping takes courage. It is a virtue that requires agency: it's something hard won, something you'll need to work at in your own way.

Perhaps there's no firmer ground for hope than the possibility that some good ultimately might come from your painful experience. In this vein, Solomon[114] provided a fitting end for our discussion of hope:

> The unexamined life is unavailable to the depressed. That is, perhaps, the greatest revelation I have had: not that depression is compelling but that the people who suffer from it may become compelling because of it. I hope that this basic fact will offer sustenance to those who suffer and will inspire patience and love in those who witness that suffering.... There is great value in specific kinds of adversity. None of us would choose to learn this way: difficulty is unpleasant. I crave the easy life and would make and have made considerable compromises in my quest for it. But I have found that there are things to be made of this lot I have in life, that there are values to be found in it, at least when one is not in its most acute grip. (pp. 438–439)

TABLE 15–1. Bases for hope

Benevolence
Loving friends
The love of my 2-year old son
The kindness of strangers
Someone's kind word or helpful act
The grocery clerk's smile

Inspiration
Knowing that my mother overcame trauma
A neighbor who overcame adversity
A friend who recovered from depression
Someone believing in me
My employer holding my job for me

Spirituality
A connection with God
My higher power
Prayer
Listing things for which I am grateful

Nature
An inspiring encounter with nature
Seeing a tiny yellow rose in the sand
A sliver of light coming in my window
The ocean, a vast expanse with no obstacles
Seeing a monarch butterfly

Strengths
Inner strength
Visualizing myself in a strong stance
Successful coping with past challenges
My ability to learn coping skills

Growth
Getting my mind back with medication
Identifying self-defeating patterns
Clarity about what's caused me trouble

Fresh starts
The prospect of a fresh start
My son's birth after my daughter's death
Knowing that things change
Awareness of the unforeseen

GLOSSARY

Agency the capacity to take action on your own behalf; implies freedom, choice, and responsibility

Ambivalent attachment a pattern of INSECURE ATTACHMENT characterized by a combination of excessive dependence and hostility

Amygdala a structure deep in the temporal lobe of the brain that rapidly registers threatening stimuli and organizes fear responses

Appraisal more or less conscious judgment of the emotional significance of a situation

Attachment the emotional bond that develops in close relationships, the archetype being the mother–infant bond

Attachment trauma trauma in ATTACHMENT relationships; often interferes with establishing and maintaining trusting relationships

Avoidant attachment a pattern of INSECURE ATTACHMENT characterized by avoiding dependence on others and coping all by oneself

Bipolar disorder formerly manic-depressive disorder, characterized by alternations between MANIC episodes and depression

Brain-derived neurotrophic factor (BDNF) a chemical that promotes the growth and health of neurons (brain cells)

Catch-22 a snag or dilemma the precludes success; in depression, the idea that all the things one must do to recover from depression (e.g., sleep well) are made difficult by the symptoms of depression (e.g., insomnia)

SMALL CAPS type indicates terms defined elsewhere in this glossary.

Continuation treatment employment of medication or psychotherapy past the point of RESPONSE or REMISSION to ensure durable RECOVERY

Cortisol a major stress hormone that regulates the stress response at normal levels and dysregulates the stress response at excess levels

Deliberate self-harm self-injury (e.g., cutting or overdosing) for the primary purpose of escaping from unbearable emotional states; not based on suicidal intent

Dependent depression depression stemming from excess dependency and triggered by rejection, abandonment, or loss

Depression tolerance the adaptive capacity to be aware of and learn from depressive feelings without succumbing to depressive ILLNESS

Dopamine a neurotransmitter involved in alerting and reward

Double depression episodes of major depression on top of DYSTHYMIA

Dysthymia a depressive disorder that is less severe but more chronic than major depression (i.e., duration of at least 2 years)

Extraversion a personality trait characterized by POSITIVE EMOTIONALITY and sociability

Flow intensely enjoyable experience based on absorption in activity that optimally balances challenge and skill

Hippocampus a structure deep in the temporal lobe of the brain that plays a central role in encoding coherent memories of complex events and facilitating their conversion into long-term autobiographical memories

Illness a state from which one cannot recover by a mere act of will, and a social role that provides a legitimate excuse from many social and occupational obligations while obligating the ill person to seek and cooperate with treatment

Insecure attachment a lack of confidence in ATTACHMENT figures as evident in AMBIVALENT ATTACHMENT and AVOIDANT ATTACHMENT

Interpersonal trauma TRAUMA inflicted deliberately or recklessly by another person (e.g., a sexual assault or accident stemming from drunk driving)

Involuntary subordination strategy   in the face of being overpowered or oppressed, submitting involuntarily for the adaptive purpose of avoiding a dangerous confrontation, resulting in a state of depression

Learned helplessness   a response to repeated uncontrollable stress; learning to be helpless, evident in a failure to learn to escape the stress once it becomes avoidable

Maintenance treatment   employment of medication or psychotherapy after RECOVERY from an episode of ILLNESS for the purpose of preventing RECURRENCE

Mania   a state of heightened activity and elevated mood associated with poor judgment that leads to behavior with adverse consequences (e.g., reckless spending)

Mentalizing   apprehending mental states in oneself and others, for example, thinking about feelings; in relationships, the experience that each person has the other person's mind in mind

Negative emotionality   a spectrum of emotion ranging from calm contentment at the low end to fear and panic at the high end

Neuroticism   a partly TEMPERAMENTAL personality trait characterized by proneness to distress and anxiety

Norepinephrine   a form of adrenaline, a neurotransmitter involved in sympathetic nervous system arousal and the fight-or-flight response

Positive emotionality   a spectrum of emotion ranging from excitement and joy at the high end to depression at the low end

Postpartum depression   a major depressive episode beginning in the few weeks after childbirth

Prefrontal cortex   the front-most part of the cerebral cortex that mediates executive functions such as deliberating, planning, and prioritizing

Psychosis   loss of touch with reality; may take the form of hallucinations (e.g., hearing voices), delusions (e.g., unrealistically believing you are being persecuted), or severely disorganized thinking

PTSD   posttraumatic stress disorder; a psychiatric disorder that may develop after exposure to potentially traumatic events, symptoms of which include reexperiencing the traumatic event (e.g., in the form of flashbacks or nightmares), hyperarousal, avoidance, and numbing of emotional responsiveness

Reassurance seeking   a common form of interpersonal behavior in depression that engenders friction in relationships

Recovery   sustained REMISSION after an episode of ILLNESS, variously defined as ranging from 2 to 6 months

Recurrence   a new episode of ILLNESS after a period of RECOVERY

Relapse   a worsening of symptoms after RESPONSE or REMISSION but prior to RECOVERY

Remission   abatement of symptoms implying that the ILLNESS remains latent, with an ongoing risk of RELAPSE

Resilience   capacity to cope effectively with adversity; enhanced by SECURE ATTACHMENT and the capacity to MENTALIZE

Response   improvement short of REMISSION after initiation of treatment, defined in research as a 50% reduction in symptoms

Rumination   mulling over depressive concerns without progress in problem solving; makes symptoms worse

Safe haven   feeling of security provided by contact with an attachment figure

Seasonal affective disorder (SAD)   diagnosed when there is a consistent conjunction of mood episodes with the seasons of the year, with onset typically in fall or winter and remission in the spring

Secure attachment   the optimal pattern of ATTACHMENT characterized by confidence in the availability and emotional responsiveness of the attachment figure

Secure base   foundation for autonomy and exploration—including exploring the mind of oneself and others—provided by a SECURE ATTACHMENT relationship

Self-critical depression   depression stemming from harsh self-criticism in conjunction with a feeling of failure

Self-dependence   the capacity to bridge the gap between separation and re-union (e.g., by self-soothing or by holding in mind a comforting memory of being with a caring person)

Self-efficacy   a feeling of being able to influence the external environment (e.g., other persons) or internal experience (e.g., emotions)

Self-love   the virtue of emotional bonding with oneself that fosters strength, vitality, and hope

Sensitization   increased emotional responsiveness to a stressful stimulus re-sulting from repeated exposure to extreme, repeated, and uncontrollable stress

Serotonin   a neurotransmitter that plays a key role in modulating the stress response and enhancing impulse control; the immediate target of SSRIS

SSRIs   selective SEROTONIN reuptake inhibitors; widely used antidepres-sants (e.g., Prozac and Zoloft)

Stoicism   ancient Greek and Roman philosophical movement advocating eliminating emotional reactions to uncontrollable events

Stress generation   the process of unwittingly engaging in behavior or cre-ating patterns of relationships that increase stress

Stress pileup   an accumulation of stress that erodes the capacity for coping, often manifested in episodes of depression

Temperament   biologically based personality characteristics evident early in life that place constraints on development (e.g., proneness to anxiety)

Therapeutic alliance   optimal patient–therapist relationship based on feel-ings of trust and acceptance coupled with active collaboration on shared goals

Trauma   lasting negative effects of exposure to extremely stressful events

Vicious circle   two factors interacting such that each one makes the other worse (e.g., depression promotes alcohol abuse which, in turn, deepens de-pression)

REFERENCES

1. Heller J: *Catch-22*. New York, Simon and Schuster, 1955.
2. Styron W: *Darkness Visible*. New York, Random House, 1990.
3. McDermott JJ: *The Writings of William James: A Comprehensive Edition*. Chicago, IL, University of Chicago Press, 1977.
4. Watson D: *Mood and Temperament*. New York, Guilford, 2000.
5. Kendler KS, Kuhn J, Prescott CA: "The Interrelationship of Neuroticism, Sex, and Stressful Life Events in the Prediction of Episodes of Major Depression." *American Journal of Psychiatry* 161:631–636, 2004.
6. Meehl PE: "Hedonic Capacity: Some Conjectures." *Bulletin of the Menninger Clinic* 39:295–307, 1975.
7. Panksepp J: *Affective Neuroscience: The Foundations of Human and Animal Emotions*. New York, Oxford University Press, 1998.
8. American Psychiatric Association: *Diagnostic and Statistical Manual of Mental Disorders*, 4th Edition, Text Revision. Washington, DC, American Psychiatric Association, 2000.
9. Hankin BL, Fraley RC, Lahey BB, et al.: "Is Depression Best Viewed as a Continuum or Discrete Category? A Taxometric Analysis of Childhood and Adolescent Depression in a Population-Based Sample." *Journal of Abnormal Psychology* 114:96–110, 2005.
10. Ruscio J, Ruscio AM: "Informing the Continuity Controversy: A Taxometric Analysis of Depression." *Journal of Abnormal Psychology* 109:473–487, 2000.
11. Judd LL, Akiskal HS, Maser JD, et al.: "Major Depressive Disorder: A Prospective Study of Residual Subthreshold Depressive Symptoms as Predictor of Rapid Relapse." *Journal of Affective Disorders* 50:97–108, 1998.
12. Nierenberg AA, Wright EC: "Evolution of Remission as the New Standard in the Treatment of Depression." *Journal of Clinical Psychiatry* 60 (suppl):7–11, 1999.
13. Wells KB, Sturm R, Sherbourne CD, et al.: *Caring for Depression*. Cambridge, MA, Harvard University Press, 1996.
14. Angst J: "Minor and Recurrent Brief Depression," in *Dysthymia and the Spectrum of Chronic Depressions*. Edited by Akiskal HS, Cassano GB. New York, Guilford, 1997, pp. 183–190.

15. Akiskal HS, Cassano GB: *Dysthymia and the Spectrum of Chronic Depressions.* New York, Guilford, 1997.

16. Keller MB, Lavori PW: "Double Depression, Major Depression, and Dysthymia: Distinct Entities or Different Phases of a Single Disorder?" *Psychopharmacology Bulletin* 20:399–402, 1984.

17. Roth A, Fonagy P: *What Works for Whom? A Critical Review of Psychotherapy Research*, 2nd Edition. New York, Guilford, 2005.

18. Haykal RF, Akiskal HS: "The Long-Term Outcome of Dysthymia in Private Practice: Clinical Features, Temperament, and the Art of Management." *Journal of Clinical Psychiatry* 60:508–518, 1999.

19. Keller MB, Shapiro RW: "'Double Depression': Superimposition of Acute Depressive Episodes on Chronic Depressive Disorders." *American Journal of Psychiatry* 139:438–442, 1982.

20. Klein DN, Taylor EB, Harding K, et al.: "Double Depression and Episodic Major Depression: Demographic, Clinical, Familial, Personality, and Socioenvironmental Characteristics and Short-Term Outcome." *American Journal of Psychiatry* 145:1226–1231, 1988.

21. Keller MB, Hirschfeld RM, Hanks DL: "Double Depression: A Distinctive Subtype of Unipolar Depression." *Journal of Affective Disorders* 45:65–73, 1997.

22. Ryder AG, Bagby RM, Dion KL: "Chronic, Low-Grade Depression in a Nonclinical Sample: Depressive Personality or Dysthymia?" *Journal of Personality Disorders* 15:84–93, 2001.

23. McDermut W, Zimmerman M, Chelminski I: "The Construct Validity of Depressive Personality Disorder." *Journal of Abnormal Psychology* 112:49–60, 2003.

24. Phillips KA, Gunderson JG, Triebwasser J, et al.: "Reliability and Validity of Depressive Personality Disorder." *American Journal of Psychiatry* 155:1044–1048, 1998.

25. Rosenthal NE, Sack DA, Gillin JC, et al.: "Seasonal Affective Disorder." *Archives of General Psychiatry* 41:72–80, 1984.

26. Magnusson A, Boivin D: "Seasonal Affective Disorder: An Overview." *Chronobiology International* 20:189–207, 2003.

27. Oren DA, Rosenthal NE: "Light Therapy," in *Treatments of Psychiatric Disorders*, Volume 2, 3rd Edition. Edited by Gabbard GO. Washington, DC, American Psychiatric Publishing, 2001, pp. 1295–1306.

28. Frank E, Prien RF, Jarrett RB, et al.: "Conceptualization and Rationale for Consensus Definitions of Terms in Major Depressive Disorder: Remission, Recovery, Relapse, and Recurrence." *Archives of General Psychiatry* 48:851–885, 1991.

29. Riso LP, Thase ME, Howland RH, et al.: "A Prospective Test of Criteria for Response, Remission, Relapse, Recovery, and Recurrence in Depressed Patients Treated With Cognitive Behavior Therapy." *Journal of Affective Disorders* 43:131–142, 1997.

30. Keller MB: "Past, Present, and Future Directions for Defining Optimal Treatment Outcome of Depression: Remission and Beyond." *Journal of the American Medical Association* 289:3152–3160, 2003.

31. Kim-Cohen J, Caspi A, Moffitt TE, et al.: "Prior Juvenile Diagnoses in Adults With Mental Disorder." *Archives of General Psychiatry* 60:709–717, 2003.

32. Lewis L, Kelly KA, Allen JG: *Restoring Hope and Trust: An Illustrated Guide to Mastering Trauma.* Baltimore, MD, Sidran Press, 2004.

33. Darwin C: *The Expression of Emotion in Man and Animals* (1872). Chicago, IL, University of Chicago Press, 1965.

34. Cannon WB: *Bodily Changes in Pain, Hunger, Fear and Rage: An Account of Recent Researches Into the Function of Emotional Excitement.* Boston, MA, Charles T. Branford, 1953.

35. Schmale AH: "Depression as Affect, Character Style, and Symptom Formation," in *Psychoanalysis and Contemporary Science: An Annual of Integrative Interdisciplinary Studies,* Volume 1. Edited by Holt RR, Peterfeund E. New York, Macmillan, 1972, pp. 327–351.

36. Price J, Sloman L, Gardner R, et al.: "The Social Competition Hypothesis of Depression." *British Journal of Psychiatry* 164:309–315, 1994.

37. Dubovsky SL: *Mind–Body Deceptions: The Psychosomatics of Everyday Life.* New York, W.W. Norton, 1997.

38. Klinger E: "Loss of Interest," in *Symptoms of Depression.* Edited by Costello CG. New York, Wiley, 1993, pp. 43–62.

39. Neese RM: "Is Depression an Adaptation?" *Archives of General Psychiatry* 57:14–20, 2000.

40. Gilbert P: *Depression: The Evolution of Powerlessness.* New York, Guilford, 1992.

41. Seligman MEP: *Helplessness: On Depression, Development and Death.* San Francisco, CA, W.H. Freeman, 1975.

42. Zetzel ER: "Depression and the Incapacity to Bear It," in *Drives, Affects, Behavior,* Volume 2. Edited by Schur M. New York, International Universities Press, 1965, pp. 243–274.

43. Martin P: *The Zen Path Through Depression.* New York, HarperCollins, 1999.

44. Michels R: "Treatment of Depression in the New Health Care Scene," in *Treatment of Depression: Bridging the 21st Century.* Edited by Weissman MM. Washington, DC, American Psychiatric Press, 2001, pp. 47–54.

45. Hammen C: *Depression.* East Sussex, UK, Psychology Press, 1997.

46. Blazer D, Kessler RC, McGonagle KA, et al.: "The Prevalence and Distribution of Major Depression in a National Community Sample: The National Comorbidity Survey." *American Journal of Psychiatry* 151:979–986, 1994.

47. Hammen C, Rudolph KD: "Childhood Depression," in *Child Psychopathology.* Edited by Mash EJ, Barkley RA. New York, Guilford, 1996, pp. 153–195.

48. Friedman RA: "Social and Occupational Adjustment in Chronic Depression," in *Diagnosis and Treatment of Chronic Depression.* Edited by Kocsis JH, Klein DN. New York, Guilford, 1995, pp. 89–102.

49. Judd LL, Akiskal HS, Zeller PJ, et al.: "Psychosocial Disability in the Long-Term Course of Unipolar Major Depressive Disorder." *Archives of General Psychiatry* 57:375–380, 2000.

50. Hirschfeld RM, Montgomery SA, Keller MB, et al.: "Social Functioning in Depression: A Review." *Journal of Clinical Psychiatry* 61:268–275, 2000.

51. Murray CJL, Lopez AD: "Executive Summary," in *The Global Burden of Disease: A Comprehensive Assessment of Mortality and Disability From Diseases, Injuries, and Risk Factors in 1990 and Projected to 2020*. Geneva, Switzerland, World Health Organization, and Boston, MA, Harvard School of Public Health, 1996, pp. 1–43.

52. Ustun TB: "The Worldwide Burden of Depression in the 21st Century," in *Treatment of Depression: Bridging the 21st Century*. Edited by Weissman MM. Washington, DC, American Psychiatric Press, 2001, pp. 35–45.

53. Kraepelin E: *Manic-Depressive Insanity and Paranoia*. Translated by Barclay RM. Edinburgh, Scotland, Livingstone, 1921.

54. Angst J: "The Course of Affective Disorders." *Psychopathology* 19:47–52, 1986.

55. Mueller TI, Leon AC: "Recovery, Chronicity, and Level of Psychopathology in Major Depression." *Psychiatric Clinics of North America* 19:85–102, 1996.

56. Oldehinkel AJ, Ormel J, Neeleman J: "Predictors of Time to Remission From Depression in Primary Care Patients: Do Some People Benefit More From Positive Life Change Than Others?" *Journal of Abnormal Psychology* 109:299–307, 2000.

57. Wilkinson P, Hawton K, Andrew B, et al.: "Does the Duration of Illness Before Treatment Affect the Time Taken to Recover on Treatment in Severely Depressed Women?" *Journal of Affective Disorders* 41:89–92, 1996.

58. Keller MB, Lavori PW, Mueller TI, et al.: "Time to Recovery, Chronicity, and Levels of Psychopathology in Major Depression." *Archives of General Psychiatry* 49:809–816, 1992.

59. Solomon DA, Keller MB, Leon AC, et al.: "Recovery From Major Depression: A 10-Year Prospective Follow-Up Across Multiple Episodes." *Archives of General Psychiatry* 54:1001–1006, 1997.

60. Keller MB: "The Long-Term Treatment of Depression." *Journal of Clinical Psychiatry* 60 (suppl):41–45, 1999.

61. O'Leary D, Costello F, Gormley N, et al.: "Remission Onset and Relapse in Depression: An 18-Month Prospective Study of Course for 100 First Admission Patients." *Journal of Affective Disorders* 159:159–171, 2000.

62. Sargeant JK, Bruce MI, Florio LP, et al.: "Factors Associated With 1-Year Outcome of Major Depression in the Community." *Archives of General Psychiatry* 47:519–526, 1990.

63. Cronkite RC, Moos RH, Twohey J, et al.: "Life Circumstances and Personal Resources as Predictors of the Ten-Year Course of Depression." *American Journal of Community Psychology* 26:255–280, 1998.

64. Keller MB: "Depression: Considerations for Treatment of a Recurrent and Chronic Disorder." *Journal of Psychopharmacology* 10 (suppl):41–44, 1996.

65. Judd LL, Akiskal HS, Maser JD, et al. "A Prospective 12-Year Study of Sub-syndromal and Syndromal Depressive Symptoms in Unipolar Major Depressive Disorders." *Archives of General Psychiatry* 1998,55:694–700.

66. Solomon DA, Keller MB, Leon AC, et al.: "Multiple Recurrences of Major Depressive Disorder." *American Journal of Psychiatry* 157:229–233, 2000.

67. Daley SE, Hammen C, Rao U: "Predictors of First Onset and Recurrence of Major Depression in Young Women During the 5 Years Following High School Graduation." *Journal of Abnormal Psychology* 109:525–533, 2000.

68. Judd LL, Paulus MP, Schettler PJ, et al.: "Does Incomplete Recovery From First Lifetime Major Depressive Episode Herald a Chronic Course of Illness?" *American Journal of Psychiatry* 157:1501–1504, 2000.

69. American Psychiatric Association: *Major Depressive Disorder: A Patient and Family Guide.* Washington, DC, American Psychiatric Association, 2000.

70. Belsher G, Costello CG: "Relapse After Recovery From Unipolar Depression: A Critical Review." *Psychological Bulletin* 104:84–96, 1988.

71. Melfi CA, Chawla AJ, Croghan TW, et al.: "The Effects of Adherence to Antidepressant Treatment Guidelines on Relapse and Recurrence of Depression." *Archives of General Psychiatry* 55:1128–1132, 1998.

72. Ilardi SS, Craighead WE, Evans DD: "Modeling Relapse in Unipolar Depression: The Effects of Dysfunctional Cognitions and Personality Disorders." *Journal of Consulting and Clinical Psychology* 65:381–391, 1997.

73. Suominen KH, Isometsa ET, Hernriksson MM, et al.: "Inadequate Treatment for Depression Both Before and After Attempted Suicide." *American Journal of Psychiatry* 155:1778–1780, 1998.

74. Hirschfeld RM, Keller MB, Panico S, et al.: "The National Depressive and Manic-Depressive Association Consensus Statement on the Undertreatment of Depression." *Journal of the American Medical Association* 277:333–340, 1997.

75. Laukkala T, Isometsa ET, Hamalainen J, et al.: "Antidepressant Treatment of Depression in the Finnish General Population." *American Journal of Psychiatry* 158:2077–2079, 2001.

76. Meyers BS, Sirey JA, Bruce MI, et al.: "Predictors of Early Recovery From Major Depression Among Persons Admitted to Community-Based Clinics." *Archives of General Psychiatry* 59:729–735, 2002.

77. Wells KB, Sturm R: "Informing the Policy Process: From Efficacy to Effectiveness Data on Pharmacotherapy." *Journal of Consulting and Clinical Psychology* 64:638–645, 1996.

78. Young AS, Klap R, Sherbourne CD, et al.: "The Quality of Care for Depressive and Anxiety Disorders in the United States." *Archives of General Psychiatry* 58:55–61, 2001.

79. Dawson R, Lavori PW, Coryell W, et al.: "Course of Treatment Received by Depressed Patients." *Journal of Psychiatric Research* 33:233–242, 1999.

80. Mueller TI, Leon AC, Keller MB, et al.: "Recurrence After Recovery From Major Depressive Disorder During 15 Years of Observational Follow-Up." *American Journal of Psychiatry* 156:1000–1006, 1999.

81. Katon WJ, Rutter CM, Ludman EJ, et al.: "A Randomized Trial of Relapse Prevention of Depression in Primary Care." *Archives of General Psychiatry* 58:241–247, 2001.

82. Lin EHB, Simon GE, Katon WJ, et al.: "Can Enhanced Acute-Phase Treatment of Depression Improve Long-Term Outcomes? A Report of Randomized Trials in Primary Care." *American Journal of Psychiatry* 156:643–645, 1999.

83. Simon GE, Manning WG, Katzelnick DJ, et al.: "Cost-Effectiveness of Systematic Depression Treatment for High Utilizers of General Medical Care." *Archives of General Psychiatry* 58:181–187, 2001.

84. Blacker D: "Maintenance Treatment of Major Depression: A Review of the Literature." *Harvard Review of Psychiatry* 4:1–9, 1996.

85. Weissman MM: *Treatment of Depression: Bridging the 21st Century*. Washington, DC, American Psychiatric Press, 2001.

86. Dennett DC: *Elbow Room: The Varieties of Free Will Worth Wanting*. Cambridge, MA, MIT Press, 1984.

87. O'Connor T: "Agent Causation," in *Agents, Causes, and Events: Essays on Indeterminism and Free Will*. Edited by O'Connor T. New York, Oxford University Press, 1995, pp. 173–200.

88. Kauffman S: *Investigations*. New York, Oxford University Press, 2000.

89. Stern DN: *The Interpersonal World of the Infant: A View From Psychoanalysis and Developmental Psychology*. New York, Basic Books, 1985.

90. Scanlon TM: *What We Owe to Each Other*. Cambridge, MA, Harvard University Press, 1998.

91. Bandura A: "Social Cognitive Theory: An Agentic Perspective." *Annual Review of Psychology* 52:1–26, 2001.

92. Bandura A, Pastorelli C, Barbaranelli C, et al.: "Self-Efficacy Pathways to Childhood Depression." *Journal of Personality and Social Psychology* 76:258–269, 1999.

93. Brown GW, Harris TO: *Social Origins of Depression: A Study of Psychiatric Disorder in Women*. New York, Free Press, 1978.

94. Ayer AJ: "Freedom and Necessity," in *Free Will*. Edited by Watson G. New York, Oxford University Press, 1982, pp. 15–23.

95. Allen JG: *Coping With Trauma: Hope Through Understanding*, 2nd Edition. Washington, DC, American Psychiatric Publishing, 2005.

96. de Botton A: *Status Anxiety*. New York, Random House, 2004.

97. Dewey J: *Human Nature and Conduct*. Carbondale, IL, Southern Illinois University Press, 1988.

98. Scarr S: "Developmental Theories for the 1990s: Development and Individual Differences." *Child Development* 63:1–19, 1992.

99. Buss AH: "Selection, Evocation, and Manipulation." *Journal of Personality and Social Psychology* 53:1214–1221, 1987.

100. Hammen C: "Stress and Depression." *Annual Review of Clinical Psychology* 1:293–319, 2005.

101. Rhodes R: *How to Write: Advice and Reflections*. New York, William Morrow, 1995.

102. Beck AT: "Beyond Belief: A Theory of Modes, Personality, and Psychopathology," in *Frontiers of Cognitive Therapy*. Edited by Salkovskis PM. New York, Guilford, 1996, pp. 1–25.

103. McKenchnie JL: *Webster's New Universal Unabridged Dictionary*. New York, Simon and Schuster, 1979.

104. Szasz TS: *The Myth of Mental Illness: Foundations of a Theory of Personal Conduct*, Revised Edition. New York, Harper and Row, 1974.

105. Allen JG, Munich RL, Rogan A: *Agency in Illness and Recovery*. Houston, TX, The Menninger Clinic, 2004.

106. Parsons T: "Illness and the Role of the Physician: A Sociological Perspective." *American Journal of Orthopsychiatry* 21:452–460, 1951.

107. Munich RL: "Efforts to Preserve the Mind in Contemporary Hospital Treatment." *Bulletin of the Menninger Clinic* 76:167–186, 2003.

108. MacIntyre A: *Dependent Rational Animals: Why Human Beings Need the Virtues*. Chicago, IL, Open Court, 1999.

109. Halleck SL: "Dissociative Phenomena and the Question of Responsibility." *International Journal of Clinical and Experimental Hypnosis* 38:298–314, 1990.

110. Dennett DC: *Freedom Evolves*. New York, Penguin, 2003.

111. Nagel T: *The Last Word*. New York, Oxford University Press, 1997.

112. Menninger KA: *Whatever Became of Sin?* New York, Hawthorn Books, 1973.

113. Brown L: *The New Shorter Oxford English Dictionary*. Oxford, UK, Clarendon Press, 1993.

114. Solomon A: *The Noonday Demon: An Atlas of Depression*. New York, Simon and Schuster, 2001.

115. Seminowicz DA, Mayberg HS, McIntosh AR, et al.: "Limbic-Frontal Circuitry in Major Depression: A Path Modeling Metanalysis." *NeuroImage* 22:409–418, 2004.

116. Goldberg E: *The Executive Brain: Frontal Lobes and the Civilized Mind*. New York, Oxford University Press, 2001.

117. Wallace J, Schneider T, McGuffin P: "Genetics of Depression," in *Handbook of Depression*. Edited by Gotlib IH, Hammen C. New York, Guilford, 2002, pp. 169–191.

118. Pliszka SR: *Neuroscience for the Mental Health Clinician*. New York, Guilford, 2003.

119. Morange M: *The Misunderstood Gene*. Translated by Cobb M. Cambridge, MA, Harvard University Press, 2001.

120. Keller EF: *The Century of the Gene*. Cambridge, MA, Harvard University Press, 2000.

121. Kendler KS, Kessler RC, Walters EE, et al.: "Stressful Life Events, Genetic Liability, and Onset of an Episode of Major Depression in Women." *American Journal of Psychiatry* 152:833–842, 1995.

122. Caspi A, Sugden K, Moffitt TE, et al.: "Influence of Life Stress on Depression: Moderation by a Polymorphism on the *5-HTT* Gene." *Science* 301:386–389, 2003.

123. Kendler KS, Neale M, Kessler R, et al.: "A Twin Study of Recent Life Events and Difficulties." *Archives of General Psychiatry* 50:789–796, 1993.

124. Kendler KS: "Social Support: A Genetic-Epidemiological Analysis." *American Journal of Psychiatry* 154:1398–1404, 1997.

125. Glover V, O'Connor TG: "Effects of Antenatal Stress and Anxiety: Implications for Developmental Psychiatry." *British Journal of Psychiatry* 180:389–391, 2002.

126. Field T: "Prenatal Effects of Maternal Depression," in *Children of Depressed Parents: Mechanisms of Risk and Implications for Treatment.* Edited by Goodman SH, Gotlib IH. Washington, DC, American Psychological Association, 2002, pp. 59–88.

127. Field T, Diego M, Hernandez-Reif M, et al.: "Right Frontal EEG and Pregnancy/Neonatal Outcomes." *Psychiatry* 65:35–47, 2002.

128. Goodman SH: "Depression and Early Adverse Experiences," in *Handbook of Depression.* Edited by Gotlib IH, Hammen C. New York, Guilford, 2002, pp. 245–267.

129. O'Connor TG, Heron J, Golding J, et al.: "Maternal Antenatal Anxiety and Children's Behavioural/Emotional Problems at 4 Years." *British Journal of Psychiatry* 180:502–508, 2002.

130. Buss AH: "Personality: Primate Heritage and Human Distinctiveness," in *Personality Structure in the Life Course: Essays on Personology in the Murray Tradition.* Edited by Zucker RA, Rabin AI, Aronoff J. New York, Springer, 1992, pp. 57–100.

131. Kagan J: "Behavioral Inhibition as a Temperamental Category," in *Handbook of Affective Sciences.* Edited by Davidson RJ, Scherer KR, Goldsmith HH. New York, Oxford University Press, 2003, pp. 320–331.

132. Kendler KS, Kessler RC, Neale MC, et al.: "The Prediction of Major Depression in Women: Toward an Integrated Etiologic Model." *American Journal of Psychiatry* 150:1139–1148, 1993.

133. Akiskal HS: "Overview of Chronic Depressions and Their Clinical Management," in *Dysthymia and the Spectrum of Chronic Depressions.* Edited by Akiskal HS, Cassano GB. New York, Guilford, 1997, pp. 1–34.

134. Akiskal HS: "Temperamental Foundation of Affective Disorders," in *Interpersonal Factors in the Origin and Course of Affective Disorders.* Edited by Mundt C, Goldstein MJ, Hahlweg K, et al. London, England, Gaskell, 1996, pp. 3–30.

135. Watson D, Clark LA: "Extraversion and Its Positive Emotional Core," in *Handbook of Personality Psychology.* Edited by Hogan R, Johnson JA, Briggs S. San Diego, CA, Academic Press, 1997, pp. 767–793.

136. James W: *The Varieties of Religious Experience.* New York, Modern Library, 1994.

137. Blackburn S: *Being Good: A Short Introduction to Ethics*. New York, Oxford University Press, 2001.
138. Peterson C: "The Future of Optimism." *American Psychologist* 55:44–55, 2000.
139. Nolen-Hoeksema S: "Gender Differences in Depression," in *Handbook of Depression*. Edited by Gotlib IH, Hammen C. New York, Guilford, 2002, pp. 492–509.
140. Harter S: *The Construction of the Self: A Developmental Perspective*. New York, Guilford, 1999.
141. Allgood-Merten B, Lewinsohn PM, Hops H: "Sex Differences and Adolescent Depression." *Journal of Abnormal Psychology* 99:55–63, 1990.
142. Stice E, Hayward C, Cameron RP, et al.: "Body-Image and Eating Disturbances Predict Onset of Depression Among Female Adolescents: A Longitudinal Study." *Journal of Abnormal Psychology* 109:438–444, 2000.
143. Kendler KS, Thornton LM, Prescott CA: "Gender Differences in the Rates of Exposure to Stressful Life Events and Sensitivity to Their Depressogenic Effects." *American Journal of Psychiatry* 158:587–593, 2001.
144. Allen JG: *Traumatic Relationships and Serious Mental Disorders*. Chichester, UK, Wiley, 2001.
145. Welner A, Marten S, Wochnick E, et al.: "Psychiatric Disorders Among Professional Women." *Archives of General Psychiatry* 36:169–173, 1979.
146. Belle D: "Poverty and Women's Health." *American Psychologist* 45:385–389, 1990.
147. Nolen-Hoeksema S: "Responses to Depression and Their Effects on the Duration of Depressive Episodes." *Journal of Abnormal Psychology* 100:569–582, 1991.
148. Freud S: *Civilization and Its Discontents* (1929). Translated by Strachey J. New York, Norton, 1961.
149. Bowlby J: *Attachment and Loss*, Volume I: *Attachment*, 2nd Edition. New York, Basic Books, 1982.
150. Ainsworth MDS, Blehar MC, Waters E, et al.: *Patterns of Attachment: A Psychological Study of the Strange Situation*. Hillsdale, NJ, Erlbaum, 1978.
151. Bowlby J: *A Secure Base: Parent–Child Attachment and Healthy Human Development*. New York, Basic Books, 1988.
152. Grossmann KE, Grossmann K, Zimmermann P: "A Wider View of Attachment and Exploration: Stability and Change During the Years of Immaturity," in *Handbook of Attachment: Theory, Research, and Clinical Applications*. Edited by Cassidy J, Shaver PR. New York, Guilford, 1999, pp. 760–786.
153. Hofer MA: "The Emerging Neurobiology of Attachment and Separation: How Parents Shape Their Infant's Brain and Behavior," in *September 11: Trauma and Human Bonds*. Edited by Coates SW, Rosenthal JL, Schechter DS. New York, Guilford, 2003, pp. 191–209.
154. Schore AN: "Effects of a Secure Attachment Relationship on Right Brain Development, Affect Regulation, and Infant Mental Health." *Infant Mental Health Journal* 22:7–66, 2001.

155. Field T, Reite M: "The Psychobiology of Attachment and Separation: A Summary," in *The Psychobiology of Attachment and Separation*. Edited by Reite M, Field T. New York, Academic Press, 1985, pp. 455–479.

156. Fonagy P: "Thinking About Thinking: Some Clinical and Theoretical Considerations in the Treatment of a Borderline Patient." *International Journal of Psycho-Analysis* 72:639–656, 1991.

157. Fonagy P, Gergely G, Jurist EL, et al.: *Affect Regulation, Mentalization, and the Development of the Self*. New York, Other Press, 2002.

158. Fox NA, Card JA: "Psychophysiological Measures in the Study of Attachment," in *Handbook of Attachment: Theory, Research, and Clinical Applications*. Edited by Cassidy J, Shaver PR. New York, Guilford, 1999, pp. 226–245.

159. Blatt SJ: *Experiences of Depression: Theoretical, Clinical, and Research Perspectives*. Washington, DC, American Psychological Association, 2004.

160. Thompson RA: "Early Attachment and Later Development," in *Handbook of Attachment: Theory, Research, and Clinical Applications*. Edited by Cassidy J, Shaver PR. New York, Guilford, 1999, pp. 265–286.

161. Belsky J: "Interactional and Contextual Determinants of Attachment Security," in *Handbook of Attachment: Theory, Research, and Clinical Applications*. Edited by Cassidy J, Shaver PR. New York, Guilford, 1999, pp. 249–264.

162. Ainsworth MDS: "Attachments Beyond Infancy." *American Psychologist* 44:709–716, 1989.

163. Lichtenberg JD: *Psychoanalysis and Motivation*. Hillsdale, NJ, Analytic Press, 1989.

164. Melson GF: "Studying Children's Attachment to Their Pets: A Conceptual and Methodological Review." *Anthrozoos* 4:91–99, 1988.

165. MacLean PD: *The Triune Brain in Evolution: Role in Paleocerebral Functions*. New York, Plenum, 1990.

166. Howes C: "Attachment Relationships in the Context of Multiple Caregivers," in *Handbook of Attachment: Theory, Research, and Clinical Applications*. Edited by Cassidy J, Shaver PR. New York, Guilford, 1999, pp. 671–687.

167. Allen JG, Huntoon J, Fultz J, et al.: "A Model for Brief Assessment of Attachment and Its Application to Women in Inpatient Treatment for Trauma-Related Psychiatric Disorders." *Journal of Personality Assessment* 76:420–446, 2001.

168. Blatt SJ, Blass RB: "Relatedness and Self-Definition: Two Primary Dimensions in Personality Development, Psychopathology, and Psychotherapy," in *Interface of Psychoanalysis and Psychology*. Edited by Barron JW, Eagle MN, Wolitzky DL. Washington, DC, American Psychological Association, 1992, pp. 399–428.

169. Schafer R: *Aspects of Internalization*. New York, International Universities Press, 1968.

170. Hatfield E, Cacioppo JT, Rapson RL: *Emotional Contagion*. Paris, France, Cambridge University Press, 1994.

171. Preston SD, de Waal FBM: "Empathy: Its Ultimate and Proximate Bases." *Behavioral and Brain Sciences* 25:1–72, 2002.

172. O'Hara MW: "The Nature of Postpartum Depressive Disorders," in *Postpartum Depression and Child Development*. Edited by Murray L, Cooper PJ. New York, Guilford, 1997, pp. 3–31.

173. Cramer B: "Psychodynamic Perspectives on the Treatment of Postpartum Depression," in *Postpartum Depression and Child Development*. Edited by Murray L, Cooper PJ. New York, Guilford, 1997, pp. 237–261.

174. Teti DM, Gelfand DM: "Maternal Cognitions as Mediators of Child Outcomes in the Context of Postpartum Depression," in *Postpartum Depression and Child Development*. Edited by Murray L, Cooper PJ. New York, Guilford, 1997, pp. 136–164.

175. Gergely G, Watson JS: "Early Social-Emotional Development: Contingency Perception and the Social Biofeedback Model," in *Early Social Cognition: Understanding Others in the First Months of Life*. Edited by Rochat P. Hillsdale, NJ, Erlbaum, 1999, pp. 101–137.

176. Tronick EZ, Weinberg MK: "Depressed Mothers and Infants: Failure to Form Dyadic States of Consciousness," in *Postpartum Depression and Child Development*. Edited by Murray L, Cooper PJ. New York, Guilford, 1997, pp. 54–81.

177. Stern DN: *The Present Moment in Psychotherapy and Everyday Life*. New York, Norton, 2004.

178. Field T: "Infants of Depressed Mothers." *Infant Behavior and Development* 18:1–13, 1995.

179. Ashman SB, Dawson G: "Maternal Depression, Infant Psychobiological Development, and Risk for Depression," in *Children of Depressed Parents: Mechanisms of Risk and Implications for Treatment*. Edited by Goodman SH, Gotlib IH. Washington, DC, American Psychological Association, 2002, pp. 37–58.

180. Papousek H, Papousek M: "Fragile Aspects of Early Social Integration," in *Postpartum Depression and Child Development*. Edited by Murray L, Cooper PJ. New York, Guilford, 1997, pp. 35–53.

181. Lyons-Ruth K, Lyubchik A, Wolfe R, et al.: "Parental Depression and Child Attachment: Hostile and Helpless Profiles of Parent and Child Behavior Among Families at Risk," in *Children of Depressed Parents: Mechanisms of Risk and Implications for Treatment*. Edited by Goodman SH, Gotlib IH. Washington, DC, American Psychological Association, 2002, pp. 89–120.

182. Dawson G, Frey K, Self J, et al.: "Frontal Brain Electrical Activity in Infants of Depressed and Nondepressed Mothers: Relation to Variations in Infant Behavior." *Development and Psychopathology* 11:589–605, 1999.

183. Campbell SB, Cohn JF: "The Timing and Chronicity of Postpartum Depression: Implications for Infant Development," in *Postpartum Depression and Child Development*. Edited by Murray L, Cooper PJ. New York, Guilford, 1997, pp. 165–197.

184. Hay DF: "Postpartum Depression and Cognitive Development," in *Postpartum Depression and Child Development*. Edited by Murray L, Cooper PJ. New York, Guilford, 1997, pp. 85–110.

185. Murray L, Cooper PJ: "The Role of Infant and Maternal Factors in Postpartum Depression, Mother–Infant Interactions, and Infant Outcomes," in *Postpartum Depression and Child Development*. Edited by Murray L, Cooper PJ. New York, Guilford, 1997, pp. 111–135.

186. Hossain Z, Field T, Gonzalez J, et al.: "Infants of 'Depressed' Mothers Interact Better With Their Nondepressed Fathers." *Infant Mental Health Journal* 15:348–357, 1994.

187. Pelaez-Nogueras M, Field T, Cigales M, et al.: "Infants of Depressed Mothers Show Less 'Depressed' Behavior With Their Nursery Teachers." *Infant Mental Health Journal* 15:358–367, 1994.

188. Gladstone TRG, Beardslee WR: "Treatment, Intervention, and Prevention With Children of Depressed Parents: A Developmental Perspective," in *Children of Depressed Parents: Mechanisms of Risk and Implications for Treatment*. Edited by Goodman SH, Gotlib IH. Washington, DC, American Psychological Association, 2002, pp. 277–305.

189. Gitlin MJ: "Pharmacological Treatment of Depression," in *Handbook of Depression*. Edited by Gotlib IH, Hammen C. New York, Guilford, 2002, pp. 360–382.

190. Weissman MM, Markowitz JC: "Interpersonal Psychotherapy for Depression," in *Handbook of Depression*. Edited by Gotlib IH, Hammen C. New York, Guilford, 2002, pp. 404–421.

191. Cooper PJ, Murray L: "The Impact of Psychological Treatments of Postpartum Depression on Maternal Mood and Infant Development, 1: Impact on Maternal Mood," in *Postpartum Depression and Child Development*. Edited by Murray L, Cooper PJ. New York, Guilford, 1997, pp. 201–220.

192. Field T: "The Treatment of Depressed Mothers and Their Infants," in *Postpartum Depression and Child Development*. Edited by Murray L, Cooper PJ. New York, Guilford, 1997, pp. 221–236.

193. Cooper PJ, Murray L, Wilson A, et al.: "Controlled Trial of the Short- and Long-Term Effect of Psychological Treatment of Postpartum Depression." *British Journal of Psychiatry* 182:412–419, 2003.

194. Murray L, Cooper PJ, Wilson A, et al.: "Controlled Trial of the Short- and Long-Term Effect of Psychological Treatment of Postpartum Depression, 2: Impact on the Mother–Child Relationship and Child Outcome." *British Journal of Psychiatry* 182:420–427, 2003.

195. Goodman SH, Gotlib IH: *Children of Depressed Parents: Mechanisms of Risk and Implications for Treatment*. Washington, DC, American Psychological Association, 2002.

196. Radke-Yarrow M, Klimes-Dougan B: "Parental Depression and Offspring Disorders: A Developmental Perspective," in *Children of Depressed Parents: Mechanisms of Risk and Implications for Treatment.* Edited by Goodman SH, Gotlib IH. Washington, DC, American Psychological Association, 2002, pp. 155–173.

197. Hammen C: "Context of Stress in Families of Children With Depressed Parents," in *Children of Depressed Parents: Mechanisms of Risk and Implications for Treatment.* Edited by Goodman SH, Gotlib IH. Washington, DC, American Psychological Association, 2002, pp. 175–199.

198. Bowlby J: *Attachment and Loss,* Volume III: *Loss, Sadness and Depression.* New York, Basic Books, 1980.

199. Bowlby J: *Attachment and Loss,* Volume II: *Separation.* New York, Basic Books, 1973.

200. Bifulco A, Harris T, Brown GW: "Mourning or Early Inadequate Care? Reexamining the Relationship of Maternal Loss in Childhood With Adult Depression and Anxiety." *Development and Psychopathology* 4:433–439, 1992.

201. Cicchetti D, Toth SL: "A Developmental Psychopathology Perspective on Child Abuse and Neglect." *Journal of the American Academy of Child and Adolescent Psychiatry* 34:541–565, 1995.

202. Walker LE: *The Battered Woman.* New York, Harper and Row, 1979.

203. Goldstein MZ: "Elder Maltreatment and Posttraumatic Stress Disorder," in *Aging and Posttraumatic Stress Disorder.* Edited by Ruskin PE, Talbott JA. Washington, DC, American Psychiatric Press, 1996, pp. 127–135.

204. Fonagy P, Target M: "Attachment and Reflective Function: Their Role in Self-Organization." *Development and Psychopathology* 9:679–700, 1997.

205. Bifulco A, Brown GW, Harris TO: "Childhood Experience of Care and Abuse (CECA): A Retrospective Interview Measure." *Journal of Child Psychology and Psychiatry* 35:1419–1435, 1994.

206. Stein HB, Allen D, Allen JG, et al.: *Supplementary Manual for Scoring Bifulco's Childhood Experiences of Care and Abuse Interview (M-CECA), Version 2.0 (Technical Report No. 00–0024).* Topeka, KS, The Menninger Clinic, Research Department, 2000.

207. Bifulco A, Moran P: *Wednesday's Child: Research Into Women's Experience of Neglect and Abuse in Childhood and Adult Depression.* London, England, Routledge, 1998.

208. Harkness KL, Monroe SM: "Childhood Adversity and the Endogenous Versus Nonendogenous Distinction in Women With Major Depression." *American Journal of Psychiatry* 159:387–393, 2002.

209. Brodsky BS, Oquendo M, Ellis SP, et al.: "The Relationship of Childhood Abuse to Impulsivity and Suicidal Behavior in Adults With Major Depression." *American Journal of Psychiatry* 158:1871–1877, 2001.

210. Bernet CZ, Stein MB: "Relationship of Childhood Maltreatment to the Onset and Course of Major Depression in Adulthood." *Depression and Anxiety* 9:169–174, 1999.

211. Bifulco A, Moran PM, Baines R, et al.: "Exploring Psychological Abuse in Childhood, II: Association With Other Abuse and Adult Clinical Depression." *Bulletin of the Menninger Clinic* 66:241–258, 2002.

212. Wolock I, Horowitz B: "Child Maltreatment as a Social Problem: The Neglect of Neglect." *American Journal of Orthopsychiatry* 54:530–542, 1984.

213. Egeland B: "Mediators of the Effects of Child Maltreatment on Developmental Adaptation in Adolescence," in *Developmental Perspectives on Trauma: Theory, Research, and Intervention*. Edited by Cicchetti D, Toth SL. Rochester, NY, University of Rochester Press, 1997, pp. 403–434.

214. Barnett D, Manly JT, Cicchetti D: "Defining Child Maltreatment: The Interface Between Policy and Research," in *Child Abuse, Child Development, and Social Policy: Advances in Applied Developmental Psychology*. Edited by Cicchetti D, Toth SL. Norwood, NJ, Ablex Publishing, 1993, pp. 7–73.

215. Bifulco A, Brown GW, Adler Z: "Early Sexual Abuse and Clinical Depression in Adult Life." *British Journal of Psychiatry* 159:115–122, 1991.

216. Garber J, Horowitz JL: "Depression in Children," in *Handbook of Depression*. Edited by Gotlib IH, Hammen C. New York, Guilford, 2002, pp. 510–540.

217. Kashani JH, Carlson GA: "Seriously Depressed Preschoolers." *American Journal of Psychiatry* 144:348–350, 1987.

218. Klein DN, Lewinsohn PM, Seeley JR, et al.: "A Family Study of Major Depressive Disorder in a Community Sample of Adolescents." *Archives of General Psychiatry* 58:13–20, 2001.

219. Lieb R, Isensee B, Hofler M, et al.: "Parental Depression and the Risk of Depression and Other Mental Disorders in Offspring." *Archives of General Psychiatry* 59:365–374, 2002.

220. Nelson DR, Hammen C, Brennan PA, et al.: "The Impact of Maternal Depression on Adolescent Adjustment: The Role of Expressed Emotion." *Journal of Consulting and Clinical Psychology* 71:935–944, 2003.

221. Lewinsohn PM, Essau CA: "Depression in Adolescents," in *Handbook of Depression*. Edited by Gotlib IH, Hammen C. New York, Guilford, 2002, pp. 541–559.

222. Fergusson DM, Woodward LJ: "Mental Health, Educational, and Social Role Outcomes of Adolescents With Depression." *Archives of General Psychiatry* 59:225–231, 2002.

223. Kasen S, Cohen P, Skodol AE, et al.: "Childhood Depression and Adult Personality Disorder." *Archives of General Psychiatry* 58:231–236, 2001.

224. Spence SH, Sheffield JK, Donovan CL: "Preventing Adolescent Depression: An Evaluation of the Problem Solving for Life Program." *Journal of Consulting and Clinical Psychology* 71:3–13, 2003.

225. Rutter M: "Resilience Concepts and Findings: Implications for Family Therapy." *Journal of Family Therapy* 21:119–144, 1999.

226. Yates TM, Egeland B, Sroufe A: "Rethinking Resilience: A Developmental Process Perspective," in *Resilience and Vulnerability: Adaptation in the Context of Childhood Adversities*. Edited by Luthar SS. New York, Cambridge University Press, 2003, pp. 243–265.

227. Luthar SS, Zelazo LB: "Research on Resilience: An Integrative Review," in *Resilience and Vulnerability: Adaptation in the Context of Childhood Adversities*. Edited by Luthar SS. New York, Cambridge University Press, 2003, pp. 510–549.

228. Hammen C: "Risk and Protective Factors for Children of Depressed Parents," in *Resilience and Vulnerability: Adaptation in the Context of Childhood Adversities*. Edited by Luthar SS. New York, Cambridge University Press, 2003, pp. 50–75.

229. Serbin LA, Karp J: "The Intergenerational Transfer of Psychosocial Risk: Mediators of Vulnerability and Resilience." *Annual Review of Psychology* 55:333–363, 2004.

230. Thase ME, Jindal R, Howland RH: "Biological Aspects of Depression," in *Handbook of Depression*. Edited by Gotlib IH, Hammen C. New York, Guilford, 2002, pp. 192–218.

231. Mazure C: "Life Stressors as Risk Factors in Depression." *Clinical Psychology: Science and Practice* 5:291–313, 1998.

232. Monroe SM, Hadjiyannakis K: "The Social Environment and Depression: Focusing on Severe Life Stress," in *Handbook of Depression*. Edited by Gotlib IH, Hammen C. New York, Guilford, 2002, pp. 314–340.

233. Allen JG: "Psychotherapy: The Artful Use of Science." *Smith College Studies in Social Work*, in press.

234. Brown GW, Bifulco A, Harris TO: "Life Events, Vulnerability and Onset of Depression: Some Refinements." *British Journal of Psychiatry* 150:30–42, 1987.

235. Brown GW, Harris TO, Hepworth C: "Loss, Humiliation and Entrapment Among Women Developing Depression: A Patient and Non-Patient Comparison." *Psychological Medicine* 25:7–21, 1995.

236. Beck AT, Rush AJ, Shaw BF, et al.: *Cognitive Therapy of Depression*. New York, Guilford, 1979.

237. Brown GW: "Loss and Depressive Disorders," in *Adversity, Stress, and Psychopathology*. Edited by Dohrenwend BP. New York, Oxford University Press, 1998, pp. 358–370.

238. Roberts JE, Gotlib IH: "Social Support and Personality in Depression: Implications From Quantitative Genetics," in *Sourcebook of Social Support and Personality*. Edited by Pierce GR, Lakey B, Sarason IG, et al. New York, Plenum, 1997, pp. 187–214.

239. Hammen C: "Generation of Stress in the Course of Unipolar Depression." *Journal of Abnormal Psychology* 100:555–561, 1991.

240. Shrout PE, Link BG, Dohrenwend BP, et al.: "Characterizing Life Events as Risk Factors for Depression: The Role of Fateful Loss Events." *Journal of Abnormal Psychology* 98:460–467, 1989.

241. Kendler KS, Karkowski LM, Prescott CA: "Causal Relationship Between Stressful Life Events and the Onset of Major Depression." *American Journal of Psychiatry* 156:837–841, 1999.

242. Weissman MM: "Advances in Psychiatric Epidemiology: Rates and Risks for Major Depression." *American Journal of Public Health* 77:445–451, 1987.

243. Whisman MA, Bruce ML: "Marital Dissatisfaction and Incidence of Major Depressive Episode in a Community Sample." *Journal of Abnormal Psychology* 108:674–678, 1999.

244. Robins CJ: "Congruence of Personality and Life Events in Depression." *Journal of Abnormal Psychology* 99:393–397, 1990.

245. Brown GW, Bifulco A, Veiel HOF, et al.: "Self-Esteem and Depression, II: Social Correlates of Self-Esteem." *Social Psychiatry and Psychiatric Epidemiology* 25:225–234, 1990.

246. Brown GW, Andrews B, Harris TO, et al.: "Social Support, Self-Esteem and Depression." *Psychological Medicine* 16:813–831, 1986.

247. Kendler KS, Gardner CO, Prescott CA: "Toward a Comprehensive Developmental Model of Major Depression in Women." *American Journal of Psychiatry* 159:1133–1145, 2002.

248. Brown GW, Harris TO: "Depression," in *Life Events and Illness*. Edited by Brown GW, Harris TO. New York, Guilford, 1989, pp. 49–93.

249. Post RM: "Transduction of Psychosocial Stress Into the Neurobiology of Recurrent Affective Disorder." *American Journal of Psychiatry* 149:999–1010, 1992.

250. Post RM, Weiss SRB, Smith MA, et al.: "Impact of Psychosocial Stress on Gene Expression: Implications for PTSD and Recurrent Affective Disorder," in *Theory and Assessment of Stressful Life Events*. Edited by Miller TW. Madison, CT, International Universities Press, 1996, pp. 37–91.

251. Brown GW, Harris TO: "Life Events and Endogenous Depression." *Archives of General Psychiatry* 51:525–534, 1994.

252. Lewinsohn PM, Allen NB, Seeley JR, et al.: "First Onset Versus Recurrence of Depression: Differential Processes of Psychosocial Risk." *Journal of Abnormal Psychology* 108:483–489, 1999.

253. Kendler KS, Thornton LM, Gardner CO: "Genetic Risk, Number of Previous Depressive Episodes, and Stressful Life Events in Predicting Onset of Major Depression." *American Journal of Psychiatry* 158:582–586, 2001.

254. Tangney JP: "Perfectionism and the Self-Conscious Emotions: Shame, Guilt, Embarrassment, and Pride," in *Perfectionism: Theory, Research, and Treatment*. Edited by Flett GL, Hewitt PL. Washington, DC, American Psychological Association, 2002, pp. 199–215.

255. Blatt SJ: "The Destructiveness of Perfectionism: Implications for the Treatment of Depression." *American Psychologist* 50:1003–1020, 1995.

256. Flett GL, Hewitt PL: "Perfectionism and Maladjustment: An Overview of Theoretical, Definitional, and Treatment Issues," in *Perfectionism: Theory, Research, and Treatment*. Edited by Flett GL, Hewitt PL. Washington, DC, American Psychological Association, 2002, pp. 5–31.

257. Flett GL, Hewitt PL, Oliver JM, et al.: "Perfectionism in Children and Their Parents: A Developmental Analysis," in *Perfectionism: Theory, Research, and Treatment*. Edited by Flett GL, Hewitt PL. Washington, DC, American Psychological Association, 2002, pp. 89–132.

258. Zerbe KJ: *The Body Betrayed: Women, Eating Disorders, and Treatment*. Washington, DC, American Psychiatric Press, 1993.

259. Antony MM, Swinson RP: *When Perfect Isn't Good Enough: Strategies for Coping With Perfectionism*. Oakland, CA, New Harbinger, 1998.

260. Shahar G, Blatt SJ, Zuroff DC, et al.: "Role of Perfectionism and Personality Disorder Features in Response to Brief Treatment of Depression." *Journal of Consulting and Clinical Psychology* 71:629–633, 2003.

261. Shahar G, Blatt SJ, Zuroff DC, et al.: "Perfectionism Impedes Social Relations and Response to Brief Treatment." *Journal of Social and Clinical Psychology* 23:140–155, 2004.

262. Eisenberg N, Losoya S, Spinrad T: "Affect and Prosocial Responding," in *Handbook of Affective Science*. Edited by Davidson RJ, Scherer KR, Goldsmith HH. New York, Oxford University Press, 2003, pp. 787–803.

263. Nussbaum MC: *Upheavals of Thought: The Intelligence of the Emotions*. Cambridge, UK, Cambridge University Press, 2001.

264. Scheff T: "Shame and Community: Social Components in Depression." *Psychiatry* 64:212–224, 2001.

265. Nathanson DL: *Shame and Pride: Affect, Sex, and the Birth of the Self*. New York, W.W. Norton, 1992.

266. Shahar G: "Personality, Shame, and the Breakdown of Social Bonds: The Voice of Quantitative Depression Research. (Commentary on 'Shame and Community: Social Components in Depression')." *Psychiatry* 64:228–239, 2001.

267. Freud S: "Mourning and Melancholia" (1917), in *The Standard Edition of the Complete Psychological Works of Sigmund Freud*. Edited by Strachey J. London, England, Hogarth Press, 1957, pp. 243–258.

268. Berkowitz L: "Affect, Aggression, and Antisocial Behavior," in *Handbook of Affective Sciences*. Edited by Davidson RJ, Scherer KR, Goldsmith HH. New York, Oxford University Press, 2003, pp. 804–823.

269. Horwitz L: "The Capacity to Forgive: Intrapsychic and Developmental Perspectives." *Journal of the American Psychoanalytic Association* 53:485–511, 2005.

270. Murphy JG: *Getting Even: Forgiveness and Its Limits*. New York, Oxford University Press, 2003.

271. Card C: *The Atrocity Paradigm: A Theory of Evil*. New York, Oxford University Press, 2002.

272. Abramson LY, Alloy LB, Hankin BL, et al.: "Cognitive Vulnerability-Stress Models of Depression in a Self-Regulatory and Psychobiological Context," in *Handbook of Depression*. Edited by Gotlib IH, Hammen C. New York, Guilford, 2002, pp. 268–294.

273. Coyne JC, Gallo SM, Klinkman MS, et al.: "Effects of Recent and Past Major Depression and Distress on Self-Concept and Coping." *Journal of Abnormal Psychology* 107:86–96, 1998.

274. Shahar G, Davidson L: "Depressive Symptoms Erode Self-Esteem in Severe Mental Illness: A Three-Wave, Cross-Lagged Study." *Journal of Consulting and Clinical Psychology* 71:890–900, 2003.

275. Ingram RE, Miranda J, Segal ZV: *Cognitive Vulnerability to Depression*. New York, Guilford, 1998.

276. Edelman GM: *Wider Than the Sky: The Phenomenal Gift of Consciousness*. New Haven, CT, Yale University Press, 2004.

277. Swanton C: *Virtue Ethics: A Pluralistic View*. New York, Oxford, 2003.

278. Kosslyn SM: *Image and Brain: The Resolution of the Imagery Debate*. Cambridge, MA, MIT Press, 1994.

279. Calvin WH: *The Cerebral Symphony: Seashore Reflections on the Structure of Consciousness*. New York, Bantam, 1989.

280. Levitan IB, Kaczmarek LK: *The Neuron: Cell and Molecular Biology*. New York, Oxford University Press, 1997.

281. Cook ND: *The Brain Code*. New York, Methuen, 1986.

282. Borod JC: "Interhemispheric and Intrahemispheric Control of Emotion: A Focus on Unilateral Brain Damage." *Journal of Consulting and Clinical Psychology* 60:339–348, 1992.

283. Mayberg HS: "Limbic-Cortical Dysregulation: A Proposed Model of Depression," in *The Neuropsychiatry of Limbic and Subcortical Disorders*. Edited by Salloway S, Malloy P, Cummings JL. Washington, DC, American Psychiatric Press, 1997, pp. 167–177.

284. Miller EK, Cohen JD: "An Integrative Theory of Prefrontal Cortex Function." *Annual Review of Neuroscience* 24:167–202, 2001.

285. Fuster JM: *Memory in the Cerebral Cortex: An Empirical Approach to Neuronal Networks in the Human and Nonhuman Primate*. Cambridge, MA, MIT Press, 1995.

286. Nauta WJH: "The Problem of the Frontal Lobe: A Reinterpretation." *Journal of Psychiatric Research* 8:167–187, 1971.

287. Damasio A: *The Feeling of What Happens: Body and Emotion in the Making of Consciousness*. New York, Harcourt Brace, 1999.

288. Barrett LF, Salovey P: *The Wisdom in Feeling: Psychological Processes in Emotional Intelligence*. New York, Guilford, 2002.

289. McEwen BS: *The End of Stress As We Know It*. Washington, DC, Joseph Henry Press, 2002.

290. Sapolsky RM: *Why Zebras Don't Get Ulcers: A Guide to Stress, Stress-Related Diseases, and Coping*. New York, W.H. Freeman, 1994.

291. Yehuda R: "Neuroendocrinology of Trauma and Posttraumatic Stress Disorder," in *Psychological Trauma*. Edited by Yehuda R. Washington, DC, American Psychiatric Press, 1998, pp. 97–131.

292. Rajkowska G, Miguel-Hidalgo JJ, Wei J, et al.: "Morphometric Evidence for Neuronal and Glial Prefrontal Cell Pathology in Major Depression." *Biological Psychiatry* 45:1085–1098, 1999.

293. Nemeroff CB: "Psychopharmacology of Affective Disorders in the 21st Century." *Biological Psychiatry* 44:517–525, 1998.

294. Shelton RC: "Cellular Mechanisms in the Vulnerability to Depression and Response to Antidepressants." *Psychiatric Clinics of North America* 23:713–729, 2000.

295. Nemeroff CB: "The Neurobiology of Depression." *Scientific American* 1998, pp. 42–49.

296. Plotsky PM, Owens MJ, Nemeroff CB: "Psychoneuroendocrinology of Depression: Hypothalamic-Pituitary-Adrenal Axis." *Psychiatric Clinics of North America* 21:293–307, 1998.

297. Dunman RS, Heninger GR, Nestler EJ: "A Molecular and Cellular Theory of Depression." *Archives of General Psychiatry* 54:597–606, 1997.

298. Graham YP, Heim C, Goodman SH, et al.: "The Effects of Neonatal Stress on Brain Development: Implications for Psychopathology." *Development and Psychopathology* 11:545–565, 1999.

299. Newport DJ, Stowe ZN, Nemeroff CB: "Parental Depression: Animal Models of an Adverse Life Event." *American Journal of Psychiatry* 159:1265–1283, 2002.

300. Kozol J: *Amazing Grace: The Lives of Children and the Conscience of a Nation.* New York, HarperCollins, 1995.

301. Gold PW, Goodwin FK, Chrousos GP: "Clinical and Biochemical Manifestations of Depression: Relation to the Neurobiology of Stress." *New England Journal of Medicine* 319:413–420, 1988.

302. Sapolsky RM: "Stress, Glucocorticoids, and Damage to the Nervous System: The Current State of Confusion." *Stress* 1:1–19, 1996.

303. Dunman RS, Malberg J, Thome J: "Neural Plasticity to Stress and Antidepressant Treatment." *Biological Psychiatry* 46:1181–1191, 1999.

304. Marek G, Dunman RS: "Neural Circuitry and Signaling in Depression," in *Brain Circuitry and Signaling in Psychiatry*. Edited by Kaplan GB, Hammer RP Jr. Washington, DC, American Psychiatric Publishing, 2002, pp. 153–178.

305. Ressler KJ, Nemeroff CB: "Role of Norepinephrine in the Pathophysiology and Treatment of Mood Disorders." *Biological Psychiatry* 46:1219–1233, 1999.

306. Insel TR, Fernald RD: "How the Brain Processes Social Information: Searching for the Social Brain." *Annual Review of Neuroscience* 27:697–722, 2004.

307. Drevets WC, Gautier C, Price JC, et al.: "Amphetamine-Induced Dopamine Release in Human Ventral Striatum Correlates With Euphoria." *Biological Psychiatry* 49:81–96, 2001.

308. Spangel R, Weiss F: "The Dopamine Hypothesis of Reward: Past and Current Status." *Trends in Neuroscience* 22:521–527, 1999.

309. Davidson RJ, Putnam KM, Larson CL: "Dysfunction in the Neural Circuitry of Emotion Regulation: A Possible Prelude to Violence." *Science* 289:591–594, 2000.

310. Brothers L: *Friday's Footprint: How Society Shapes the Human Mind*. New York, Oxford University Press, 1997.

311. Hyman SE, Nestler EJ: "Initiation and Adaptation: A Paradigm for Understanding Psychotropic Drug Action." *American Journal of Psychiatry* 153:151–162, 1996.

312. Healy D: "The Antidepressant Drama," in *Treatment of Depression: Bridging the 21st Century*. Edited by Weissman MM. Washington, DC, American Psychiatric Press, 2001, pp. 7–34.

313. Binder J, Price CJ: "Functional Neuroimaging of Language," in *Handbook of Functional Neuroimaging of Cognition*. Edited by Cabeza R, Kingstone A. Cambridge, MA, MIT Press, 2001, pp. 187–251.

314. Davidson RJ: "Affective Style, Psychopathology, and Resilience: Brain Mechanisms and Plasticity." *American Psychologist* 55:1196–1214, 2000.

315. Davidson RJ, Pizzagalli D, Nitschke JB: "The Representation and Regulation of Emotion in Depression: Perspectives From Affective Neuroscience," in *Handbook of Depression*. Edited by Gotlib IH, Hammen C. New York, Guilford, 2002, pp. 219–244.

316. Davidson RJ, Pizzagalli D, Nitschke JB, et al.: "Parsing the Subcomponents of Emotion and Disorders of Emotion: Perspectives from Affective Neuroscience," in *Handbook of Affective Sciences*. Edited by Davidson RJ, Scherer KR, Goldsmith HH. New York, Oxford University Press, 2003, pp. 8–24.

317. Davidson RJ: "Affective Style and Affective Disorders: Perspectives From Affective Neuroscience." *Cognition and Emotion* 12:307–330, 1998.

318. Dawson G: "Development of Emotional Expression and Emotion Regulation in Infancy: Contributions of the Frontal Lobe," in *Human Behavior and the Developing Brain*. Edited by Dawson G, Fischer KW. New York, Guilford, 1994, pp. 346–379.

319. LeDoux J: *The Emotional Brain*. New York, Simon and Schuster, 1996.

320. Drevets WC, Videen TO, Price JL, et al.: "A Functional Anatomical Study of Unipolar Depression." *Journal of Neuroscience* 12:3628–3641, 1992.

321. Drevets WC: "Prefrontal Cortical-Amygdalar Metabolism in Major Depression." *Annals of the New York Academy of Sciences* 877:614–637, 1999.

322. Drevets WC: "Neuroimaging and Neuropathological Studies of Depression: Implications for the Cognitive-Emotional Features of Mood Disorders." *Current Opinion in Neurobiology* 11:240–249, 2001.

323. Drevets WC: "Neuroimaging Studies of Mood Disorders." *Biological Psychiatry* 48:813–829, 2000.

324. Dougherty D, Rauch SL: "Neuroimaging and Neurobiological Models of Depression." *Harvard Review of Psychiatry* 5:138–159, 1997.

325. Videbech P: "PET Measurements of Brain Glucose Metabolism and Blood Flow in Major Depressive Disorder: A Critical Review." *Acta Psychiatrica Scandinavica* 101:11–20, 2000.

326. Elliott R, Baker C, Rogers RD, et al.: "Prefrontal Dysfunction in Depressed Patients Performing a Complex Planning Task: A Study Using Positron Emission Tomography." *Psychological Medicine* 27:931–942, 1997.

327. Gallagher HL, Happe F, Brunswick N, et al.: "Reading the Mind in Cartoons and Stories: An fMRI Study of 'Theory of Mind' in Verbal and Nonverbal Tasks." *Neuropsychologia* 38:11–21, 2000.

328. Klin A, Schultz R, Cohen DJ: "Theory of Mind in Action: Developmental Perspectives on Social Neuroscience," in *Understanding Other Minds: Perspectives From Developmental Cognitive Neuroscience*, 2nd Edition. Edited by Baron-Cohen S, Tager-Flusberg H, Cohen DJ. New York, Oxford University Press, 2000, pp. 357–388.

329. Stone VE: "The Role of the Frontal Lobes and the Amygdala in Theory of Mind," in *Understanding Other Minds: Perspectives From Developmental Cognitive Neuroscience*, 2nd Edition. Edited by Baron-Cohen S, Tager-Flusberg H, Cohen DJ. New York, Oxford University Press, 2000, pp. 253–273.

330. Drevets WC, Raichle ME: "Reciprocal Suppression of Regional Cerebral Blood Flow During Emotional Versus Higher Cognitive Processes: Implications for Interactions Between Emotion and Cognition." *Cognition and Emotion* 12:353–385, 1998.

331. Mayberg HS: "Modulating Dysfunctional Limbic-Cortical Circuits in Depression: Towards Development of Brain-Based Algorithms for Diagnosis and Optimised Treatment." *British Medical Bulletin* 65:193–207, 2003.

332. Mayberg HS, Liotti M, Brannan SK, et al.: "Reciprocal Limbic-Cortical Function and Negative Mood: Converging PET Findings in Depression and Normal Sadness." *American Journal of Psychiatry* 156:675–682, 1999.

333. Mayberg HS, Brannan SK, Tekell JL, et al.: "Regional Metabolic Effects of Fluoxetine in Major Depression: Serial Changes and Relationship to Clinical Response." *Biological Psychiatry* 48:830–843, 2000.

334. Mayberg HS, Silva JA, Brannan SK, et al.: "The Functional Neuroanatomy of the Placebo Effect." *American Journal of Psychiatry* 159:728–737, 2002.

335. Brody AL, Saxena S, Stoessel P, et al.: "Regional Brain Metabolic Changes in Patients With Major Depression Treated With Either Paroxetine or Interpersonal Therapy: Preliminary Findings." *Archives of General Psychiatry* 58:631–640, 2001.

336. Martin SD, Martin E, Rai SS, et al.: "Brain Blood Flow Changes in Depressed Patients Treated With Interpersonal Psychotherapy or Venlafaxine Hydrochloride: Preliminary Findings." *Archives of General Psychiatry* 58:641–648, 2001.

337. Coryell W, Endicott J, Maser JD, et al.: "Long-Term Stability of Polarity Distinctions in the Affective Disorders." *American Journal of Psychiatry* 152:385–390, 1995.

338. Johnson SL, Kizer A: "Bipolar and Unipolar Depression: A Comparison of Clinical Phenomenology and Psychosocial Predictors," in *Handbook of Depression*. Edited by Gotlib IH, Hammen C. New York, Guilford, 2002, pp. 141–165.

339. Hales RE, Yudofsky SC: *Synopsis of Psychiatry*. Washington, DC, American Psychiatric Press, 1996.

340. Hammen C, Gitlin M: "Stress Reactivity in Bipolar Patients and Its Relation to Prior History of Disorder." *American Journal of Psychiatry* 154:856–857, 1997.

341. Malkoff-Schwartz S, Frank E, Anderson B, et al.: "Stressful Life Events and Social Rhythm Disruption in the Onset of Manic and Depressive Bipolar Episodes." *Archives of General Psychiatry* 55:702–707, 1998.

342. Malkoff-Schwartz S, Frank E, Anderson BP, et al.: "Social Rhythm Disruption and Stressful Life Events in the Onset of Bipolar and Unipolar Episodes." *Psychological Medicine* 30:1005–1016, 2000.

343. Johnson SL, Sandrow D, Meyer B, et al.: "Increases in Manic Symptoms After Life Events Involving Goal Attainment." *Journal of Abnormal Psychology* 109:721–727, 2000.

344. Bellak L: "Basic Aspects of Ego Function Assessment," in *The Broad Scope of Ego Function Assessment*. Edited by Bellak L. New York, Wiley, 1984, pp. 6–30.

345. Goldberg JF, Harrow M, Whiteside JE: "Risk for Bipolar Illness in Patients Initially Hospitalized for Unipolar Depression." *American Journal of Psychiatry* 158:1265–1270, 2001.

346. Swann AC: "Mixed or Dysphoric Manic States: Psychopathology and Treatment." *Journal of Clinical Psychiatry* 56 (suppl):6–10, 1995.

347. Krasuski JS, Janicak PG: "Mixed States: Current and Alternate Diagnostic Models." *Psychiatric Annals* 24:371–379, 1994.

348. Krasuski JS, Janicak PG: "Mixed States: Issues of Terminology and Conceptualization." *Psychiatric Annals* 24:269–277, 1994.

349. Perugi G, Micheli C, Akiskal HS, et al.: "Polarity of First Episode, Clinical Characteristics, and Course of Manic Depressive Illness: A Systematic Retrospective Investigation of 320 Bipolar I Patients." *Comprehensive Psychiatry* 41:13–18, 2000.

350. Delgado PL, Gelenberg AJ: "Antidepressant and Antimanic Medications," in *Treatments of Psychiatric Disorders*, Volume 2, 3rd Edition. Edited by Gabbard GO. Washington, DC, American Psychiatric Publishing, 2001, pp. 1137–1179.

351. Reilly Harrington NA, Alloy LB, et al.: "Cognitive Styles and Life Events Interact to Predict Bipolar and Unipolar Symptomatology." *Journal of Abnormal Psychology* 108:567–578, 1999.

352. Johnson SL, Winett CA, Meyer B, et al.: "Social Support and the Course of Bipolar Disorder." *Journal of Abnormal Psychology* 108:558–566, 1999.

353. Mineka S, Watson D, Clark LA: "Comorbidity of Anxiety and Unipolar Mood Disorders." *Annual Review of Psychology* 49:377–412, 1998.

354. Brown C, Schulberg HC, Madonia MJ, et al.: "Treatment Outcomes for Primary Care Patients With Major Depression and Lifetime Anxiety Disorders." *American Journal of Psychiatry* 153:1293–1300, 1996.

355. Joiner TE, Steer RA, Beck AT, et al.: "Physiological Hyperarousal: Construct Validity of a Central Aspect of the Tripartite Model of Depression and Anxiety." *Journal of Abnormal Psychology* 108:290–298, 1999.

356. Kessler RC, Sonnega A, Bromet E, et al.: "Posttraumatic Stress Disorder in the National Comorbidity Survey." *Archives of General Psychiatry* 52:1048–1060, 1995.

357. Breslau N, Davis G, Adreski P, et al.: "Epidemiological Findings on Posttraumatic Stress Disorder and Co-Morbid Disorders in the General Population," in *Adversity, Stress, and Psychopathology*. Edited by Dohrenwend BP. New York, Oxford University Press, 1998, pp. 319–330.

358. Mueller TI, Lavori PW, Keller MB, et al.: "Prognostic Effect of the Variable Course of Alcoholism on the 10-Year Course of Depression." *American Journal of Psychiatry* 151:701–706, 1994.

359. Goldstein A: *Addiction: From Biology to Drug Policy*. New York, Oxford University Press, 2001.

360. Changeux J-P: "Drug Use and Abuse," in *The Brain*. Edited by Edelman GM, Changeux J-P. New Brunswick, NJ, Transaction, 2001, pp. 145–165.

361. Edell D: *Eat, Drink, and Be Merry*. New York, HarperCollins, 1999.

362. Holahan CJ, Moos RH, Holahan CK, et al.: "Drinking to Cope and Alcohol Use and Abuse in Unipolar Depression: A 10-Year Model." *Journal of Abnormal Psychology* 112:159–165, 2003.

363. Windle M, Davies PT: "Depression and Heavy Alcohol Use Among Adolescents: Concurrent and Prospective Relations." *Development and Psychopathology* 11:823–844, 1999.

364. Hyman SE, Nestler EJ: *The Molecular Foundations of Psychiatry*. Washington, DC, American Psychiatric Press, 1993.

365. Swendsen JD, Tennen H, Carney MA, et al.: "Mood and Alcohol Consumption: An Experience Sampling Test of the Self-Medication Hypothesis." *Journal of Abnormal Psychology* 109:198–204, 2000.

366. Sorg BA, Kalivas PW: "Stress and Neuronal Sensitization," in *Neurobiological and Clinical Consequences of Stress: From Normal Adaptation to Posttraumatic Stress Disorder*. Edited by Friedman MJ, Charney DS, Deutch AY. Philadelphia, PA, Lippincott-Raven, 1995, pp. 83–102.

367. Stine SM, Kosten TR: "Complications of Chemical Abuse and Dependency," in *Neurobiological and Clinical Consequences of Stress: From Normal Adaptation to Posttraumatic Stress Disorder*. Edited by Friedman MJ, Charney DS, Deutch AY. Philadelphia, PA, Lippincott-Raven, 1995, pp. 447–464.

368. Hasin D, Tsai W-Y, Endicott J, et al.: "Five-Year Course of Major Depression: Effects of Comorbid Alcoholism." *Journal of Affective Disorders* 41:63–70, 1996.

369. Kessing LV: "The Effect of Comorbid Alcoholism on Recurrence in Affective Disorder: A Case Register Study." *Journal of Affective Disorders* 53:49–55, 1999.

370. Greenfield SF, Weiss RD, Munez LR, et al.: "The Effect of Depression on Return to Drinking: A Prospective Study." *Archives of General Psychiatry* 55:259–265, 1998.

371. Hasin D, Liu X, Nunes E, et al.: "Effects of Major Depression on Remission and Relapse of Substance Dependence." *Archives of General Psychiatry* 59:375–380, 2002.

372. Regan C: *Intoxicating Minds: How Drugs Work.* New York, Columbia University Press, 2001.

373. Marlatt GA, Barrett K: "Relapse Prevention," in *Treatments of Psychiatric Disorders*, Volume 1, 3rd Edition. Edited by Gabbard GO. Washington, DC, American Psychiatric Publishing, 2001, pp. 863–878.

374. McKellar J, Stewart E, Humphreys K: "Alcoholics Anonymous Involvement and Positive Alcohol-Related Outcomes: Cause, Consequence, or Just a Correlate? A Prospective 2-Year Study of 2,319 Alcohol-Dependent Men." *Journal of Consulting and Clinical Psychology* 71:302–308, 2003.

375. Kelly JF, McKellar JD, Moos RH: "Major Depression in Patients With Substance Use Disorders: Relationship to 12-Step Involvement and Substance Use Outcomes." *Addiction* 98:499–508, 2003.

376. Rutter M: "Temperament, Personality, and Personality Disorder." *British Journal of Psychiatry* 150:443–458, 1987.

377. Gunderson JG: "The Borderline Patient's Intolerance of Aloneness: Insecure Attachments and Therapist Availability." *American Journal of Psychiatry* 153:752–758, 1996.

378. Dolan-Sewell RT, Krueger RF, Shea MT: "Co-Occurrence With Syndrome Disorders," in *Handbook of Personality Disorders: Theory, Research, and Treatment.* Edited by Livesley WJ. New York, Guilford, 2001, pp. 84–104.

379. Zanarini MC, Frankenburg FR, DeLuca CJ, et al.: "The Pain of Being Borderline: Dysphoric States Specific to Borderline Personality Disorder." *Harvard Review of Psychiatry* 6:201–207, 1998.

380. Fonagy P, Target M, Gergely G: "Attachment and Borderline Personality Disorder: A Theory and Some Evidence." *Psychiatric Clinics of North America* 23:103–122, 2000.

381. Millon T: *Disorders of Personality: DSM-IV and Beyond.* New York, Wiley, 1996.

382. Shea MT, Widiger TA, Klein MH: "Comorbidity of Personality Disorders and Depression: Implications for Treatment." *Journal of Consulting and Clinical Psychology* 60:857–868, 1992.

383. Gabbard GO: *Psychodynamic Psychiatry in Clinical Practice*, 4th Edition. Washington, DC, American Psychiatric Publishing, 2005.

384. Perry JC, Banon E, Ianni F: "Effectiveness of Psychotherapy for Personality Disorders." *American Journal of Psychiatry* 156:1312–1321, 1999.

385. Target M: "Outcome Research on the Psychosocial Treatment of Personality Disorders." *Bulletin of the Menninger Clinic* 62:215–230, 1998.

386. Clary GL, Krishnan KRR: "Treatment of Mood Disorders in the Medically Ill Patient," in *Treatment of Psychiatric Disorders*, Volume 2, 3rd Edition. Edited by Gabbard GO. Washington, DC, American Psychiatric Publishing, 2001, pp. 1389–1415.
387. McEwen BS: "Mood Disorders and Allostatic Load." *Biological Psychiatry* 54:200–207, 2003.
388. Harris EC, Barraclough B: "Suicide as an Outcome for Mental Disorders: A Meta-Analysis." *British Journal of Psychiatry* 170:205–228, 1997.
389. Angst J, Angst F, Stassen HH: "Suicide Risk in Patients With Major Depressive Disorder." *Journal of Clinical Psychiatry* 60 (suppl):57–62, 1999.
390. Jamison KR: *Night Falls Fast: Understanding Suicide*. New York, Random House, 1999.
391. Favazza AR, Rosenthal RJ: "Diagnostic Issues in Self-Mutilation." *Hospital and Community Psychiatry* 44:134–140, 1993.
392. Roy A, Nielsen D, Rylander G, et al.: "Genetics of Suicide in Depression." *Journal of Clinical Psychiatry* 60 (suppl):12–17, 1999.
393. Blumenthal SJ: "An Overview and Synopsis of Risk Factors, Assessment, and Treatment of Suicidal Patients Over the Life Cycle," in *Suicide Over the Life Cycle: Risk Factors, Assessment, and Treatment of Suicidal Patients*. Edited by Blumenthal SJ, Kupfer DJ. Washington, DC, American Psychiatric Press, 1990, pp. 685–723.
394. Bronisch T: "The Relationship Between Suicidality and Depression." *Archives of Suicide Research* 2:235–254, 1996.
395. Soloff PH, Lynch KG, Kelly TM, et al.: "Characteristics of Suicide Attempts of Patients With Major Depressive Episode and Borderline Personality Disorder: A Comparative Study." *American Journal of Psychiatry* 157:601–608, 2000.
396. Williams M: *Cry of Pain: Understanding Suicide and Self-Harm*. New York, Penguin Books, 1997.
397. Baumeister RF: "Suicide as Escape From Self." *Psychological Review* 97:90–113, 1990.
398. Dement WC: *The Promise of Sleep*. New York, Random House, 1999.
399. Hauri P, Linde S: *No More Sleepless Nights*. New York, Wiley, 1996.
400. Foster RG, Kreitzman L: *Rhythms of Life: The Biological Clocks That Control the Daily Lives of Every Living Thing*. New Haven, CT, Yale University Press, 2004.
401. Van Moffaert MMMP: "Sleep Disorders and Depression: The 'Chicken and Egg' Situation." *Journal of Psychosomatic Research* 38:9–13, 1994.
402. Benca RM, Obermeyer WH, Thisted RA, et al.: "Sleep and Psychiatric Disorders: A Meta-Analysis." *Archives of General Psychiatry* 49:651–668, 1992.
403. Cartwright RD: "Sleeping Problems," in *Symptoms of Depression*. Edited by Costello CG. New York, Wiley, 1993, pp. 243–257.
404. Kessler RC: "Epidemiology of Depression," in *Handbook of Depression*. Edited by Gotlib IH, Hammen C. New York, Guilford, 2002, pp. 23–42.

405. Maes M, Meltzer HY, Suy E, et al.: "Sleep Disorders and Anxiety as Symptom Profiles of Sympathoadrenal System Hyperactivity in Major Depression." *Journal of Affective Disorders* 27:197–207, 1993.

406. Sandor P, Shapiro CM: "Sleep Patterns in Depression and Anxiety: Theory and Pharmacological Effects." *Journal of Psychosomatic Research* 38:125–139, 1994.

407. Allen JG, Console DA, Brethour JR Jr, et al.: "Screening for Trauma-Related Sleep Disturbance in Women Admitted for Specialized Inpatient Treatment." *Journal of Trauma and Dissociation* 1:59–86, 2000.

408. Breslau N, Roth T, Rosenthal L, et al.: "Sleep Disturbance and Psychiatric Diagnosis: A Longitudinal Epidemiological Study of Young Adults." *Biological Psychiatry* 39:411–418, 1996.

409. Perlis ML, Giles DE, Buysse DJ, et al.: "Self-Reported Sleep Disturbance as a Prodromal Symptom in Recurrent Depression." *Journal of Affective Disorders* 42:209–212, 1997.

410. Ehlers CL, Frank E, Kupfer DJ: "Social Zeitgebers and Biological Rhythms." *Archives of General Psychiatry* 45:948–952, 1988.

411. Southmayd SE, Cairns J, David MM: "Sleep Disturbance in Depression Reconsidered." *Canadian Journal of Psychiatry* 36:366–373, 1991.

412. Benson H: *The Relaxation Response*. New York, William Morrow, 1975.

413. Neylan TC: "Treatment of Sleep Disturbances in Depressed Patients." *Journal of Clinical Psychiatry* 56:56–61, 1995.

414. Thayer RE, Newman JR, McClain TM: "Self-Regulation of Mood: Strategies for Changing a Bad Mood, Raising Energy, and Reducing Tension." *Journal of Personality and Social Psychology* 67:910–925, 1994.

415. Dunn AL, Dishman RK: "Exercise and the Neurobiology of Depression," in *Exercise and Sport Sciences Reviews*. Edited by Holloszy JO. Baltimore, MD, Williams and Wilkins, 1991, pp. 41–98.

416. Babyak M, Blumenthal JA, Herman S, et al.: "Exercise Treatment for Major Depression: Maintenance Therapeutic Benefit at 10 Months." *Psychosomatic Medicine* 62:633–638, 2000.

417. Fredrickson B, Levenson RW: "Positive Emotions Speed Recovery From the Cardiovascular Sequelae of Negative Emotions." *Cognition and Emotion* 12:191–220, 1998.

418. Lewinsohn PM: "A Behavioral Approach to Depression," in *The Psychology of Depression: Contemporary Research and Theory*. Edited by Friedman RJ, Katz MM. New York, Wiley, 1974, pp. 157–178.

419. Lewinsohn PM, Munoz RF, Youngren MA, et al.: *Control Your Depression*. New York, Simon and Schuster, 1986.

420. Fredrickson B: "The Value of Positive Emotions." *American Scientist* 91:330–335, 2003.

421. Folkman S, Moskowitz JT: "Positive Affect and the Other Side of Coping." *American Psychologist* 55:647–654, 2000.

422. Ekman P: *Emotions Revealed*. New York, Holt, 2003.

423. Bechara A, Damasio H, Tranel D, et al.: "Deciding Advantageously Before Knowing the Advantageous Strategy." *Science* 275:1293–1295, 1997.

424. Beck AT: "Cognitive Therapy: A 30-Year Retrospective." *American Psychologist* 46:368–375, 1991.

425. Taylor SE: *Positive Illusions: Creative Self-Deception and the Healthy Mind.* New York, Basic Books, 1989.

426. Thase ME, Beck AT: "An Overview of Cognitive Therapy," in *Cognitive Therapy With Inpatients: Developing a Cognitive Milieu.* Edited by Wright JH, Thase ME, Beck AT, et al. New York, Guilford, 1993, pp. 3–33.

427. Mineka S, Rafaeli E, Yovel I: "Cognitive Biases in Emotional Disorders: Information Processing and Social-Cognitive Perspectives," in *Handbook of Affective Sciences.* Edited by Davidson RJ, Scherer KR, Goldsmith HH. New York, Oxford University Press, 2003, pp. 976–1009.

428. Peterson C, Buchanan GM, Seligman MEP: "Explanatory Style: History and Evolution of the Field," in *Explanatory Style.* Edited by Buchanan GM, Seligman MEP. Hillsdale, NJ, Erlbaum, 1995, pp. 1–20.

429. Rose DT, Abramson LY, Hodulik CJ, et al.: "Heterogeneity of Cognitive Style Among Depressed Inpatients." *Journal of Abnormal Psychology* 103:419–429, 1994.

430. Abramson LY, Metalsky GI, Alloy LB: "Hopelessness Depression: A Theory-Based Subtype of Depression." *Psychological Review* 96:358–372, 1989.

431. Alloy LB, Abramson LY, Whitehouse WG, et al.: "Depressogenic Cognitive Styles: Predictive Validity, Information Processing and Personality Characteristics, and Developmental Origins." *Behavior Research and Therapy* 37:503–531, 1999.

432. Lyubomirsky S, Nolen-Hoeksema S: "Self-Perpetuating Properties of Dysphoric Rumination." *Journal of Personality and Social Psychology* 65:339–349, 1993.

433. Nolen-Hoeksema S: "The Role of Rumination in Depressive Disorders and Mixed Anxiety/Depressive Symptoms." *Journal of Abnormal Psychology* 109:504–511, 2000.

434. Lyubomirsky S, Nolen-Hoeksema S: "Effects of Self-Focused Rumination on Negative Thinking and Interpersonal Problem Solving." *Journal of Personality and Social Psychology* 69:176–190, 1995.

435. Lyubomirsky S, Tucker KL, Caldwell ND, et al.: "Why Ruminators are Poor Problem Solvers: Clues From the Phenomenology of Dysphoric Rumination." *Journal of Personality and Social Psychology* 77:1041–1060, 1999.

436. Nolen-Hoeksema S, Davis CG: "'Thanks for Sharing That': Ruminators and Their Social Support Networks." *Journal of Personality and Social Psychology* 77:801–814, 1999.

437. Arean PA, Perri MG, Nezu AM, et al.: "Comparative Effectiveness of Social Problem-Solving Therapy and Reminiscence Therapy as Treatment for Depression in Older Adults." *Journal of Consulting and Clinical Psychology* 61:1003–1010, 1993.

438. Haverkamp R, Arean PA, Hegel MT, et al.: "Problem-Solving Treatment for Complicated Depression in Late Life: A Case Study in Primary Care." *Perspectives in Psychiatric Care* 40:45–52, 2004.

439. Brewin CR, Reynolds M, Tata P: "Autobiographical Memory Processes and the Course of Depression." *Journal of Abnormal Psychology* 108:511–517, 1999.

440. Williams JMG: "Depression and the Specificity of Autobiographical Memory," in *Remembering Our Past: Studies in Autobiographical Memory*. Edited by Rubin DC. Cambridge, UK, Cambridge University Press, 1996, pp. 244–267.

441. Pillemer DB: *Momentous Events, Vivid Memories*. Cambridge, MA, Harvard University Press, 1998.

442. Kuyken W, Brewin CR: "Autobiographical Memory Functioning in Depression and Reports of Early Abuse." *Journal of Abnormal Psychology* 104:585–591, 1995.

443. Brittlebank AD, Scott J, Williams JMG, et al.: "Autobiographical Memory in Depression: State or Trait Marker?" *British Journal of Psychiatry* 162:118–121, 1993.

444. Watkins E, Teasdale JD: "Rumination and Overgeneral Memory in Depression: Effects of Self-Focus and Analytic Thinking." *Journal of Abnormal Psychology* 110:353–357, 2000.

445. Williams JMG, Teasdale JD, Segal ZV, et al.: "Mindfulness-Based Cognitive Therapy Reduces Overgeneral Autobiographical Memory in Formerly Depressed Patients." *Journal of Abnormal Psychology* 109:150–155, 2000.

446. Williams JMG, Scott J: "Autobiographical Memory in Depression." *Psychological Medicine* 18:689–695, 1988.

447. Mackinger HF, Pachinger MM, Leibetseder MM, et al.: "Autobiographical Memories in Women Remitted From Major Depression." *Journal of Abnormal Psychology* 109:331–334, 2000.

448. Long AA: *Epictetus: A Stoic and Socratic Guide to Life*. New York, Oxford University Press, 2002.

449. Aurelius M: *Meditations*. Translated by Hays G. New York, The Modern Library, 2002.

450. Lebell S: *Epictetus: The Art of Living*. New York, HarperCollins, 1995.

451. Ellsworth PC, Scherer KR: "Appraisal Processes in Emotion," in *Handbook of Affective Sciences*. Edited by Davidson RJ, Scherer KR, Goldsmith HH. New York, Oxford University Press, 2003, pp. 572–595.

452. Burns DD: *Feeling Good*. New York, Avon, 1980.

453. Zuroff DC, Blatt SJ, Sanislow CAI, et al.: "Vulnerability to Depression: Reexamining State Dependence and Relative Stability." *Journal of Abnormal Psychology* 108:76–89, 1999.

454. Lewinsohn PM, Joiner TE, Rohde P: "Evaluation of Cognitive Diathesis-Stress Models in Predicting Major Depressive Disorder in Adolescents." *Journal of Abnormal Psychology* 110:203–215, 2001.

455. Bothwell R, Scott J: "The Influence of Cognitive Variables on Recovery in Depressed Inpatients." *Journal of Affective Disorders* 43:207–212, 1997.

456. Williams JMG, Healy D, Teasdale JD, et al.: "Dysfunctional Attitudes and Vulnerability to Persistent Depression." *Psychological Medicine* 20:375–381, 1990.

457. Alloy LB, Abramson LY, Hogan ME, et al.: "The Temple-Wisconsin Cognitive Vulnerability to Depression Project: Lifetime History of Axis I Psychopathology in Individuals at High and Low Cognitive Risk for Depression." *Journal of Abnormal Psychology* 109:403–418, 2000.

458. Gibb BE, Alloy LB, Abramson LY, et al.: "Cognitive Vulnerability to Depression: A Taxometric Analysis." *Journal of Abnormal Psychology* 113:81–89, 2004.

459. Hollon SD, Haman KL, Brown LL: "Cognitive-Behavioral Treatment of Depression," in *Handbook of Depression*. Edited by Gotlib IH, Hammen C. New York, Guilford, 2002, pp. 383–403.

460. Segal ZV, Williams JMG, Teasdale JD: *Mindfulness-Based Cognitive Therapy for Depression: A New Approach to Preventing Relapse*. New York, Guilford, 2002.

461. Segal ZV, Gemar M, Williams S: "Differential Cognitive Response to a Mood Challenge Following Successful Cognitive Therapy or Pharmacotherapy for Depression." *Journal of Abnormal Psychology* 108:3–10, 1999.

462. Teasdale JD, Segal ZV, Williams JMG: "How Does Cognitive Therapy Prevent Depressive Relapse and Why Should Attentional Control (Mindfulness) Training Help?" *Behavior Research and Therapy* 33:25–39, 1995.

463. Hahn TN: *The Miracle of Mindfulness: A Manual on Meditation*. Boston, MA, Beacon Press, 1975.

464. Kabat-Zinn J: *Full Catastrophe Living: Using the Wisdom of Your Body and Mind to Face Stress, Pain, and Illness*. New York, Delta, 1990.

465. Kabat-Zinn J, Massion AO, Kristeller J, et al.: "Effectiveness of a Meditation-Based Stress Reduction Program in the Treatment of Anxiety Disorders." *American Journal of Psychiatry* 149:936–943, 1992.

466. Kabat-Zinn J: *Wherever You Go, There You Are: Mindfulness Meditation in Everyday Life*. New York, Hyperion, 1994.

467. Teasdale JD, Segal ZV, Williams JMG, et al.: "Prevention of Relapse/Recurrence in Major Depression by Mindfulness-Based Cognitive Therapy." *Journal of Consulting and Clinical Psychology* 68:615–623, 2000.

468. Hahn TN: *Peace is Every Step: The Path of Mindfulness in Everyday Life*. New York, Bantam Books, 1991.

469. Antoni MH, Millon CM, Millon T: "The Role of Psychological Assessment in Health Care: The MBHI, MBMC, and Beyond," in *The Millon Inventories: Clinical and Personality Assessment*. Edited by Millon T. New York, Guilford, 1997, pp. 409–448.

470. Stein H, Allen JG, Hill J: "Roles and Relationships: A Psychoeducational Approach to Reviewing Strengths and Difficulties in Adulthood Functioning." *Bulletin of the Menninger Clinic* 67:281–313, 2003.

471. Baumeister RF, Leary MR: "The Need to Belong: Desire for Interpersonal Attachment as a Fundamental Human Motivation." *Psychological Bulletin* 117:497–529, 1995.

472. Nezlek JB, Hampton CP, Shean GD: "Clinical Depression and Day-to-Day Social Interaction in a Community Sample." *Journal of Abnormal Psychology* 109:11–19, 2000.

473. Coyne JC, Burchill SAL, Stiles WB: "An Interactional Perspective on Depression," in *Handbook of Social and Clinical Psychology*. Edited by Synder CR, Forsyth DR. New York, Pergamon, 1991, pp. 327–349.

474. Segrin C, Dillard JP: "(Non)Depressed Persons' Cognitive and Affective Reactions to (Un)Successful Interpersonal Influence." *Communication Monographs* 58:115–134, 1991.

475. Joiner TE: "Depression in Its Interpersonal Context," in *Handbook of Depression*. Edited by Gotlib IH, Hammen C. New York, Guilford, 2002, pp. 295–313.

476. Swann WB Jr, Rentfrow PJ, Guinn JS: "Self-Verification: The Search for Coherence," in *Handbook of Self and Identity*. Edited by Leary M, Tagney J. New York, Guilford, 2002, pp. 367–383.

477. Segrin C, Abramson LY: "Negative Reactions to Depressive Behaviors: A Communication Theories Analysis." *Journal of Abnormal Psychology* 103:655–668, 1994.

478. Coyne JC: "Toward an Interactional Description of Depression." *Psychiatry* 39:28–40, 1976.

479. Potthoff JG, Holahan CJ, Joiner TE: "Reassurance Seeking, Stress Generation, and Depressive Symptoms: An Integrative Model." *Journal of Personality and Social Psychology* 68:664–670, 1995.

480. Coyne JC: "Interpersonal Processes in Depression," in *Depression and Families: Impact and Treatment*. Edited by Keitner GI. Washington, DC, American Psychiatric Press, 1990, pp. 31–53.

481. Silver RC, Wortman CB, Crofton C: "The Role of Coping in Support Provision: The Self-Presentational Dilemma of Victims of Life Crises," in *Social Support: An Interactional View*. Edited by Sarason BR, Sarason IG, Pierce GR. New York, Wiley, 1990, pp. 397–426.

482. Beach SRH, Fincham FD, Katz J: "Marital Therapy in the Treatment of Depression: Toward a Third Generation of Therapy and Research." *Clinical Psychology Review* 18:635–661, 1998.

483. Benazon NR: "Predicting Negative Spousal Attitudes Toward Depressed Persons: A Test of Coyne's Interpersonal Model." *Journal of Abnormal Psychology* 109:550–554, 2000.

484. Keller MB, Boland RJ: "Implications of Failing to Achieve Successful Long-Term Maintenance Treatment of Recurrent Unipolar Major Depression." *Biological Psychiatry* 44:348–360, 1998.

485. Harkness KL, Monroe SM, Simons AD, et al.: "The Generation of Life Events in Recurrent and Nonrecurrent Depression." *Psychological Medicine* 29:135–144, 1999.

486. Leff J, Vaughn C: *Expressed Emotion in Families: Its Significance for Mental Illness*. New York, Guilford, 1985.

487. Hooley JM: "Expressed Emotion and Depression," in *Depression and Families: Impact and Treatment*. Edited by Keitner GI. Washington, DC, American Psychiatric Press, 1990, pp. 57–83.

488. Davila J, Hammen C, Burge D, et al.: "Poor Interpersonal Problem Solving as a Mechanism of Stress Generation in Depression Among Adolescent Women." *Journal of Abnormal Psychology* 104:592–600, 1995.

489. Klerman GL, Weissman MM, Rounsaville BJ, et al.: *Interpersonal Psychotherapy of Depression*. New York, Basic Books, 1984.

490. Weissman MM, Markowitz JC, Klerman GL: *Comprehensive Guide to Interpersonal Psychotherapy*. New York, Basic Books, 2000.

491. Gabbard GO: "Psychodynamic Psychotherapies," in *Treatments of Psychiatric Disorders*, Volume 2, 3rd Edition. Edited by Gabbard GO. Washington, DC, American Psychiatric Publishing, 2001, pp. 1227–1245.

492. Gabbard GO, Westen D: "Rethinking Therapeutic Action." *International Journal of Psycho-Analysis* 84:823–841, 2003.

493. Menninger KA, Holzman PS: *Theory of Psychoanalytic Technique*, 2nd Edition. New York, Basic Books, 1973.

494. Busch FN, Rudden M, Shapiro T: *Psychodynamic Treatment of Depression*. Washington, DC, American Psychiatric Publishing, 2004.

495. Fonagy P, Roth A, Higgitt A: "Psychodynamic Psychotherapies: Evidence-Based Practice and Clinical Wisdom." *Bulletin of the Menninger Clinic* 69:1–58, 2005.

496. Coyne JC, Kessler RC, Tal M, et al.: "Living With a Depressed Person." *Journal of Consulting and Clinical Psychology* 55:347–352, 1987.

497. Beach SRH, Jones DJ: "Marital and Family Therapy for Depression in Adults," in *Handbook of Depression*. Edited by Gotlib IH, Hammen C. New York, Guilford, 2002, pp. 422–440.

498. Hirschfeld RM: "Antidepressants in the United States: Current Status and Future Needs," in *Treatment of Depression: Bridging the 21st Century*. Edited by Weissman MM. Washington, DC, American Psychiatric Press, 2001, pp. 123–134.

499. Kramlinger K: *Mayo Clinic on Depression*. Rochester, MN, Mayo Clinic, 2001.

500. Papolos D, Papolos J: *Overcoming Depression*, 3rd Edition. New York, HarperCollins, 1997.

501. Lissman TL, Boehnlein JK: "A Critical Review of Internet Information About Depression." *Psychiatric Services* 52:1046–1050, 2001.

502. Rosenbaum JF, Fava M, Nierenberg AA, et al.: "Treatment-Resistant Mood Disorders," in *Treatment of Psychiatric Disorders*, Volume 2, 3rd Edition. Washington, DC, American Psychiatric Publishing, 2001, pp. 1307–1387.

503. March J, Silva S, Petrycki S, et al.: "Fluoxetine, Cognitive-Behavioral Therapy, and Their Combination for Adolescents With Depression: Treatment for Adolescents With Depression Study (TADS) Randomized Controlled Trial." *Journal of the American Medical Association* 292:807–820, 2004.

504. Licinio J, Wong M-L: "Depression, Antidepressants and Suicidality: A Critical Appraisal." *Nature Reviews* 4:165–171, 2005.

505. U.S. Food and Drug Administration: *Public Health Advisory: Suicidality in Children and Adolescents Being Treated With Antidepressant Medications.* Washington, DC, U.S. Food and Drug Administration, Center for Drug Evaluation and Research, 2004.

506. Whittington CJ, Kendall T, Fonagy P, et al.: "Selective Serotonin Reuptake Inhibitors in Childhood Depression: Systematic Review of Published Versus Unpublished Data." *The Lancet* 363:1341–1345, 2004.

507. Rush AJ, Kupfer DJ: "Strategies and Tactics in the Treatment of Depression," in *Treatments of Psychiatric Disorders,* Volume 2, 3rd Edition. Edited by Gabbard GO. Washington, DC, American Psychiatric Publishing, 2001, pp. 1417–1439.

508. Thase ME, Sachs GS: "Bipolar Depression: Pharmacotherapy and Related Therapeutic Strategies." *Biological Psychiatry* 48:558–572, 2000.

509. Weiner RD, Krystal AD: "Electroconvulsive Therapy," in *Treatments of Psychiatric Disorders,* Volume 2, 3rd Edition. Edited by Gabbard GO. Washington, DC, American Psychiatric Press, 2001, pp. 1267–1293.

510. American Psychiatric Association: *Practice Guideline for the Treatment of Patients With Major Depressive Disorder,* 2nd Edition. Washington, DC, American Psychiatric Association, 2000.

511. Trivedi MH, Rush AJ, Crismon L, et al.: "Clinical Results for Patients With Major Depressive Disorder in the Texas Medication Algorithm Project." *Archives of General Psychiatry* 61:669–680, 2004.

512. Thase ME, Bhargava M, Sachs GS: "Treatment of Bipolar Depression: Current Status, Continued Challenges, and the STEP-BD Approach," *Psychiatric Clinics of North America* 26:495–518, 2003.

513. Kupfer DJ, Frank E, Perel JM, et al.: "Five-Year Outcome for Maintenance Therapies in Recurrent Depression." *Archives of General Psychiatry* 49:769–773, 1992.

514. Byrne SE, Rothschild AJ: "Loss of Antidepressant Efficacy During Maintenance Therapy: Possible Mechanisms and Treatments." *Journal of Clinical Psychiatry* 59:279–288, 1998.

515. Sackeim HA, Lisanby SH: "Physical Treatments in Psychiatry: Advances in Electroconvulsive Therapy, Transcranial Magnetic Stimulation, and Vagus Nerve Stimulation," in *Treatment of Depression: Bridging the 21st Century.* Edited by Weissman MM. Washington, DC, American Psychiatric Press, 2001, pp. 151–174.

516. Fink M: *Electroshock: Healing Mental Illness.* New York, Oxford University Press, 1999.

517. Sackeim HA, Prudic J, Devanand DP, et al.: "A Prospective, Randomized, Double-Blind Comparison of Bilateral and Right Unilateral Electroconvulsive Therapy at Different Stimulus Intensities." *Archives of General Psychiatry* 57:425–434, 2000.

518. Rush AJ, George MS, Sackheim HA, et al.: "Vagus Nerve Stimulation (VNS) for Treatment-Resistant Depressions: A Multicenter Study." *Biological Psychiatry* 47:276–286, 2000.

519. Elkin I, Shea MT, Watkins JT, et al.: "National Institute of Mental Health Treatment of Depression Collaborative Research Program: General Effectiveness of Treatments." *Archives of General Psychiatry* 46:971–982, 1989.

520. Elkin I, Gibbons RD, Shea MT, et al.: "Science is Not a Trial (But It Can Sometimes Be a Tribulation)." *Journal of Consulting and Clinical Psychology* 64:92–103, 1996.

521. Jacobson NS, Hollon SD: "Cognitive-Behavior Therapy Versus Pharmacotherapy: Now That the Jury's Returned Its Verdict, It's Time to Present the Rest of the Evidence." *Journal of Consulting and Clinical Psychology* 64:74–80, 1996.

522. Shea MT, Elkin I, Imber SD, et al.: "Course of Depressive Symptoms Over Follow-Up: Findings From the National Institute of Mental Health Treatment of Depression Collaborative Research Program." *Archives of General Psychiatry* 49:782–787, 1992.

523. Blatt SJ, Zuroff DC, Bondi CM, et al.: "Short- and Long-Term Effects of Medication and Psychotherapy in the Brief Treatment of Depression: Further Analyses of Data From the NIMH TDCRP." *Psychotherapy Research* 10:215–234, 2000.

524. Zuroff DC, Blatt SJ, Krupnick JL, et al.: "Enhanced Adaptive Capacities After Brief Treatment for Depression." *Psychotherapy Research* 13:99–115, 2003.

525. Olfson M, Marcus SC, Druss B, et al.: "National Trends in the Outpatient Treatment of Depression." *Journal of the American Medical Association* 287:203–209, 2002.

526. Casacalenda N, Perry JC, Looper K: "Remission in Major Depressive Disorder: A Comparison of Pharmacotherapy, Psychotherapy, and Control Conditions." *American Journal of Psychiatry* 159:1354–1360, 2002.

527. Antonuccio DO, Danton WG, DeNelsky GY: "Psychotherapy Versus Medication for Depression: Challenging the Conventional Wisdom With Data." *Professional Psychology: Research and Practice* 26:574–585, 1995.

528. Beutler LE, Clarkin JF, Bongar B: *Guidelines for the Systematic Treatment of the Depressed Patient.* New York, Oxford University Press, 2000.

529. Keller MB, McCullough JP, Klein DN, et al.: "A Comparison of Nefazodone, the Cognitive Behavioral-Analysis System of Psychotherapy, and Their Combination for the Treatment of Chronic Depression." *New England Journal of Medicine* 342:1462–1470, 2000.

530. McCullough JP: *Treatment for Chronic Depression: Cognitive Behavioral Analysis System of Psychotherapy.* New York, Guilford, 2000.

531. Gabbard GO, Kay J: "The Fate of Integrated Treatment: Whatever Happened to the Biopsychosocial Psychiatrist?" *American Journal of Psychiatry* 158:1956–1963, 2001.

532. Hollon SD, Fawcett J: "Combined Medication and Psychotherapy," in *Treatments of Psychiatric Disorders*, Volume 2, 3rd Edition. Edited by Gabbard GO. Washington, DC, American Psychiatric Publishing, 2001, pp. 1247–1266.

533. Fava GA, Grandi S, Zielezny M, et al.: "Four-Year Outcome for Cognitive Behavioral Treatment of Residual Symptoms in Major Depression." *American Journal of Psychiatry* 153:945–947, 1996.

534. Fava GA, Rafanelli C, Grandi S, et al.: "Six-Year Outcome for Cognitive Behavioral Treatment of Residual Symptoms in Major Depression." *American Journal of Psychiatry* 155:1443–1445, 1998.

535. Fava GA, Rafanelli C, Grandi S, et al.: "Prevention of Recurrent Depression With Cognitive Behavioral Therapy." *Archives of General Psychiatry* 55:816–820, 1998.

536. Luborsky L, Singer B, Luborsky L: "Comparative Studies of Psychotherapies: Is It True That 'Everyone Has Won and All Must Have Prizes'?" *Archives of General Psychiatry* 32:995–1008, 1975.

537. Smith ML, Glass GV: "Meta-Analysis of Psychotherapy Outcome Studies." *American Psychologist* 32:752–760, 1977.

538. Jones EE, Pulos SM: "Comparing the Process in Psychodynamic and Cognitive-Behavioral Therapies." *Journal of Consulting and Clinical Psychology* 61:306–316, 1993.

539. Ablon JS, Jones EE: "Psychotherapy Process in the National Institute of Mental Health Treatment of Depression Collaborative Research Program." *Journal of Consulting and Clinical Psychology* 67:64–75, 1999.

540. Ablon JS, Jones EE: "Validity of Controlled Clinical Trials of Psychotherapy: Findings from the NIMH Treatment of Depression Collaborative Research Program." *American Journal of Psychiatry* 159:775–783, 2002.

541. Jacobson NS, Dobson KS, Truax PA, et al.: "A Component Analysis of Cognitive-Behavioral Treatment for Depression." *Journal of Consulting and Clinical Psychology* 64:295–304, 1996.

542. Rogers CR: "The Necessary and Sufficient Conditions of Therapeutic Personality Change." *Journal of Consulting and Clinical Psychology* 60:827–832, 1992.

543. Burns DD, Auerbach A: "Therapeutic Empathy in Cognitive-Behavioral Therapy: Does It Really Make a Difference?" in *Frontiers of Cognitive Therapy*. Edited by Salkovskis PM. New York, Guilford, 1996, pp. 135–164.

544. Luborsky L: "Helping Alliances in Psychotherapy," in *Successful Psychotherapy*. Edited by Claghorn JL. New York, Brunner/Mazel, 1976, pp. 92–116.

545. Colson DB, Horwitz L, Allen JG, et al.: "Patient Collaboration as a Criterion for the Therapeutic Alliance." *Psychoanalytic Psychology* 5:259–268, 1988.

546. Frank E, Kupfer DJ, Perel JM, et al.: "Three-Year Outcomes for Maintenance Therapies in Recurrent Depression." *Archives of General Psychiatry* 47:1093–1099, 1990.

547. Pruyser PW: "Maintaining Hope in Adversity." *Bulletin of the Menninger Clinic* 51:463–474, 1987.

548. Peterson C, Chang EC: "Optimism and Flourishing," in *Flourishing: Positive Psychology and the Life Well-Lived*. Edited by Keyes CL, Haidt J. Washington, DC, American Psychiatric Press, 2003, pp. 55–79.

549. Groopman J: *The Anatomy of Hope: How People Prevail in the Face of Illness*. New York, Random House, 2004.

550. Menninger KA: "Hope." *Bulletin of the Menninger Clinic* 51:447–462, 1987.

551. McGinn C: *Mindsight: Image, Dream, Meaning*. Cambridge, MA, Harvard University Press, 2004.

552. Erikson EH: *Childhood and Society*. New York, Norton, 1963.

553. Csikszentmihalyi M: *Flow: The Psychology of Optimal Experience*. New York, HarperCollins, 1990.

554. Snyder CR, Cheavens J, Michael ST: "Hoping," in *Coping: The Psychology of What Works*. Edited by Snyder CR. New York, Oxford University Press, 1999, pp. 205–231.

SUGGESTED READINGS

GENERAL LITERATURE

Allen JG: *Coping With Trauma: Hope Through Understanding*, 2nd Edition. Washington, DC, American Psychiatric Publishing, 2005.

Antony MM, Swinson RP: *When Perfect Isn't Good Enough: Strategies for Coping With Perfectionism*. Oakland, CA: New Harbinger, 1998.

Bifulco A, Moran P: *Wednesday's Child: Research Into Women's Experience of Neglect and Abuse in Childhood, and Adult Depression*. London, England, Routledge, 1998.

Bowlby J: *A Secure Base: Parent–Child Attachment and Healthy Human Development*. New York, Basic Books, 1988.

Burns DD: *Feeling Good*. New York, Avon, 1980.

Cronkite K: *On the Edge of Darkness: America's Most Celebrated Actors, Journalists and Politicians Chronicle Their Most Arduous Journey*. New York, Dell, 1994.

Dement WC: *The Promise of Sleep*. New York, Random House, 1999.

Groopman J: *The Anatomy of Hope: How People Prevail in the Face of Illness*. New York, Random House, 2004.

Hammen C: *Depression*. East Sussex, UK, Psychology Press, 1997.

Jamison KR: *An Unquiet Mind*. New York, Random House, 1995.

Jamison KR: *Night Falls Fast: Understanding Suicide*. New York, Random House, 1999.

Lewinsohn PM, Munoz RF, Youngren MA, et al.: *Control Your Depression*. New York, Simon and Schuster, 1986.

Lewis L, Kelly KA, Allen JG: *Restoring Hope and Trust: An Illustrated Guide to Mastering Trauma*. Baltimore, MD, Sidran Press, 2004.

Martin P: *The Zen Path Through Depression*. New York, HarperCollins, 1999.

McEwen B: *The End of Stress As We Know It*. Washington, DC, Joseph Henry Press, 2002.

Solomon A: *The Noonday Demon: An Atlas of Depression*. New York, Simon and Schuster, 2001.

Styron W: *Darkness Visible*. New York, Random House, 1990.

Whybrow P: *A Mood Apart: Depression, Mania, and Other Afflictions of the Self*. New York, BasicBooks, 1997.

Williams M: *Cry of Pain: Understanding Suicide and Self-Harm*. New York, Penguin Books, 1997.

Yudofsky SC: *Fatal Flaws: Navigating Destructive Relationships With People With Disorders of Personality and Character*. Washington, DC, American Psychiatric Publishing, 2005.

PROFESSIONAL LITERATURE

Allen JG: *Traumatic Relationships and Serious Mental Disorders*. Chichester, UK, Wiley, 2001.

Beutler LE, Clarkin JF, Bongar B: *Guidelines for the Systematic Treatment of the Depressed Patient*. New York, Oxford University Press, 2000.

Blatt SJ: *Experiences of Depression: Theoretical, Clinical, and Research Perspectives*. Washington, DC, American Psychological Association, 2004.

Bowlby J: *Attachment and Loss*, Volume III: *Loss, Sadness and Depression*. New York, Basic Books, 1980.

Brown GW, Harris TO: *Social Origins of Depression: A Study of Psychiatric Disorder in Women*. New York, Free Press, 1978.

Busch FN, Rudden M, Shapiro T: *Psychodynamic Treatment of Depression*. Washington, DC, American Psychiatric Publishing, 2004.

Flett GL, Hewitt PL (eds): *Perfectionism: Theory, Research, and Treatment*. Washington, DC, American Psychological Association, 2002.

Gabbard GO (ed.): *Treatments of Psychiatric Disorders*, 3rd Edition. Washington, DC, American Psychiatric Publishing, 2001.

Gilbert P: *Depression: The Evolution of Powerlessness*. New York, Guilford, 1992.

Goodman SH, Gotlib IH (eds.): *Children of Depressed Parents: Mechanisms of Risk and Implications for Treatment*. Washington, DC, American Psychological Association, 2002.

Gotlib IH, Hammen C (eds.): *Handbook of Depression*. New York, Guilford, 2002.

McCullough JP: *Treatment for Chronic Depression: Cognitive Behavioral Analysis System of Psychotherapy*. New York, Guilford, 2000.

Roth A, Fonagy P: *What Works for Whom? A Critical Review of Psychotherapy Research*, 2nd Edition. New York, Guilford, 2005.

Segal ZV, Williams JMG, Teasdale JD: *Mindfulness-Based Cognitive Therapy for Depression: A New Approach to Preventing Relapse*. New York, Guilford, 2002.

Watson D: *Mood and Temperament*. New York, Guilford, 2000.

Weissman MM, Markowitz JC, Klerman GL: *Comprehensive Guide to Interpersonal Psychotherapy*. New York, Basic Books, 2000.

Wells KB, Sturm R, Sherbourne CD, et al.: *Caring for Depression*. Cambridge, MA, Harvard University Press, 1996.

APPENDIX
INTERNET RESOURCES

*Information on Depression and
Related Topics*

About Depression
www.depression.about.com

American Association of Suicidology
www.suicidology.org

American Foundation for Suicide Prevention
www.afsp.org

American Psychiatric Association
www.psych.org

American Psychiatric Publishing, Inc.
www.appi.org

American Psychological Association
www.apa.org

Anxiety Disorders Association of America
www.adaa.org

Association for Advancement of Behavior Therapy
www.aabt.org

Depression and Bipolar Support Alliance
www.dbsalliance.org

Depression.com (funded by GlaxoSmithKline)
www.depression.com

Depression.org (sponsored by the American Society of Clinical Psychopharmacology)
www.depression.org

Dr. Ivan's Depression Central
www.psycom.net/depression.central.html

The Mayo Clinic
www.mayoclinic.com

The Menninger Clinic
www.MenningerClinic.com

Mental Health Screening
www.mentalhealthscreening.org

National Alliance on Mental Illness (NAMI)
www.nami.org

National Institute of Mental Health
www.nimh.nih.gov

National Mental Health Association
www.nmha.org

Psychiatric Times
www.psychiatrictimes.com

Psychology Information Online: Depression
www.psychologyinfo.com/depression/

Sidran Foundation
sidran.org

Stress, Anxiety, and Depression Resource Center
www.stress-anxiety-depression.org

Zoloft
www.zoloft.com

INDEX

A

Abandonment
  borderline personality disorder
    and, 166
  by caregivers, 222
  feelings of failure and, 74
  insecure attachment and, 68–69
  suicidal states and, 169–170
Abuse. *See* Childhood maltreatment;
  Trauma
ACTH (adrenocorticotropic
  hormone), 134
Activity, 183–184
Activity scheduling, 183, 186, 241
Addiction, 159, 162, 165
  substance abuse, 158–166. *See also*
    specific drugs
Adolescent depression, 87–89
  antidepressant medication and,
    228, 238–239
  predisposing factor, 15
  prevalence of, 25
  recurrence of, 29–30
  self-esteem and, 60, 119–120
  stress pileup and, 103
  substance abuse and, 160
Adrenocorticotropic hormone
  (ACTH), 134
Agency, 33–48
  becoming depressed and, 38–40

case example, 33–34
cognitive therapy and, 199
constraints and, 34, 36–37
definition of, 33, 35
degrees of, 37–38, 45–47
hope and, 251, 253, 257
hospitalization and, 244
medication and, 233
moral judgment and, 44–45
prefrontal cortex and, 132–133
problem solving and, 197, 216
psychotherapy and, 216, 242
seeking system and, 140
self-efficacy, 36
Aggression, 36, 40, 152, 155
Agitation, 10, 229
Alcohol, 159–165
  catalyst for depression, 161, 163
  course of depression and, 163–164
  depressive disorder and, 161
  developmental impact, 160
  drinking to cope, 159
  sleep disturbance and, 179–180
  suicide and, 171
  treatment, 165
Alienation, 109, 214–215, 244
Amphetamines, 139, 162
Amygdala, 131–132, 144
Anger, 114–118
  adaptive functions of, 19, 114–115